Noncolorectal, Nonneuroendocrine Liver Metastases

Isidoro Di Carlo
Editor

Noncolorectal, Nonneuroendocrine Liver Metastases

Diagnosis and Current Therapies

Foreword by Masatoshi Makuuchi

Springer

Editor
Isidoro Di Carlo, MD, PhD, FACS
Department of Surgical Sciences Organ Transplantation
and Advanced Technologies
University of Catania
Cannizzaro Hospital
Catania
Italy

ISBN 978-3-319-09292-8 ISBN 978-3-319-09293-5 (eBook)
DOI 10.1007/978-3-319-09293-5
Springer Cham Heidelberg New York Dordrecht London

Library of Congress Control Number: 2014956271

Printed on acid-free paper

Springer is part of Springer Science+Business Media (www.springer.com)

Foreword

In the last three decades, hepatic surgery for liver metastases from colorectal or neuroendocrine cancer has undergone radical development and gained widespread acceptance. Knowledge of the segmental and subsegmental liver anatomy and hepatic regeneration has expanded markedly, ability to evaluate the functional reserve has improved, and new surgical instruments and procedures have been introduced. As a consequence, surgery for liver metastases from colorectal or neuroendocrine cancer is now considered safe and is performed on a daily basis.

In our own experience, it proved possible to remove at first attempt 97 colorectal liver metastases and 185 neuroendocrine liver metastases. Repeat resection was performed whenever recurrence was detected, including six times in one patient with colorectal liver metastases and up to four times in patients with neuroendocrine liver metastases. At repeat resection, a total of 268 further tumors were removed. The results of surgery have also improved dramatically every year.

In contrast, however, noncolorectal, nonneuroendocrine liver metastases require further study and refinement of treatment owing to their rarity compared with colorectal and neuroendocrine metastases. The treatment varies depending on the primary malignancy and disease stage, and liver resection is indicated in only a limited number of cases. It is currently scarcely possible to say that established guidelines exist.

It was against this background that Professor Isidoro Di Carlo accepted the challenge of addressing the issues surrounding the resection of noncolorectal, nonneuroendocrine liver metastases in this book. The co-authors, who are all top world surgeons, consider all possible primary malignancies in individual chapters.

One doctor will have very few opportunities to experience the resection of noncolorectal, nonneuroendocrine liver metastases. Therefore, this book, which covers all state-of-the-art surgeries of liver metastases from primary malignancies in 15 organs, is very important. I would like to recommend that all surgeons and hepatologists specializing in hepatic surgery read it thoroughly and refer to it each time they encounter noncolorectal or nonneuroendocrine liver metastasis. I believe this book will shed much light on the still unclear field of liver metastasis.

Tokyo, Japan — Masatoshi Makuuchi, MD

Preface

Unlike in the case of metastases from colorectal and neuroendocrine tumors, the advantages of hepatic resection for metastases from non-colorectal non-neuroendocrine (NCRNNE) cancer have not been well proven to date. Nevertheless, interest in these metastases is continuously increasing in the medical community, as evidenced by the significant increase in publications over the past 30 years. This trend is in part due to refinement of diagnostic methods and progress in oncology, but it is especially attributable to the safety with which liver surgery, whether open, laparoscopic or robotic, can now be performed.

It has already been demonstrated that highly selected patients can achieve long-term survival after resection of liver metastases from NCRNNE cancer. However, it is difficult to compare and draw conclusions from published series owing to differences in respect of the primary malignancy. Indeed, the full spectrum of this disease remains to be explored.

This was the motivation for editing the present text: to provide a reliable point of reference for all specialists involved in the care of this disease. In order to achieve this goal, I asked the most renowned hepatic surgeons in the world to describe comprehensively their personal experiences and to summarize the currently available literature. Since liver metastases from some primary tumors are very rare, with limited experience reported by hepatic surgeons, I also engaged other specialists to achieve a complete coverage of the disease. In this way, all NCRNNE liver metastases have been described and for each one the reader is supplied with current answers concerning diagnosis and treatment.

I would like to express my gratitude to all the authors of each chapter. Without their skills and experience this book would not have been possible. I will conclude in expressing my personal deep gratitude, and that of all coauthors, for the great privilege of having Professor Masatoshi Makuuchi's presenting this volume.

Catania, Italy
October 2014

Isidoro Di Carlo, MD, PhD, FACS

Contents

Contributors

Anya Adair, MD Department of Surgery, Royal Infirmary of Edinburgh, Edinburgh, UK

Luca Aldrighetti, MD Hepatobiliary Surgery Unit, IRCCS San Raffaele Hospital, Milan, MI, Italy

Thomas A. Aloia, MD Department of Surgical Oncology, The University of Texas MD Anderson Cancer Center, Houston, TX, USA

Matteo Cescon, MD General Surgery and Transplantation, S. Orsola – Malpighi Hospital, University of Bologna, Bologna, Italy

Federica Cipriani, MD Hepatobiliary Surgery Unit, IRCCS San Raffaele Hospital, Milan, MI, Italy

David Cosgrove, MD Department of Medical Oncology, Johns Hopkins Hospital, Baltimore, MD, USA

Koert P. de Jong, MD Department of Hepato-Pancreato-Biliary Surgery and Liver Transplantation, University Medical Centre Groningen, University of Groningen, Groningen, The Netherlands

Isidoro Di Carlo, MD, PhD Department of Surgical Sciences, Organ Trasplantation and Advanced Technologies, University of Catania, Cannizzaro Hospital, Catania, Italy

Giorgio Ercolani, MD General Surgery and Transplantation, S. Orsola – Malpighi Hospital, University of Bologna, Bologna, Italy

Jin He, MD, PhD Department of Surgery, Johns Hopkins Hospital, Baltimore, MD, USA

Joseph M. Herman, MD, MSc Department of Radiation Oncology, Johns Hopkins Hospital, Baltimore, MD, USA

Hishaam Ismael, MD Hepatobiliary Surgery Section, Department of Surgical Oncology, MD Anderson Cancer Center, Houston, TX, USA

Kazunori Kihara, MD Department of Urology, Tokyo Medical and Dental University Graduate School, Tokyo, Japan

Schelto Kruijff, MD Department of Hepato-Pancreato-Biliary Surgery and Liver Transplantation, University Medical Centre Groningen, University of Groningen, Groningen, The Netherlands

Luigi Manfrè, MD Department of Minimal Invasive Spinal Therapy, Cannizzaro Hospital, Catania, Italy

Arianeb Mehrabi, MD Department of General, Visceral and Transplant Surgery, Ruprecht-Karls University of Heidelberg, Heidelberg, Baden-Württemberg, Germany

Chetan Merchant, MD Section of Colon and Rectal Surgery, Department of Surgery, Weill Cornell Medical College and New York Presbyterian Hospital, New York, NY, USA

Flavia Neri, MD General Surgery and Transplantation, S. Orsola – Malpighi Hospital, University of Bologna, Bologna, Italy

Arash Nickkholgh, MD Department of General, Visceral and Transplant Surgery, Ruprecht-Karls University of Heidelberg, Heidelberg, Baden-Württemberg, Germany

Timothy M. Pawlik, MD, MPH, PhD Division of Surgical Oncology, Department of Surgery, Johns Hopkins Hospital, Baltimore, MD, USA

Antonio Daniele Pinna, MD General Surgery and Transplantation, S. Orsola – Malpighi Hospital, University of Bologna, Bologna, Italy

Enrico Pinotti, MD Hepatobiliary Surgery Unit, IRCCS San Raffaele Hospital, Milan, MI, Italy

Francesca Ratti, MD Hepatobiliary Surgery Unit, IRCCS San Raffaele Hospital, Milan, MI, Italy

Matteo Ravaioli, MD General Surgery and Transplantation, S. Orsola – Malpighi Hospital, University of Bologna, Bologna, Italy

Akio Saiura, MD, PhD Department of Gastroenterological Surgery, Cancer Institute Hospital, Japanese Foundation for Cancer Research, Ariake Hospital, Koto-ku, Tokyo, Japan

Charbel Sandroussi, MD Hepatobiliary and Upper Gastrointestinal Surgery, Royal Prince Alfred Hospital, Camperdown, NSW, Australia

Rupali N. Shah, MD Department of Otolaryngology—Head and Neck Surgery, University of North Carolina at Chapel Hill, Chapel Hill, NC, USA

Parul J. Shukla, MD Department of Surgery, Weill Cornell Medical College and New York Presbyterian Hospital, New York, NY, USA

Department of Surgical GastroenterologyTata Memorial Hospital, Parel, Mumbai, India

Satyan B. Sreenath, MD Department of Otolaryngology—Head and Neck Surgery, University of North Carolina at Chapel Hill, Chapel Hill, NC, USA

Manabu Tatokoro, MD Department of Urology, Tokyo Medical and Dental University Graduate School, Tokyo, Japan

Adriana Toro, MD, PhD Department of Surgery, Taormina Hospital, Messina, Italy

Anouk N.A. van der Horst-Schrivers, MD Department of Endocrinology, University Medical Centre Groningen, University of Groningen, Groningen, The Netherlands

HaiTao Wang, MD Department of Interventional Oncology, Tianjin Key Laboratory of Cancer Prevention and Therapy, Tianjin, China

Department of Interventional Oncology, Tianjin Medical University Cancer Institute and Hospital, National Clinical Research Center for Cancer, Tianjin, China

Medical Oncology, Research Group of Evidence-based Clinical Oncology, Tianjin, China

Stephen J. Wigmore, MD Department of Surgery, Royal Infirmary of Edinburgh, Edinburgh, UK

YanHong Yao, MD Department of Interventional Oncology, Tianjin Medical University Cancer Institute and Hospital, National Clinical Research Center for Cancer, Tianjin, China

Research Group of Evidence-based Clinical Oncology, Tianjin, China

Adam M. Zanation, MD Department of Otolaryngology—Head and Neck Surgery, University of North Carolina at Chapel Hill, Chapel Hill, NC, USA

Department of Neurosurgery, University of North Carolina at Chapel Hill, Chapel Hill, NC, USA

Jiao Zhang, MD Department of Interventional Oncology, Tianjin Medical University Cancer Institute and Hospital, National Clinical Research Center for Cancer, Tianjin, China

Department of Interventional Oncology, Tianjin Key Laboratory of Cancer Prevention and Therapy, Tianjin, China

Liver Metastases from Adrenocortical Carcinomas

1

Adriana Toro and Isidoro Di Carlo

1.1 Introduction

Hepatic resection is still recognized as the best treatment for colorectal and neuroendocrine liver metastases. However, the liver is also a target for primary metastases for tumors originating from many other sites. Liver metastases that are not colorectal nor neuroendocrine in origin have lacked a well-defined indication, approach, and outcome for liver resection [1]. However, literature reports of highly selected patients with favorable safety and outcomes suggest that hepatic resection represents the only possibility of curative treatment in these patients [2].

Adrenocortical carcinoma (ACC) is a rare and highly aggressive endocrine neoplasm with a worldwide incidence of approximately 0.5–2 per million population and has a poor prognosis [3]. The 5-year survival rates are 58–66 % and 0–24 % in patients with intra-adrenal and extra-adrenal ACC, respectively [4]. The liver is one of the organs most frequently involved [5]. Between 17 and 70 % of patients with ACC have synchronous metastases at the time of diagnosis [6], and more than half of patients with ACC will develop a distant metastasis [7]. Interest in ACC liver metastases has recently increased; many more articles on ACC liver metastases have been published on PubMed in the last 12 years than in the 50 previous years [8].

Although surgical resection is the only curative treatment for these patients, the 5-year survival rate is approximately 40 % [7]. Because adjuvant treatments,

A. Toro, MD, PhD
Department of Surgery, Taormina Hospital, Messina, Italy
e-mail: atoroct@gmail.com

I. Di Carlo, MD, PhD, FACS (✉)
Department of Surgical Sciences, Organ Transplantation, and Advanced Technologies, University of Catania, Cannizzaro Hospital, via Messina 826, Catania 95126, Italy
e-mail: idicarlo@unict.it

I. Di Carlo (ed.), *Noncolorectal, Nonneuroendocrine Liver Metastases: Diagnosis and Current Therapies*, DOI 10.1007/978-3-319-09293-5_1

including the adrenolytic drug mitotane, chemotherapy, and radiotherapy, are of limited effectiveness, the 5-year survival rate for patients with metastatic disease is less than 20 %, with a median survival between 6 and 20 months [9].

After an increase in the number of surgical resections and re-resections of adrenal tumors, survival rates reported in the literature improved dramatically. However, data related to the long-term outcomes of liver resection for ACC metastases are scarce, and, thus, the prognostic factors remain ill-defined [9].

1.2 Epidemiology

Although ACC may occur at any age, the maximum incidence occurs between 40 and 50 years of age [8]. ACC occur 1.5 times more frequently in women than men [5]. Although ACC do not typically occur in children, a high incidence has been recorded in some countries, such as Brazil. In southern Brazil, there is a high prevalence (0.27 %) of a specific TP53 germline mutation (R337H) [10] that is strictly related to the incidence of these tumors.

Recent increases in understanding the molecular mechanisms of ACC development permitted beneficial advancements [5]. Recently, the role of the activation of the Wnt/ß-catenin pathway in adrenal cortex tumorigenesis was elucidated, in part through ß-catenin gene (*CTNNB1*) mutation [7]. Wnt/ß-catenin can be used as a prognostic factor in resected primary ACC because it is associated with tumors that are more aggressive [5]. Additionally, p53, a protein that regulates the cell cycle in response to DNA damage, has been investigated in adrenocortical tumorigenesis. The p53 tumor-suppressor gene (*TP53*) is located at 17q13 and loss of heterozygosity in this locus has been reported in almost 80 % of ACC. Additionally, poorer outcomes are found in the up to 30 % of cases that have an inactivating mutation in the TP53 gene, similar to results reported for other tumors [11].

In 2004, the first tumor classification for ACC was proposed by the Union International Contre le Cancer (UICC). This classification divided tumors into four stages dependent on the stages of tumor, node, and metastasis (TNM). Stage I are tumors with a size of ≤5 cm ($T_1N_0M_0$); stage II are tumors with a size of >5 cm ($T_2N_0M_0$); stage III are tumors that infiltrate the surrounding adipose tissue ($T_3N_0M_0$) or invade at least one lymph node ($T_{1-2}N_1M_0$); and stage IV are tumors that infiltrate surrounding adipose tissue and at invade at least one lymph node ($T_3N_1M_0$), that invade adjacent organs ($T_4N_{0-1}M_0$), or that have distant metastases ($T_{1-4}N_0M_1$).

In 2008, the European Network of the Study for the Study of Adrenal Tumors (ENSAT) proposed a modification for stages III and IV of the UICC classification. The new staging system of ACC consists of four stages: stage I are tumors with a size of ≤5 cm ($T_1N_0M_0$); stage II are tumors with a size of >5 cm ($T_2N_0M_0$); stage III are tumors characterized by infiltration into the surrounding tissue and regional lymph nodes ($T_{1-4}N_1M_0$) or that have a tumor thrombus in the vena cava/renal vein ($T_{3-4}N_0M_0$); and stage IV is restricted to tumors that have a distant metastasis ($T_{1-4}N_{0-1}M_1$). The staging system for ACC is given in Table 1.1 and the 5-year stage-dependent survival is 81, 61, 50, and 13 % for stages I–IV, respectively [7].

Table 1.1 Comparison between UICC classification and ENSAT classification

Stage	UICC classification	ENSAT classification
I	Tumors with a size of ≤5 cm	Tumors with a size of ≤5 cm
II	Tumors with a size of >5 cm	Tumors with a size of >5 cm
III	Tumors that infiltrate the surrounding adipose tissue or invade at least one lymph node	Infiltration in surrounding tissue, positive regional lymph nodes, or a tumor thrombus in the vena cava/renal vein
IV	Infiltration of surrounding adipose tissue and at least one positive lymph node, tumor invasion into adjacent organs, or the presence of distant metastases	Distant metastasis

Number, size of metastasis, tumor presentation (synchronous or metachronous with a long disease-free interval), biologic characteristics of the primary tumor (node positive, Weiss score, Ki-67, and mitotic index), and possibility of achieving a radical resection (R0/R1 vs. R2) [11] are considered the common prognostic factors of liver metastases from ACC. In the case of metachronous metastases, the best prognosis is achieved in patients who develop metachronous metastases after a disease-free survival longer than 1 year and who have a complete resection. On the other hand, patients with synchronous metastases have poor prognoses because recurrence occurs rapidly and survival is very short [12].

1.3 Diagnosis

ACC can be functional and nonfunctional; functional ACC may produce only hormonal precursor excess, because they may not be able to complete the steroidogenesis process. Elevated levels of hormones associated with clinical symptoms have clinical relevance. Excess of mineral corticosteroids is not usually encountered; on the other hand, excesses of the corticosteroids androgen and estrogen are frequently responsible for clinical symptoms.

When patients have no clinical symptoms, before the classification of an ACC as nonfunctioning, they should be screened for steroid precursors (especially dehydroepiandrosterone sulfate (DHEAS), through serum and urine assays) to avoid an incorrect diagnosis [13]. Clinically, symptomatic ACCs can lead to symptoms because of an abdominal mass or a hormonal excess, such as Cushing's syndrome, virilization, feminization, or Conn's syndrome. A complete diagnosis for ACC must evaluate the clinical history, physical examination, laboratory tests, and radiological examinations.

The preoperative laboratory workup for suspected ACC comprises assessment of basal cortisol, adrenocorticotropic hormone (ACTH), DHEAS, 17-hydroxyprogesterone, androstenedione, testosterone, and estradiol levels as well as a dexamethasone suppression test and measurement of urinary free cortisol excretion. The ratio of aldosterone to renin is measured in patients with hypertension or hypokalemia.

Radiological imaging is used in making the diagnosis and in staging the tumor. Computed tomography (CT), ultrasound, and magnetic resonance imaging (MRI) are the most common examinations used for both diagnosis and staging. The chest and abdomen are examined first because the lung and liver are the most common site of metastases from ACC. Metastases can be detected with these methods when the diameter is >1 cm.

The detection of liver metastases using multislice spiral computed tomography (MSCT) can be difficult because of the hypervascularization of the metastases. The arterial filling phase of hypervascularized hepatic metastases of ACC occurs within a few seconds, as demonstrated by echo-enhanced ultrasound. Because liver contrast-enhanced CT is performed 60 s after intravenous injection of a contrast agent, the hypervascularization of the ACC metastases does not allow good visualization of the enhancement phase. Lesions <1 cm cannot be diagnosed in the portal phase if the wash out of the contrast agent is not complete. One solution to this problem might be the use of multiphase MSCT with a shorter acquisition interval that might be able to detect small lesions. However, this procedure carries risks because of high radiation exposure of the metastases. The arterial filling phase of hypervascularized hepatic metastases of ACC occurs within a few seconds, as demonstrated by echo-enhanced ultrasound. Because liver contrast-enhanced CT is performed 60 s after intravenous injection of a contrast agent, the hypervascularization of the ACC metastases does not allow good visualization of the enhancement phase. Lesions <1 cm cannot be diagnosed in the portal phase if the wash out of the contrast agent is not complete. One solution to this problem might be the use of multiphase MSCT with a shorter acquisition interval that might be able to detect small lesions. However, this procedure carries risks because of high radiation exposure [14].

Ultrasound, in both the conventional and echo-enhanced modes, is a sensitive and useful method especially in follow-up examinations. At this stage, when the primary tumor has been removed, the use of ultrasound can permit the diagnosis of small lesions earlier than other methods. This is particularly useful when a single lesion located in the liver can be diagnosed; however, when multiple metastases exist, merely detecting a few additional lesions may not affect overall management [14].

The use of MRI to detect liver metastases of ACC has not been used extensively to date because of lack of capacity, high costs, and the rarity of liver metastases in this disease. To differentiate benign and malignant adrenal tumors, [^{18}F]fluorodeoxyglucose (FDG)–position emission tomography (PET) and PET/CT imaging have been used, but the results have not been useful and no clear indication for these techniques in liver metastases has yet been identified [15].

^{11}C-Metomidate (MTO)-PET is a new adrenal imaging technique that has been used to differentiate tumors of cortical origin from those of noncortical origin. Metomidate tracers specifically bind to adrenocortical CYP11B enzymes, which catalyze the final steps of steroid synthesis. Additional evaluation is needed and application to liver metastases has not been reported [16].

The diagnostic accuracy of fine-needle biopsy is low [17] and violation of the tumor capsule may promote needle track metastases. Fine-needle biopsy can be used to establish a diagnosis, but only after the failure of other diagnostic methods.

1.4 Treatment

ACC is a rare disease with a poor prognosis. Conclusions in the literature are varied, but all reports agree that surgical resection, when possible, represents the only effective treatment for the primary tumor and for isolated metastases [1, 11, 12]. Effective management of liver metastases from ACC, in selected patients, is associated with long-term survival, but the outcome depends on patient selection and on the primary tumor [18].

1.4.1 Surgery

When feasible, a surgical approach is recommended for the treatment of liver metastases for ACC. An aggressive surgical approach in selected patients with liver metastases can lead to long-term survival, with a median overall survival of 31.5 months and a 5-year survival of 39 % [11]. It is important to note, however, that none of these patients survived without recurrence [11].

Review of the literature reveals that there is limited experience related to the management of ACC liver metastases; from 1978 until now, only 219 cases have been reported (Table 1.2). This is one of the reasons for the absence of uniform guidelines. In fact, published studies regarding ACC liver metastases analyze clinical case reports or liver metastasis from multiple primary sites [12]; few manuscripts focus on ACC liver metastases alone. In a multi-institutional analysis of 420 patients with metastases of the liver from primary tumors that were not colorectal nor neuroendocrine in origin, only 5 patients (1.2 %) had metastases from ACC [1]. Although stage IV adrenocortical cancer is associated with a dismal prognosis (5-year survival <15 %), in this series of five patients who underwent liver resections for adrenocortical metastases, 33 % had acceptable outcomes. Three patients died approximately 3, 5, and 10 years after their liver resections and two patients were alive 9 and 13 years after their metastasectomies. Patients with adrenocortical liver metastases who appear to have favorable tumor biology should be given careful consideration for hepatic resection [1].

The rarity of ACC combined with the fact that most patients with metastatic disease are not candidates for resection make it difficult to study a large cohort. However, despite the lack of a clear indication for surgery, surgery represents the only treatment choice for metastatic liver disease. Patients with synchronous metastases have poorer results and their survival is inconsistent. On the other hand, patients with metachronous metastases developed after a disease-free survival of longer than 1 year can achieve good results after a complete resection. Another application of surgery is in debulking of tumors. To be beneficial in large symptomatic tumors in which chemotherapy failed to shrink the mass, debulking procedures have to achieve a resection of 80–90 % of the tumor. An alternative indication is in tumors in which secretion is not controlled by usual therapies; in this group of patients, not only can survival be prolonged, but the overall quality of life can be improved.

Table 1.2 Patients with metastases of adrenocortical carcinoma (ACC) treated with surgical procedures

Author	Year	Number of patients	Sex (male/female)	Age (years)	Time to primary tumor syn/met (months)	Number of MTS	Disease-free interval (months)	Survival (months)	Outcome
Foster [19]	1978	2	–	–	–	–	–	–	–
Cobourn [20]	1987	2	–	–	–	–	–	–	–
Iwatsuki [21]	1988	4	–	–	–	–	–	–	–
Harrison [22]	1997	7	–	–	–	–	–	–	–
Berney [23]	1998	1	Female	27	met (36)	2	135	135	Alive
Lang [24]	1999	6	–	–	–	–	–	–	–
Hemming [25]	2000	3	–	–	–	–	–	–	–
Langer [26]	2000	2	–	–	syn	1	–	1	Dead
			–	–	met (?)	1	–	4	Dead
Takada [27]	2001	1	–	–	–	–	–	–	–
Laurent [28]	2001	1	–	–	met (22)	–	–	42	Dead
Williams [29]	2002	1	–	–	met (20)	3	18	27	Dead
Karavias [30]	2002	6	Male	74	syn	1	–	1	Alive
				68	met (9)	1	–	10	Dead
				66	syn	3	–	36	Alive
				60	syn	con	–	60	Alive
				51	syn	con	–	36	Alive
				56	syn	con	–	36	Alive
Nermoen [31]	2004	1	Female	39	syn	2	27	48	Alive
Di Carlo [32]	2004	1	Female	32	met (36)	1	38	38	Alive
Weitz [2]	2005	15	–	–	–	–	–	–	–

Author	Year	Number of patients	Sex (male/female)	Age (years)	Time to primary tumor syn/met (months)	Number of MTS	Disease-free interval (months)	Survival (months)	Outcome
Ercolani [33]	2005	3	Male	18	syn	4	–	11	Dead
			–	22	met (6)	6	6	10	Dead
			–	51	syn	3	–	6	Dead
Adam [18]	2006	28	–	–	–	–	–	–	–
Assié [9]	2007	41	–	–	–	–	–	–	–
Bauditz [14]	2008	7	Female	67	met (?)	–	–	19	Dead
			Male	60	met (?)	–	–	77	Alive
			Female	24	met (?)	–	–	8	Alive
			Male	61	met (?)	–	–	21	Alive
			Male	44	met (?)	–	–	19	Dead
			Female	58	met (?)	–	–	4	Dead
			Female	28	met (?)	–	–	25	Dead
Ripley [34]	2011	19	–	–	–	–	–	–	–
Langan [35]	2012	10	2 female/8 male	47	syn 5 pt/met 5 pt (19.5)	1 MTS 7 pt; 2 MTS 2 pt; 3–4 MTS 1 pt	23.5	24	–
Datrice [36]	2012	23	–	–	–	–	–	–	–
Mawardi [37]	2012	1	Male	73	met (288)	1	288	60	Alive
Gaujoux [11]	2012	28	20 female/8 male	45	syn 11 pt/ met 17 pt	2	27.7	31.5	25 dead/3 alive

(continued)

Table 1.2 (continued)

Author	Year	Number of patients	Sex (male/female)	Age (years)	Time to primary tumor syn/met (months)	Number of MTS	Disease-free interval (months)	Survival (months)	Outcome
Groeschi [1]	2012	5	–	–	–	–	–	–	–
Huang [38]	2013	1	Male	65	syn	con	–	2	Dead
Total		219							

Syn synchronous, *met* metachronous, *MTS* metastases, *pt* patients, *Con* metastases from contact

In cases of bilateral liver metastases from ACC, a two-stage hepatectomy can be performed to resect both of the metastases. Cryotherapy has been reported as a bridging therapy to prevent the progression of the remaining tumor [29].

An additional reason that surgical treatment represents the treatment of choice is because chemotherapy is not well established. Mitotane is currently used alone or in combination with other chemotherapeutic agents; however, there is no evidence for its efficacy [12, 39].

One of the most important prognostic factors for liver metastasis surgery is the response to preoperative chemotherapy. One suggested use for mitotane is in the neoadjuvant setting to select patients for surgery [40]. A valid rationale to treat patients who have ACC metastases with either adjuvant or neoadjuvant chemotherapy is the very high rate of early recurrence. However, this rationale is limited by the absence of effective chemotherapeutic agents and the lack of evidence of benefit [41].

1.4.2 Chemotherapy

Chemotherapy is used with minimal impact, yielding a 30 % response rate at best. Mitotane, an adrenolytic drug, is the most commonly used chemotherapeutic agent. Mitotane was initially thought to have promising response rates but a doubtful effect on survival [42]. Other chemotherapy regimens (streptozotocin, or the combination of etoposide, doxorubicin, and cisplatin (EDP) [43]) have response rates of approximately 25 %, but a clear definition of the first-line therapy is not yet standardized [44]. However, because of the unclear results of chemotherapy, future treatments could be addressed to targeted therapies, especially against Wnt/ß-catenin [45].

1.4.3 Transarterial Chemoembolization

Another promising alternative for the treatment of liver metastatic ACC is the use of transarterial chemoembolization. With this technique, a median survival of 11 months in patients with progressive disease has been reported [46].

Liver transcatheter arterial chemoembolization (TACE) is useful to reach antitumor activity. TACE has two potential benefits in liver metastases from ACC, in the control of hormonal secretion and in tumor necrosis that may shrink the mass. Liver metastases from ACC have the high arterial support characteristics described for hepatocellular carcinomas or neuroendocrine liver metastases and, thus, TACE may be promising in this metastatic condition.

However, the rationale for treatment can explain the encouraging and favorable results reported in the literature [46]. The degree of lipiodol uptake and the size of the hepatic metastases are predictors of response. Lesions <3 cm can have a better uptake of lipiodol and a better objective response. Early treatment when the liver metastases are <3 cm is also recommended [47].

Table 1.3 Patients with metastases of adrenocortical carcinoma (ACC) treated with radiofrequency ablation

Author	Year	Number of patients	Sex male/female	Age (years)	Time to primary tumor syn/met (months)	Number of MTS	Disease-free interval (months)	Survival (months)	Outcome
Wood [48]	2003	5	–	–	–	–	–	–	–
Bauditz [14]	2009	1	female	30	18 met	2	–	–	–
Ripley [34]	2011	8	–	–	–	–	–	–	–

Syn synchronous, *met* metachronous, *MTS* metastases

1.4.4 Radiofrequency Ablation

Radiofrequency ablation (RFA) has been advocated by some authors for the treatment of liver metastases of ACC, but evidence for improvement in local control or improved survival is lacking [34]. In the literature, only 14 cases from 2003 are reported (Table 1.3). RFA may be an alternative to surgery in some patients with metastatic ACC of smaller size, but clinical data are scarce. Percutaneous RFA for ACC liver metastases is relatively easy to repeat and has a lower morbidity and lower cost than a surgical procedure, but it has all of the limitations and inconveniences of this technique. Thus, with superficial tumors, subcapsular complications such as bleeding or gastrointestinal complications have been reported. Furthermore, tumors located close to great vessels have a "sink" effect and incomplete treatment of the tumor may be recorded [48]. Hypervascular tumors may also have blood stream-induced cooling not only from adjacent vessels but also from the highly arterial vascularization of the tumor itself. For this reason, in these cases, standard protocols are not sufficient and prolonged ablations associated with high temperature have to be adopted for the complete ablation of these tumors. For a similar reason, better results are achieved in small-sized lesions. RFA could be used in patients who have clear contraindications to surgery.

References

1. Groeschl RT, Nachmany I, Steel JL, Reddy SK, Glazer ES, de Jong MC, Pawlik TM, Geller DA, Tsung A, Marsh JW, Clary BM, Curley SA, Gamblin TC (2012) Hepatectomy for noncolorectal non-neuroendocrine metastatic cancer: a multi-institutional analysis. J Am Coll Surg 214:769–777
2. Weitz J, Blumgart LH, Fong Y, Jarnagin WR, D'Angelica M, Harrison LE, DeMatteo RP (2005) Partial hepatectomy for metastases from noncolorectal, nonneuroendocrine carcinoma. Ann Surg 241:269–276
3. Allolio B, Fassnacht M (2006) Clinical review: adrenocortical carcinoma: clinical update. J Clin Endocrinol Metab 91:2027–2037
4. Icard P, Goudet P, Charpenay C, Andreassian B, Carnaille B, Chapuis Y, Cougard P, Henry JF, Proye C (2001) Adrenocortical carcinomas: surgical trends and results of a 253-patient series from the French Association of Endocrine Surgeons study group. World J Surg 25:891–897
5. Bilimoria KY, Shen WT, Elaraj D, Bentrem DJ, Winchester DJ, Kebebew E, Sturgeon C (2008) Adrenocortical carcinoma in the United States: treatment utilization and prognostic factors. Cancer 113:3130–3136
6. Stojadinovic A, Ghossein RA, Hoos A, Nissan A, Marshall D, Dudas M, Cordon-Cardo C, Jaques DP, Brennan MF (2002) Adrenocortical carcinoma: clinical, morphologic, and molecular characterization. J Clin Oncol 20:941–950
7. Fassnacht M, Johanssen S, Quinkler M, Bucsky P, Willenberg HS, Beuschlein F, Terzolo M, Mueller HH, Hahner S, Allolio B, German Adrenocortical Carcinoma Registry Group; European Network for the Study of Adrenal Tumors (2009) Limited prognostic value of the 2004 International Union Against Cancer staging classification for adrenocortical carcinoma: proposal for a revised TNM classification. Cancer 115:243–250
8. Fassnacht M, Kroiss M, Allolio B (2013) Update in adrenocortical carcinoma. J Clin Endocrinol Metab 98:4551–4564

9. Assié G, Antoni G, Tissier F, Caillou B, Abiven G, Gicquel C, Leboulleux S, Travagli JP, Dromain C, Bertagna X, Bertherat J, Schlumberger M, Baudin E (2007) Prognostic parameters of metastatic adrenocortical carcinoma. J Clin Endocrinol Metab 92:148–154
10. Custódio G, Komechen H, Figueiredo FR, Fachin ND, Pianovski MA, Figueiredo BC (2012) Molecular epidemiology of adrenocortical tumors in southern Brazil. Mol Cell Endocrinol 351:44–51
11. Gaujoux S, Al-Ahmadie H, Allen PJ, Gonen M, Shia J, D'Angelica M, Dematteo R, Fong Y, Blumgart L, Jarnagin WR (2012) Resection of adrenocortical carcinoma liver metastasis: is it justified? Ann Surg Oncol 19:2643–2651
12. Di Carlo I, Toro A, Sparatore F, Cordio S (2006) Liver resection for hepatic metastases from adrenocortical carcinoma. HPB (Oxford) 8:106–109
13. Schulick RD, Brennan MF (1999) Adrenocortical carcinoma. World J Urol 17:26–34
14. Bauditz J, Quinkler M, Beyersdorff D, Wermke W (2008) Improved detection of hepatic metastases of adrenocortical cancer by contrast-enhanced ultrasound. Oncol Rep 19:1135–1139
15. Tenenbaum F, Groussin L, Foehrenbach H, Tissier F, Gouya H, Bertherat J, Dousset B, Legmann P, Richard B, Bertagna X (2004) 18F-fluorodeoxyglucose positron emission tomography as a diagnostic tool for malignancy of adrenocortical tumours? Preliminary results in 13 consecutive patients. Eur J Endocrinol 150:789–792
16. Zettinig G, Mitterhauser M, Wadsak W, Becherer A, Pirich C, Vierhapper H, Niederle B, Dudczak R, Kletter K (2004) Positron emission tomography imaging of adrenal masses: (18) F-fluorodeoxyglucose and the 11beta-hydroxylase tracer (11)C-metomidate. Eur J Nucl Med Mol Imaging 31:1224–1230
17. Else T, Williams AR, Sabolch A, Jolly S, Miller BS, Hammer GD (2014) Adjuvant therapies and patient and tumor characteristics associated with survival of adult patients with adrenocortical carcinoma. J Clin Endocrinol Metab 99:455–461
18. Adam R, Chiche L, Aloia T, Elias D, Salmon R, Rivoire M, Jaeck D, Saric J, Le Treut YP, Belghiti J, Mantion G, Mentha G, Association Française de Chirurgie (2006) Hepatic resection for noncolorectal nonendocrine liver metastases: analysis of 1,452 patients and development of a prognostic model. Ann Surg 244:524–535
19. Foster JH (1978) Survival after liver resection for secondary tumors. Am J Surg 135:389–394
20. Cobourn CS, Makowka L, Langer B, Taylor BR, Falk RE (1987) Examination of patient selection and outcome for hepatic resection for metastatic disease. Surg Gynecol Obstet 165:239–246
21. Iwatsuki S, Starzl TE (1988) Personal experience with 411 hepatic resections. Ann Surg 208:421–434
22. Harrison LE, Brennan MF, Newman E, Fortner JG, Picardo A, Blumgart LH, Fong Y (1997) Hepatic resection for noncolorectal, nonneuroendocrine metastases: a fifteen-year experience with ninety-six patients. Surgery 121:625–632
23. Berney T, Mentha G, Roth AD, Morel P (1998) Results of surgical resection of liver metastases from non-colorectal primaries. Br J Surg 85:1423–1427
24. Lang H, Nussbaum KT, Weimann A, Raab R (1999) Liver resection for non-colorectal, non-neuroendocrine hepatic metastases. Chirurg 70:439–446
25. Hemming AW, Sielaff TD, Gallinger S, Cattral MS, Taylor BR, Greig PD, Langer B (2000) Hepatic resection of noncolorectal nonneuroendocrine metastases. Liver Transpl 6:97–100
26. Langer P, Bartsch D, Moebius E, Rothmund M, Nies C (2000) Adrenocortical carcinoma – our experience with 11 cases. Langenbecks Arch Surg 385:393–397
27. Takada Y, Otsuka M, Seino K, Taniguchi H, Koike N, Kawamoto T, Koda K, Adachi S, Yuzawa K, Nozue M, Todoroki T, Fukao K (2001) Hepatic resection for metastatic tumors from noncolorectal carcinoma. Hepatogastroenterology 48:83–86
28. Laurent C, Rullier E, Feyler A, Masson B, Saric J (2001) Resection of noncolorectal and nonneuroendocrine liver metastases: late metastases are the only chance of cure. World J Surg 25:1532–1536
29. Williams RN, White SA, Lloyd DM (2002) Two stage subtotal hepatectomy for metastatic adrenal adenocarcinoma, a case report. Hepatogastroenterology 49:535–537

30. Karavias DD, Tepetes K, Karatzas T, Felekouras E, Androulakis J (2002) Liver resection for metastatic non-colorectal non-neuroendocrine hepatic neoplasms. Eur J Surg Oncol 28:135–139
31. Nermoen I, Foss A, Holte H, Mathisen Ø, Brekke IB, Line PD, Bergan A (2004) Surgical treatment of hormone-producing adrenocortical carcinoma with liver metastases. Tidsskr Nor Laegeforen 124:3061–3063
32. Di Carlo I, Barbagallo F, Toro A, Sofia M, Cordio S, Grasso G (2004) Primary adrenocortical carcinoma and delayed metastasis: is the surgery alone the right treatment? Case report. Hepatogastroenterology 51:343–345
33. Ercolani G, Grazi GL, Ravaioli M, Ramacciato G, Cescon M, Varotti G, Del Gaudio M, Vetrone G, Pinna AD (2005) The role of liver resections for noncolorectal, nonneuroendocrine metastases: experience with 142 observed cases. Ann Surg Oncol 12:459–466
34. Ripley RT, Kemp CD, Davis JL, Langan RC, Royal RE, Libutti SK, Steinberg SM, Wood BJ, Kammula US, Fojo T, Avital I (2011) Liver resection and ablation for metastatic adrenocortical carcinoma. Ann Surg Oncol 18:1972–1979
35. Langan RC, Ripley RT, Davis JL, Prieto PA, Datrice N, Steinberg SM, Bratslavsky G, Rudloff U, Kammula US, Stojadinovic A, Avital I (2012) Liver directed therapy for renal cell carcinoma. J Cancer Educ 3:184–190
36. Datrice NM, Langan RC, Ripley RT, Kemp CD, Steinberg SM, Wood BJ, Libutti SK, Fojo T, Schrump DS, Avital I (2012) Operative management for recurrent and metastatic adrenocortical carcinoma. J Surg Oncol 105:709–713
37. Mawardi M, Al-Judaibi B, Marotta P (2012) Hepatic metastasis from adrenocortical carcinoma fifteen years after primary resection. Saudi J Gastroenterol 18:140–142
38. Huang CJ, Wang TH, Lo YH, Hou KT, Won JG, Jap TS, Kuo CS (2013) Adrenocortical carcinoma initially presenting with hypokalemia and hypertension mimicking hyperaldosteronism: a case report. BMC Res Notes 6:405
39. Hahner S, Fassnacht M (2005) Mitotane for adrenocortical carcinoma treatment. Curr Opin Investig Drugs 6:386–394
40. Gonzalez RJ, Tamm EP, Ng C, Phan AT, Vassilopoulou-Sellin R, Perrier ND, Evans DB, Lee JE (2007) Response to mitotane predicts outcome in patients with recurrent adrenal cortical carcinoma. Surgery 142:867–875
41. Berruti A, Fassnacht M, Baudin E, Hammer G, Haak H, Leboulleux S, Skogseid B, Allolio B, Terzolo M (2010) Adjuvant therapy in patients with adrenocortical carcinoma: a position of an international panel. J Clin Oncol 28:e401–e402
42. Grubbs EG, Callender GG, Xing Y, Perrier ND, Evans DB, Phan AT, Lee JE (2010) Recurrence of adrenal cortical carcinoma following resection: surgery alone can achieve results equal to surgery plus mitotane. Ann Surg Oncol 17:263–270
43. Glover AR, Ip JC, Zhao JT, Soon PS, Robinson BG, Sidhu SB (2013) Current management options for recurrent adrenocortical carcinoma. Onco Targets Ther 6:635–643
44. Abraham J, Bakke S, Rutt A, Meadows B, Merino M, Alexander R, Schrump D, Bartlett D, Choyke P, Robey R, Hung E, Steinberg SM, Bates S, Fojo T (2002) A phase II trial of combination chemotherapy and surgical resection for the treatment of metastatic adrenocortical carcinoma: continuous infusion doxorubicin, vincristine, and etoposide with daily mitotane as a P-glycoprotein antagonist. Cancer 94:2333–2343
45. Doghman M, Cazareth J, Lalli E (2008) The T cell factor/beta-catenin antagonist PKF115-584 inhibits proliferation of adrenocortical carcinoma cells. J Clin Endocrinol Metab 93:3222–3225
46. Cazejust J, De Baère T, Auperin A, Deschamps F, Hechelhammer L, Abdel-Rehim M, Schlumberger M, Leboulleux S, Baudin E (2010) Transcatheter arterial chemoembolization for liver metastases in patients with adrenocortical carcinoma. J Vasc Interv Radiol 21:1527–1532
47. Roche A, Girish BV, de Baère T, Baudin E, Boige V, Elias D, Lasser P, Schlumberger M, Ducreux M (2003) Trans-catheter arterial chemoembolization as first-line treatment for hepatic metastases from endocrine tumors. Eur Radiol 13:136–140
48. Wood BJ, Abraham J, Hvizda JL, Alexander HR, Fojo T (2003) Radiofrequency ablation of adrenal tumors and adrenocortical carcinoma metastases. Cancer 97:554–560

12. [illegible]

Liver Metastases from Breast Cancer

2

Arash Nickkholgh and Arianeb Mehrabi

2.1 Incidence

Breast cancer (BC) accounts for 1.38 million cancer diagnoses and 458,000 cancer deaths in women annually, making it the most frequently diagnosed cancer and the leading cause of cancer death in women worldwide [1]. Among women diagnosed with BC, only a minority presents with distant metastasis (Stage IV disease). However, the disease has a predilection to metastasize systemically; nearly 30 % of women initially diagnosed with early stage disease will ultimately develop metastatic lesions, often months or even years later [2]. Data from a large US autopsy study concerning metastatic patterns of cancers during a 29-year period revealed that, among all cancers, BC contributed the greatest proportion of metastases to the broadest range of sites. Among others, liver constitutes the third most frequent site of metastasis from BC, after the lymph nodes and lung, with 9.5 % of all detected metastases from BC [3]. In the majority of patient series, isolated liver metastasis (BCLM) has been reported to occur in 5–25 % of all women with BC [4].

2.2 Natural History

The interval from the initial diagnosis of primary BC to the development of BCLM has been reported to range from 23 to 77 months (median 40 months) [5]. The prognosis and clinical course in patients with metastatic BC may vary due to host factors as well as biological characteristics of the disease. Among other tumor characteristics, the site of metastasis seems to be the most significant independent

A. Nickkholgh, MD • A. Mehrabi, MD (✉)
Department of General, Visceral and Transplant Surgery,
Ruprecht-Karls University of Heidelberg, Im Neuenheimer Feld 110,
69120 Heidelberg, Baden-Württemberg, Germany
e-mail: arash.nickkholgh@med.uni-heidelberg.de;
arianeb.mehrabi@med.uni-heidelberg.de

I. Di Carlo (ed.), *Noncolorectal, Nonneuroendocrine Liver Metastases: Diagnosis and Current Therapies*, DOI 10.1007/978-3-319-09293-5_2

Table 2.1 Site-specific survival analysis for metastatic breast cancer ($n = 1{,}038$)

Site of metastasis	*n*	Median survival (mo)	95 % CI	HR	95 % CI	*p*
LN/skin	158	43.0	33.0–53.0	1	1	–
Bone	404	33.2	31.0–38.9	1.62	1.16–2.24	0.004
Lung	184	22.4	18.0–28.0	2.01	1.41–2.88	0.0001
Liver	123	12.0	9.0–15.0	4.30	2.92–6.34	<0.0001
Multiple	143	9.0	7.0–11.0	4.87	3.35–7.06	<0.0001
Brain	26	3.0	1.0–8.0	15.00	8.17–27.50	<0.0001

Modified with permission from Largillier et al. [8]
mo month, *CI* confidence interval, *HR* hazard ratio

prognostic factor, with the visceral site of metastasis associated with a significant poorer prognosis compared to non-visceral site of metastasis [6, 7].

In a large cohort study of 1,038 women with metastatic BC over a 25-year period (1980–2005) from Nice, France, BCLM, as well as brain or multiple sites of metastasis, age at initial diagnosis >50 years, negative hormone receptor (HR) status, the presence of chemotherapy, higher histological grading (Scarff-Bloom-Richardson (SBR) grades 2 and 3 vs. SBR grade 1), and large primary tumor size (>20 mm vs. ≤20 mm) were found in a multivariate analysis to be unfavorable independent prognostic factors able to predict specific survival following the first metastatic occurrence [8].

An Australian autopsy study identifying 945 metastatic deposits in 197 autopsies performed on women who died of BC over a 50-year period showed that younger age (≤49 years), surgical excision of the primary tumor, and downregulation of estrogen receptors (ER) and/or progesterone receptors (PR) were associated with metastasis to the liver; clonal heterogeneity of the primary tumor was shown to be important in developing metastatic propensity [9]. Amplification of the human epidermal growth factor 2 receptor (HER-2)/neu gene has been also shown to be a significant predictor of both overall survival and time to relapse in patients with BC [10, 11]. The so-called triple-negative BC phenotype, which lacks both ER and PR and also HER2 expression and is particularly common in younger women [12, 13], is likely to be accompanied by earlier distant, hematogenous metastases and relatively short relapse-free and overall survival times [14].

In the abovementioned French cohort, a site-specific median survival was shown to be 43 months for lymph node and skin metastases, 33 months for bone metastases, 22 months for lung metastases, 12 months for BCLM, 9 months for multiple metastatic sites, and 3 months for brain metastases (Table 2.1) [8].

2.3 Diagnosis

Conventional imaging modalities yield different accuracies in the diagnosis of BCLM (Fig. 2.1). Although ultrasound (US) has limited screening value and is highly examiner dependent, intraoperative US has become crucial for many surgeons to intraoperatively localize BCLM. Enhanced computed tomography (CT)

(Fig. 2.1b) yields a sensitivity, specificity, and accuracy of 70, 85, and 82 %, respectively [15, 16]. However, the accuracy is much lower with lesions <1 cm. Magnetic resonance imaging (MRI) (Fig. 2.1c) has a high sensitivity of 80–92 % and a specificity of 85 %. For lesions around 1 cm, MRI is more accurate than CT [17]. More recently, the integration of functional imaging, i.e., positron emission tomography (PET) with 2-deoxy-2-[F-18]fluoro-D-glucose (FDG), to conventional imaging has increased the diagnostic accuracy. In a recent meta-analysis, FDG-PET/CT has reported to have a pooled sensitivity and specificity of 96 and 95 %, respectively, for the detection of distant metastases from BC [18]. Several international guidelines currently recommend the inclusion of FDG-PET or PET/CT to the conventional radiologic modalities for the staging of BC and for the detection of distant metastases [19]. However, the impact of increased sensitivity of FDG-PET on patient care and outcome has not been demonstrated. The data regarding prediction of treatment response are insufficient to reach any conclusion. Several prospective, adequately powered clinical trials are currently in progress to define the exact role of this modality in the management of patients with

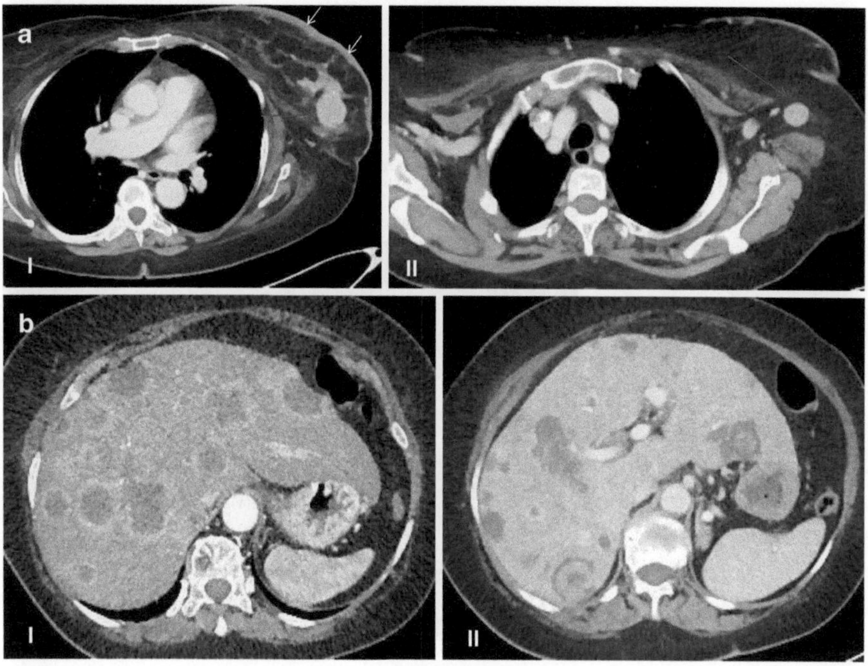

Fig. 2.1 (**a**) Computed tomography scan of the primary breast cancer (**a**-*I*, *red arrow*) and lymph node metastasis (**a**-*II*, *red arrow*). Note the thickening of the cutis (**a**-*I*, *yellow arrows*) suggesting an inflammatory carcinoma of the breast. (**b**) Dynamic contrast-enhanced computed tomography of liver metastases of breast cancer depicting arterial (**b**-*I*) and portal venous (**b**-*II*) phases. (**c**) Dynamic contrast-enhanced magnetic resonance imaging (*MRI*) of liver metastases of breast cancer depicting arterial (**c**-*I*), portal venous (**c**-*II*), and late (**c**-*III*) phases (Courtesy of Prof. Dr. Lars Grenacher, Department of Diagnostic and Interventional Radiology, Ruprecht-Karls University of Heidelberg, Germany)

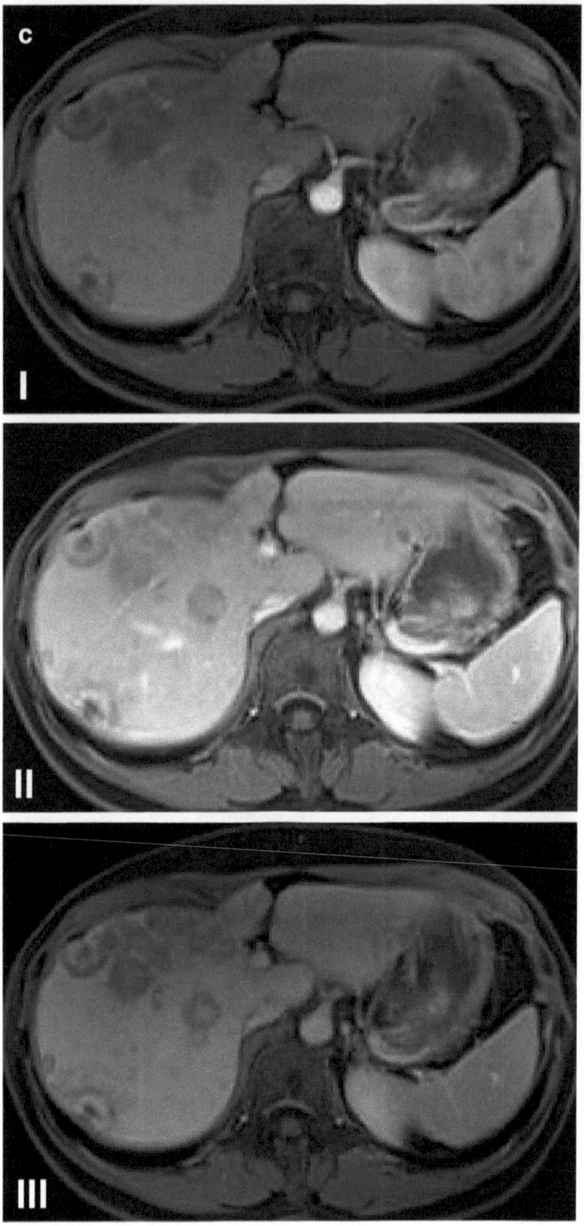

Fig. 2.1 (continued)

BC [20]. Furthermore, some new PET biomarkers for receptor expression, cell proliferation, and angiogenesis have been already introduced, the definitive role of which has to be verified through prospective trials for the purpose of treatment monitoring [21].

2.4 Treatment

Stage IV BC is almost always incurable. Despite remarkable evolution in the systemic therapy of BC, including immunologic agents (trastuzumab), hormonal therapy (selective estrogen receptor modulators and aromatase inhibitors), and more effective chemotherapeutic protocols, the prognosis of the patients with stage IV BC is still dismal; the median survival of patients with hepatic metastases ranges from 1 to 25 months [22]. In shadow of this poor prognosis, the consideration of stage IV BC as a systemic disease, and lack of an internationally accepted consensus on therapy of metastatic BC, palliative less aggressive treatments with low toxicity profiles have been generally preferred to aggressive systemic and locoregional treatments [23].

Regarding an aggressive locoregional treatment in the setting of a metastatic BC, there are two different dilemmas to the presenting clinical scenario.

2.4.1 First, the Role of Aggressive Locoregional Therapy of the Primary Site in Women Presenting with Stage IV Metastatic BC

Using the data from the National Cancer Data Base (NCDB) of the American College of Surgeons (ACS) in a total of 16,023 patients with stage IV disease between 1990 and 1993, Khan and her colleagues showed in a multivariate proportional hazards model that women treated with surgical resection of the primary tumor with free margins compared with those not surgically treated to have superior 3-year survivals with a hazard ratio of 0.61 (95 % confidence interval, 0.58–0.65) [24]. The authors recommended that the role of local therapy plus systemic therapy in women with stage IV BC be compared with systemic therapy alone in a randomized trial. Since then, at least 14 cohorts have been published in the literature [25–37], including an analysis of 1988–2003 Surveillance, Epidemiology, and End Results (SEER) program data [38], to evaluate the role of the resection of primary site in the setting of the metastatic BC, almost all of which verified the findings of Khan et al. Five clinical studies (clinical trials or observational studies) regarding the issue are currently recruiting patients [39].

2.4.2 Second, the Role of Liver Resection for Metastatic BC to the Liver

The first report concerning major liver resection for metastatic BC in the literature dates back to 1963 on Alexander Brunschwig's small cohort of patients from the Memorial Sloan Kettering Cancer Center (then the Memorial Hospital for the Treatment of Cancer and Allied Diseases) undergoing hepatic lobectomy for metastatic cancer including one patient receiving a left hemihepatectomy and partial [extra-anatomical] resection of the metastases to the right lobe due to BCLM years after the first operation for the primary tumor [40]. The patient survived 20 months after the liver resection. The author believed that the patients had achieved "although usually brief" palliation "in some instances" and that these operations [should be] "indicated essentially for palliation, and rather rigid criteria for selection of patients is necessary," provided that "the metastases be macroscopically limited to one lobe of the liver." A decade later, James H. Foster from Hartford, Connecticut, personally visited 98 hospitals to gather data on patients undergoing liver resection for solid tumors of all types, including secondaries. Together with his own small cohort, a literature review, and data from the Liver Tumor Survey (LTS), he presented a series of 345 operative survivors, about whom follow-up information was available [41]. The series included only five cases of BCLM, with one intraoperative death and a median postoperative survival of 6 months; 2-year survival was zero. The author described the results as "discouraging" and that the resection of liver metastases "cannot be recommended" except for the metastasis from a colorectal primary or from Wilms' tumor. He, however, added that in cases of a long disease-free interval, the patient's good general condition, the absence of accompanying diseases, and the surgeon's experience and dexterity in hepatic resection, "liver resection may occasionally be indicated," including the palliative resection of bulky tumors, functioning endocrine tumors, or in some rare cases to control hemorrhage from rupture of a necrotic tumor into the peritoneal cavity. In 1991, Elias et al. published the first series concerning specifically the liver resection for isolated BCLM [42]. From the 22 patients with BCLM undergoing explorative laparotomy, liver resection was possible in 12 patients, with a median survival time of 37 ± 9 months after resection. Although the median survival time was twice as much as those with conservative treatment, the authors considered the procedure as having "doubtful benefit" and rather serving as a "cytoreductive surgical treatment," with the main limiting factor being the relatively low effectiveness of chemotherapy. They recommended that the chemotherapeutic protocols be radically modified.

Since then, many centers have published their experiences with the surgical resection for BCLM, some of which with unexpectedly promising results, trying to evaluate safety and effectiveness of liver resection for BCLM, to define indications for liver resection, to identify prognostic factors affecting survival, and to set management guidelines for surgical approach (Table 2.2) [4, 5, 43–71]. As shown in Table 2.2, through aggressive combination therapy including liver resection, these studies achieved median survivals ranging from 15 to 91 months, with 5-year survival rates ranging from 11 to 61 %. In our own series of 41 consecutive patients undergoing liver resection for BCLM between 1999 and 2008 at the Department of General, Visceral and Transplant Surgery at the Ruprecht-Karls University of Heidelberg, a median overall survival from the primary tumor of 211 months and a 10-year survival rate from primary tumor of 76 % could be achieved following liver resection [48]. Adam et al. [52] in a study of 454 patients undergoing hepatic resection for BCLM even succeeded to show a 10-year survival rate of 22 % after liver resection. Twenty one out of 29 studies report a postoperative mortality rate of 0 % (complication rate of 21 %; range, 0–44 %), suggesting that liver resection for BCLM can, in the majority of patients, be performed safely. Some series have

Table 2.2 Patient series evaluating outcome after liver resection for BCLM

Author	Country	yr published	Study period	*n*	Postoperative mortality (%)	Median survival (mo)	5-yr survival (%)
Weinrich [43]	Germany	2014	2001–2007	21	0	53	33
Dittmar [44]	Germany	2013	1997–2010	34	0	36	28
Mariani [45]	France	2013	1988–2007	100	0	91	50
Polistina [46]	Italy	2013	2004–2011	12	0	13.5	11.5
Abbott [47]	United States	2012	1997–2010	86	0	57	44
Chua [5]	Australia	2011	2000–2011	553	0	40	40
Hoffmann [48]	Germany	2010	1999–2008	41	0	58	48
Thelen [49]	Germany	2008	1988–2006	39	0	16–74	42
Caralt [4]	Spain	2008	1988–2006	12	0	36	33
Lubrano [50]	France	2008	1989–2004	16	0	42	33
Adam [51]	France	2006	1984–2004	85	0	32	37
Adam [52]	France	2006	1983–2004	454	NR	45	41
Martinez [53]	United States	2006	1995–2004	20	NR	32	33
Sakamoto [54]	Japan	2005	1985–2003	34	0	36	21
Weitz [55]	United states	2005	1981–2002	29	0	48	NR
Yedibela [56]	Germany	2005	1978–2001	24	7	33	43
d'Annibale [57]	Italy	2005	1984–1999	18	0	32	30
Ercolani [58]	Italy	2005	1990–2003	21	0	42	25
Vlastos [59]	United States	2004	1991–2002	31	0	63	61
Arena [60]	Italy	2004	NR	17	NR	36	41
Elias [61]	France	2003	1986–2000	44	0	34	34
Carlini [62]	Italy	2002	1990–1999	17	0	53	46

(continued)

Table 2.2 (continued)

Author	Country	yr published	Study period	*n*	Postoperative mortality (%)	Median survival (mo)	5-yr survival (%)
Pocard [63]	France	2001	1988–1999	65	0	47	NR
Yoshimoto [64]	Japan	2000	1985–1998	25	NR	34	NR
Selzner [65]	United States	2000	1987–1999	17	6	25	22
Maksan [66]	Germany	2000	1984–1998	9	0	NR	51
Kondo [67]	Japan	2000	1990–1999	6	0	36	40
Raab [68]	Germany	1998	1983–1993	34	3	27	18
Elias [69]	France	1995	1986–1994	21	0	26	22
Lorenz [70]	Germany	1995	1982–1991	8	NR	15	12
Schneebaum [71]	United States	1994	1982–1990	6	NR	42	NR

Series including ≥5 patients undergoing liver resection for BCLM
yr year, *mo* month, *NR* not reported

yielded such promising results that Howlader et al. more recently claimed that the outcomes of liver resection for BCLM were comparable to those for colorectal cancer and suggested that liver resection be incorporated into the management guidelines [72]. It should be however pointed out that almost all of the studies mentioned in Table 2.2 are retrospective single-center case series of highly selected patients with limited hepatic metastases and no to minimal residual extrahepatic disease without a control group, thus allowing to yield only a level 4 evidence regarding the definitive role and survival benefit for the surgical resection of BCLM.

More recently, Mariani et al. have shown for the first time in a case-matched control study in highly selected patients that medical treatment combined with surgical resection of BCLM appears to provide a survival benefit compared with medical treatment alone [45]. In the "medical treatment plus surgical resection" arm, only the patients with stable disease or disease responding to medical treatment were included. The patients had (except for bone metastases) no extrahepatic distant metastasis and had ≤4 resectable BCLMs. This group of patients ($n=51$) was matched with the control "medical treatment alone" arm ($n=51$) for age, year of the primary disease diagnosis, time to metastasis, TNM stage, hormone receptor status, and BC tumor pathology. The "medical treatment plus surgical resection" was associated with significantly improved survival (81 % vs. 51 % at 36 months, RR=3.04, CI: 1.87–4.92, $p<0.0001$). Hence, Mariani et al. have already upgraded the level of evidence for the effectiveness of surgical resection for BCLM from level 4 to 3b. However, this growing body of evidence should be further evaluated in terms of definitive survival and quality of life advantages through controlled randomized clinical trials.

2.4.3 Analysis of Prognostic Factors

A variety of potential prognostic factors have been analyzed in the abovementioned case series in the context of liver resection for BCLM in an attempt to better define the subgroups that mostly benefit from this procedure. These include equivocal conclusions regarding prognostic value of demographics (age, gender), extrahepatic extent of disease as well as response to neoadjuvant chemotherapy, primary tumor biology (HR status), HER2 status, primary tumor surgical pathology (site, TNM, grading, surgical procedure), BCLM characteristics (synchronicity vs. metachronicity, number and size of metastases, HR status, invasion of adjacent structures), and surgical technical variables (histological margins, R_0 vs. $R_{1/2}$; type of resection, major vs. minor; and repeat hepatectomy) [73].

The positive or negative prognostic potentials of many of the abovementioned variables in some studies could not be documented in other studies. Moreover, some seemingly important prognostic factors have been documented to conversely affect the survival: while some authors have demonstrated that HR-negative BCLM is a negative predictor of overall survival [47, 48, 53, 61], others have shown the contrary [50]. Therefore, according to the current data, few generalizations concerning the prognostic value of a certain factor or another can be made. The reason most likely lies within the relatively small size of the available case series.

2.4.4 Selection Criteria and Timing of the Liver Resection for BCLM

In the context of highly selected series of patients undergoing liver surgery for BCLM, three general selection criteria have been applied by almost all centers performing liver surgery for BCLM. These include: (1) acceptable perioperative risk, (2) technically feasible liver resection, and (3) no to minimal residual extrahepatic disease. In our center, the selection criteria have been technical feasibility (≤5 metastases, no vascular invasion, potential feasibility to achieve R_0 resection), general performance status (Karnofsky index of 80 % or higher), and control of previously diagnosed extrahepatic metastases in a state of complete remission (no longer detectable after therapy) or stable disease (no change in size and no new lesions) for >12 months [48].

However, as mentioned previously, due to the equivocal data regarding the prognostic factors influencing survival after resection for BCLM, no strict selection criteria can be applied yet. One challenge regarding the patient selection concerns the extrahepatic disease at the time of surgery. As a matter of fact, isolated BCLM occurs only in a subset of patients with BC. Although some authors have demonstrated that in case of a stable disease, the presence of limited extrahepatic disease (including the presence of positive hilar lymph nodes) does not negatively affect survival after liver resection for BCLM [51, 64, 65], others have shown that the presence of even minimal extrahepatic residue actually significantly reduces survival [45, 48]. The same applies to the extent of resection: although it has been shown in some series, including our own series, that the positive resection margin ($R_{1/2}$ situation) is an independent prognostic factor that negatively affects survival [48, 49, 51], some other studies have shown that R situation does not affect the survival after resection [61].

Regarding the appropriate timing for the liver resection, Abbott et al. from Texas MD Anderson Cancer Center have recently shown the radiologic response of BCLM to chemotherapy immediately prior to surgical intervention to be the most reliable predictor of survival in patients undergoing resection for BCLM: patients with progressive disease under chemotherapy immediately prior to hepatectomy had a significantly lower median survival compared to those having at least a partial response [47]. This finding denotes the importance of a careful evaluation of response to chemotherapy, as the timing of liver resection is critical: the absence of radiologic response of BCLM to chemotherapy should prompt the surgeon to perform liver resection before the disease progression in the liver ensues.

2.4.5 Local Ablative Modalities

Radiofrequency ablation (RFA) is so far the most frequently employed local ablative modality for BCLM [73]. RFA can be performed with safety and with satisfying long-term outcome. Currently, there are a handful of small retrospective case series of BCLM ablation with RFA, reporting median overall survivals of 30–60 months and 5-year overall survivals of 30–38 % [59, 74]. Candidates for RFA are generally patients in whom a surgical resection cannot be performed due to poor general condition, inadequate estimated postoperative hepatic reserve, close proximity of the tumor to vital structures precluding R_0 resections, or bilobar BCLM. Intraoperative RFA may also be combined with liver resection in bilobar BCLM. Size criteria vary greatly, and local recurrence and treatment failure do occur more frequently due to incomplete peripheral ablations [75]. As the majority of reported series are small and represent diverse patient populations, prospective randomized trials are needed to determine the exact role of RFA in the management of BCLM.

Laser-induced interstitial thermotherapy (LITT) has been performed in a large series of patients ($n=232$) during a 10-year period, with a median survival of 52 months and 5-year overall survival of 41 % [76]. High-intensity focused ultrasound (HIFU) [77], microwave ablation [78], and percutaneous cryoablation [79] have also been used for the ablation of BCLM.

Percutaneous computed tomography-guided high-dose-rate brachytherapy [80] and stereotactic body radiotherapy (SBRT)/HT (helical tomotherapy) have been shown to have a good local control rate of BCLM [81]. Robotic radiosurgery with image-guided real-time tumor tracking of liver neoplasm has been described in the literature [82]. Most recently, a multi-institutional RCT comparing RFA and SBRT for hepatic oligometastasis (≤4 metastases) (RAS01-Trial, NCT01233544) has been initiated [83].

2.4.6 Non-ablative Liver-Directed Modalities

Transarterial chemoembolization (TACE) has been applied for BCLM with response rates ranging from 35.7 to 62.5 % and the average median overall survival of 27.9 months (range, 18.5–47 months) [84–87]. There is no consensus on the type of the chemotherapeutic agent of choice.

Isolated hepatic perfusion and percutaneous hepatic infusion to improve efficacy and limit unnecessary systemic toxicity by selectively delivering high-dose therapeutic agents into the hepatic arterial system are under clinical evaluation for patients with diffuse isolated BCLM [88, 89].

Radioembolization [90, 91] or radiochemoembolization using TACE followed by embolization with large radioisotope particles has been shown to be safe and provide different degrees of partial response or stable disease, but no complete response [92, 93].

2.4.7 Systemic Therapy

More than 100 randomized trials have compared more than a dozen of different chemotherapeutic agents. Response rates range between 12 and 83 % [94]. Even

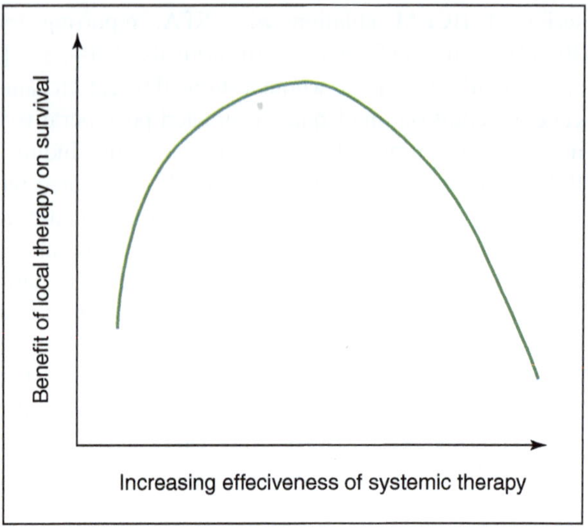

Fig. 2.2 The parabolic relationship between local therapy and systemic therapy of the metastatic breast cancer on survival (With permission from Punglia et al. [98])

with aggressive systemic chemotherapy alone, the median survival for patients with isolated BCLM has been only from 1 to 25 months (see above), with time to progression of 8–10 months in two more recent trials [95]; only rarely do the patients survive 5 years [96]. In view of the recent growing body of evidence presented here, the combination of aggressive local treatment and systemic therapy may improve survival in patients with resectable BCLM. Although stage IV BC is a systemic disease and liver surgery should still be considered as a "cytoreductive" rather than a "curative" resection, the combination of surgery may be beneficial due to the following reasons:

1. According to log-kill model, systemic chemotherapy destroys a constant fraction of cells. Therefore, performing a "cytoreductive" surgery may increase the odds that repetitive cycles of chemotherapy can significantly reduce the tumor load toward zero.
2. "Cytoreduction" may provide an immunologic benefit [97].

Punglia et al. have proposed a parabolic synergism between the effectiveness of the local therapy and systemic therapy (Fig. 2.2), so that the survival benefit yielded through local therapy (to a certain threshold of effectiveness) increases with increasingly effective systemic therapy [98].

2.4.8 Alternative Approaches

Novel therapies such as TALL-104 T cells [99] or high-dose chemotherapy with autologous stem cell transplantation for stage IV oligometastatic BC [100] are encouraging but need validation in prospective randomized studies.

2.4.9 Supportive Care and Palliative Treatment

Integration of supportive care and palliative treatment into mainstream healthcare service provision has emerged as the "gold standard" in comparative analysis of palliative care development [101]. Programs dealing with BC should provide a continuum through introducing supportive care during initial treatment, continuing supportive care after initial curative treatment, and ensuring supportive care and palliative end-of-life care for metastatic BC. Pain management should be a priority in supportive care for metastatic BC and end-of-life palliative care. Regular pain assessments and the proper use of pharmacologic and non-pharmacologic interventions are recommended [102]. Results of randomized trials recommend that psychosocial support be available to patients with metastatic BC. However, the optimal type, timing, and duration of such interventions are not clear [23]. Symptomatic anemia and/or leukopenia may be caused or aggravated by cytotoxic treatment and should be diagnosed, investigated, and corrected [23].

References

1. Jemal A, Bray F, Center MM, Ferlay J, Ward E, Forman D (2011) Global cancer statistics. CA Cancer J Clin 61:69–90
2. Redig AJ, McAllister SS (2013) Breast cancer as a systemic disease: a view of metastasis. J Intern Med 274:113–126
3. Disibio G, French SW (2008) Metastatic patterns of cancers: results from a large autopsy study. Arch Pathol Lab Med 132:931–993
4. Caralt M, Bilbao I, Cortés J et al (2008) Hepatic resection for liver metastases as part of the "oncosurgical" treatment of metastatic breast cancer. Ann Surg Oncol 15:2804–2810
5. Chua TC, Saxena A, Liauw W et al (2011) Hepatic resection for metastatic breast cancer: a systematic review. Eur J Cancer 47:2282–2290
6. Solomayer EF, Diel IJ, Meyberg GC et al (2000) Metastatic breast cancer: clinical course, prognosis and therapy related to the first site of metastasis. Breast Cancer Res Treat 59:271–278
7. Cutler SJ, Ardyce JA, Taylor SG III (1969) Classification of patients with disseminated cancer of the breast. Cancer 24:861–869
8. Largillier R, Ferrero JM, Doyen J et al (2008) Prognostic factors in 1,038 women with metastatic breast cancer. Ann Oncol 19:2012–2019
9. Cummings MC, Simpson PT, Reid LE et al (2014) Metastatic progression of breast cancer: insights from 50 years of autopsies. J Pathol 232:23–31
10. Slamon DJ, Clark GM, Wong SG et al (1987) Human breast cancer: correlation of relapse and survival with amplification of the HER-2/neu oncogene. Science 235:177–182
11. Tiwari RK, Borgen PI, Wong GY et al (1992) HER-2/neu amplification and overexpression in primary human breast cancer is associated with early metastasis. Anticancer Res 12:419–425
12. Bauer KR, Brown M, Cress RD et al (2007) Descriptive analysis of estrogen receptor (ER)-negative, progesterone receptor (PR)-negative, and HER2-negative invasive breast cancer, the so-called triple-negative phenotype: a population-based study from the California cancer Registry. Cancer 109:1721–1728
13. Dent R, Trudeau M, Pritchard KI et al (2007) Triple-negative breast cancer: clinical features and patterns of recurrence. Clin Cancer Res 13:4429–4434
14. Haffty BG, Yang Q, Reiss M et al (2006) Locoregional relapse and distant metastasis in conservatively managed triple negative early-stage breast cancer. J Clin Oncol 24:5652–5657

15. Bipat S, Leewen MS, Comans EFI et al (2005) Colorectal liver metastases: CT, MR imaging, and PET for diagnosis-meta-analysis. Radiology 237:123–131
16. Kinkel K, Lu Y, Both M et al (2002) Detection of hepatic metastases from cancers of the gastrointestinal tract by using noninvasive imaging methods (US, CT, MR imaging, PET): a meta-analysis. Radiology 224:748–756
17. Ward J, Robinson PJ, Guthrie JA et al (2005) Liver metastases in candidates for hepatic resection: comparison of helical CT and gadolinium- and SPIO-enhanced MR imaging. Radiology 237:170–180
18. Hong S, Li J, Wang S (2013) 18FDG PET-CT for diagnosis of distant metastases in breast cancer patients. A meta-analysis. Surg Oncol 22:139–143
19. Fletcher JW, Djulbegovic B, Soares HP et al (2008) Recommendations on the use of 18F-FDG PET in oncology. J Nucl Med 49:480–508
20. Hodgson NC, Gulenchyn KY (2008) Is there a role for positron emission tomography in breast cancer staging? J Clin Oncol 26:712–720
21. Gaeta CM, Vercher-Conejero JL, Sher AC et al (2013) Recurrent and metastatic breast cancer PET, PET/CT, PET/MRI: FDG and new biomarkers. Q J Nucl Med Mol Imaging 57:352–366
22. Lermite E, Marzano E, Chéreau E et al (2010) Surgical resection of liver metastases from breast cancer. Surg Oncol 19:e79–e84
23. Beslija S, Bonneterre J, Burstein H et al (2007) Second consensus on medical treatment of metastatic breast cancer. Ann Oncol 18:215–225
24. Khan SA, Stewart AK, Morrow M (2002) Does aggressive local therapy improve survival in metastatic breast cancer? Surgery 132:620–627
25. Babiera GV, Rao R, Feng L et al (2005) Effect of primary tumor extirpation in breast cancer patients who present with stage IV disease and an intact primary tumor. Ann Surg Oncol 13:776–782
26. Rapiti E, Verkooijen HM, Vlastos G et al (2006) Complete excision of primary breast tumor improves survival of patients with metastatic breast cancer at diagnosis. J Clin Oncol 24:2743–2749
27. Fields RC, Donna BJ, Trinkaus K et al (2007) Surgical resection of the primary tumor is associated with increased long-term survival in patients with stage IV breast cancer after controlling for site of metastasis. Ann Surg Oncol 14:3345–3351
28. Hazard HW, Gorla SR, Scholtens D et al (2008) Surgical resection of the primary tumor, chest wall control, and survival in women with metastatic breast cancer. Cancer 113:2011–2019
29. Rao R, Feng LMS, Kuerer HM et al (2008) Timing of surgical intervention for the intact primary in stage IV breast cancer patients. Ann Surg Oncol 15:1696–1702
30. Blanchard DK, Shetty PB, Hilsenbeck SG, Elledge RM (2008) Association of surgery with improved survival in stage IV breast cancer patients. Ann Surg 247:732–738
31. Cady B, Nathan NR, Michaelson JS et al (2008) Matched pair analyses of stage IV breast cancer with or without resection of primary breast site. Ann Surg Oncol 15:3384–3395
32. Ruiterkamp J, Ernst MF, van de Poll-Franse LV et al (2009) Surgical resection of the primary tumour is associated with improved survival in patients with distant metastatic breast cancer at diagnosis. Eur J Surg Oncol 35:1146–1151
33. Bafford AC, Burstein HJ, Barkley CR (2009) Breast surgery in stage IV breast cancer: impact of staging and patient selection on overall survival. Breast Cancer Res Treat 115:7–12
34. Shien T, Kinoshita T, Shimizu C et al (2009) Primary tumor resection improves the survival of younger patients with metastatic breast cancer. Oncol Rep 21:827–832
35. Leung AM, Vu HN, Nguyen KA et al (2009) Effects of surgical excision on survival of patients with stage IV breast cancer. J Surg Res 161:83–88
36. Neuman HB, Morrogh M, Gonen M et al (2010) Stage IV breast cancer in the era of targeted therapy: does surgery of the primary tumor matter? Cancer 116:1226–1233
37. Ruiterkamp J, Ernst MF, de Munck L et al (2011) Improved survival of patients with primary distant metastatic breast cancer in the period of 1995–2008. A nationwide population-based study in the Netherlands. Breast Cancer Res Treat 128:495–503

38. Gnerlich J, Jeffe DB, Deshpande AD et al (2007) Surgical removal of the primary tumor increases overall survival in patients with metastatic breast cancer. Analysis of the 1988–2003 SEER data. Ann Surg Oncol 14:2187–2194
39. Ruiterkamp J, Ernst MF (2011) The role of surgery in metastatic breast cancer. Eur J Cancer 47(Suppl 3):6–22
40. Brunschwig A (1963) Hepatic lobectomy for metastatic cancer. Cancer 16:277–282
41. Foster JH (1978) Survival after liver resection for secondary tumors. Am J Surg 135:389–394
42. Elias D, Lasser P, Spielmann M et al (1991) Surgical and chemotherapeutic treatment of hepatic metastases from carcinoma of the breast. Surg Gynecol Obstet 172:461–464
43. Weinrich M, Weiß C, Schuld J, Rau BM (2014) Liver resections of isolated liver metastasis in breast cancer: results and possible prognostic factors. HPB Surg. Epub 2014 Jan 19
44. Dittmar Y, Altendorf-Hofmann A, Schüle S et al (2013) Liver resection in selected patients with metastatic breast cancer: a single-centre analysis and review of literature. J Cancer Res Clin Oncol 139:1317–1325
45. Mariani P, Servois V, De Rycke Y et al (2013) Liver metastases from breast cancer: surgical resection or not? A case-matched control study in highly selected patients. Eur J Surg Oncol 39:1377–1383
46. Polistina F, Costantin G, Febbraro A et al (2013) Aggressive treatment for hepatic metastases from breast cancer: results from a single center. World J Surg 37:1322–1332
47. Abbott DE, Brouquet A, Mittendorf EA et al (2012) Resection of liver metastases from breast cancer: estrogen receptor status and response to chemotherapy before metastasectomy define outcome. Surgery 151:710–716
48. Hoffmann K, Franz C, Hinz U et al (2010) Liver resection for multimodal treatment of breast cancer metastases: identification of prognostic factors. Ann Surg Oncol 17:1546–1554
49. Thelen A, Benckert C, Jonas S et al (2008) Liver resection for metastases from breast cancer. J Surg Oncol 97:25–29
50. Lubrano J, Roman H, Tarrab S et al (2008) Liver resection for breast cancer metastasis: does it improve survival? Surg Today 38:293–299
51. Adam R, Aloia T, Krissat J et al (2006) Is liver resection justified for patients with hepatic metastases from breast cancer? Ann Surg 244:897–907
52. Adam R, Chiche L, Aloia T et al (2006) Hepatic resection for noncolorectal nonendocrine liver metastases: analysis of 1,452 patients and development of a prognostic model. Ann Surg 244:524–535
53. Martinez SR, Young SE, Giuliano AE, Bilchik AJ (2006) The utility of estrogen receptor, progesterone receptor, and Her-2/neu status to predict survival in patients undergoing hepatic resection for breast cancer metastases. Am J Surg 191:281–283
54. Sakamoto Y, Yamamoto J, Yoshimoto M et al (2005) Hepatic resection for metastatic breast cancer: prognostic analysis of 34 patients. World J Surg 29:524–527
55. Weitz J, Blumgart LH, Fong Y et al (2005) Partial hepatectomy for metastases from noncolorectal, nonneuroendocrine carcinoma. Ann Surg 241:269–276
56. Yedibela S, Gohl J, Graz V et al (2005) Changes in indication and results after resection of hepatic metastases from noncolorectal primary tumors: a single-institutional review. Ann Surg Oncol 12:778–785
57. d'Annibale M, Piovanello P, Cerasoli V et al (2005) Liver metastases from breast cancer: the role of surgical treatment. Hepatogastroenterology 52:1858–1862
58. Ercolani G, Grazi GL, Ravaioli M et al (2005) The role of liver resections for noncolorectal, nonneuroendocrine metastases: experience with 142 observed cases. Ann Surg Oncol 12:459–466
59. Vlastos G, Smith DL, Singletary SE et al (2004) Long-term survival after an aggressive surgical approach in patients with breast cancer hepatic metastases. Ann Surg Oncol 11:869–874
60. Arena E, Ferrero S (2004) Surgical treatment of liver metastases from breast cancer. Minerva Chir 59:7–15
61. Elias D, Maisonnette F, Druet-Cabanac M et al (2003) An attempt to clarify indications for hepatectomy for liver metastases from breast cancer. Am J Surg 185:158–164

62. Carlini M, Lonardo MT, Carboni F et al (2002) Liver metastases from breast cancer: results of surgical resection. Hepatogastroenterology 49:1597–1601
63. Pocard M, Pouillart P, Asselain B et al (2001) Hepatic resection for breast cancer metastases: results and prognosis (65 cases). Ann Chir 126:413–420
64. Yoshimoto M, Tada T, Saito M et al (2000) Surgical treatment of hepatic metastases from breast cancer. Breast Cancer Res Treat 59:177–184
65. Selzner M, Morse MA, Vredenburgh JJ et al (2000) Liver metastases from breast cancer: long-term survival after curative resection. Surgery 127:383–389
66. Maksan SM, Lehnert T, Bastert G et al (2000) Curative liver resection for metastatic breast cancer. Eur J Surg Oncol 26:209–212
67. Kondo S, Katoh H, Omi M et al (2000) Hepatectomy for metastases from breast cancer offers the survival benefit similar to that in hepatic metastases from colorectal cancer. Hepatogastroenterology 47:1501–1503
68. Raab R, Nussbaum KT, Behrend M et al (1998) Liver metastases of breast cancer: results of liver resection. Anticancer Res 18:2231–2233
69. Elias D, Lasser PH, Montrucolli D et al (1995) Hepatectomy for liver metastases from breast cancer. Eur J Surg Oncol 21:510–513
70. Lorenz M, Wiesner J, Staib-Sebler E, Encke A (1995) Regional therapy breast cancer liver metastases. Zentralbl Chir 120:786–790
71. Schneebaum S, Walker MJ, Young D et al (1994) The regional treatment of liver metastases from breast cancer. J Surg Oncol 55:26–31
72. Howlader M, Heaton N, Rela M (2011) Resection of liver metastases from breast cancer: towards a management guideline. Int J Surg 9:285–291
73. Bergenfeldt M, Jensen BV, Skjoldbye B, Nielsen D (2011) Liver resection and local ablation of breast cancer liver metastases–a systematic review. Eur J Surg Oncol 37:549–557
74. Lawes D, Chopada A, Gillams A et al (2006) Radiofrequency ablation (RFA) as a cytoreductive strategy for hepatic metastasis from breast cancer. Ann R Coll Surg Engl 88:639–642
75. Covey AM, Sofocleous CT (2008) Radiofrequency ablation as a treatment strategy for liver metastases from breast cancer. Semin Interv Radiol 25:406–412
76. Mack MG, Straub R, Eichler K et al (2004) Breast cancer metastases in liver: laser-induced interstitial thermotherapy-local tumor control rate and survival data. Radiology 233:400–409
77. Orsi F, Arnone P, Chen W, Zhang L (2010) High intensity focused ultrasound ablation: a new therapeutic option for solid tumors. J Cancer Res Ther 6:414–420
78. Lorentzen T, Skjoldbye BO, Nolsoe CP (2011) Microwave ablation of liver metastases guided by contrast-enhanced ultrasound: experience with 125 metastases in 39 patients. Ultraschall Med 32:492–496
79. Zhang W, Yu H, Guo Z et al (2014) Percutaneous cryoablation of liver metastases from breast cancer: initial experience in 17 patients. Clin Radiol 69:231–238
80. Collettini F, Golenia M, Schnapauff D et al (2012) Percutaneous computed tomography-guided high-dose-rate brachytherapy ablation of breast cancer liver metastases: initial experience with 80 lesions. J Vasc Interv Radiol 23:618–626
81. Habermehl D, Herfarth KK, Bermejo JL et al (2013) Single-dose radiosurgical treatment for hepatic metastases – therapeutic outcome of 138 treated lesions from a single institution. Radiat Oncol 8:175
82. Stintzing S, Hoffmann RT, Heinemann V et al (2010) Radiosurgery of liver tumors: value of robotic radiosurgical device to treat liver tumors. Ann Surg Oncol 17:2877–2883
83. Hoyer M, Swaminath A, Bydder S et al (2012) Radiotherapy for liver metastases: a review of evidence. Int J Radiat Oncol Biol Phys 82:1047–1057
84. Duan XF, Dong NN, Zhang T, Li Q (2011) Treatment outcome of patients with liver-only metastases from breast cancer after mastectomy: a retrospective analysis. J Cancer Res Clin Oncol 137:1363–1370
85. Giroux MF, Baum RA, Soulen MC (2004) Chemoembolization of liver metastasis from breast carcinoma. J Vasc Interv Radiol 15:289–291

86. Li XP, Meng ZQ, Guo WJ, Li J (2005) Treatment for liver metastases from breast cancer: results and prognostic factors. World J Gastroenterol 11:3782–3787
87. Vogl TJ, Naguib NN, Nour-Eldin NE et al (2010) Transarterial chemoembolization (TACE) with mitomycin C and gemcitabine for liver metastases in breast cancer. Eur Radiol 20:173–180
88. Ang C, Jhaveri K, Patel D et al (2013) Hepatic arterial infusion and systemic chemotherapy for breast cancer liver metastases. Breast J 19:96–99
89. Nielsen DL, Nørgaard H, Vestermark LW et al (2012) Intrahepatic and systemic therapy with oxaliplatin combined with capecitabine in patients with hepatic metastases from breast cancer. Breast 21:556–561
90. Smits ML, Prince JF, Rosenbaum CE et al (2013) Intra-arterial radioembolization of breast cancer liver metastases: a structured review. Eur J Pharmacol 709:37–42
91. Coldwell D, Sangro B, Salem R et al (2012) Radioembolization in the treatment of unresectable liver tumors: experience across a range of primary cancers. Am J Clin Oncol 35:167–177
92. Buijs M, Kamel IR, Vossen JA et al (2007) Assessment of metastatic breast cancer response to chemoembolization with contrast agent enhanced and diffusion-weighted MR imaging. J Vasc Interv Radiol 18:957–963
93. Akhlaghpoor S, Aziz-Ahari A, Amoui M, Tolooee S et al (2012) Short-term effectiveness of radiochemoembolization for selected hepatic metastases with a combination protocol. World J Gastroenterol 18:5249–5259
94. Rodes Brown S, Martin RC 2nd (2012) Management of liver dominant metastatic breast cancer: surgery, chemotherapy, or hepatic arterial therapy – benefits and limitations. Minerva Chir 67:297–308
95. Atalay G, Biganzoli L, Renard F et al (2003) Clinical outcome of breast cancer patients with liver metastases alone in the anthracycline-taxane era: a retrospective analysis of two prospective, randomised metastatic breast cancer trials. Eur J Cancer 39:2439–2449
96. Wyld L, Gutteridge E, Pinder SE et al (2003) Prognostic factors for patients with hepatic metastases from breast cancer. Br J Cancer 89:284–290
97. Kavanaugh DY, Carbone DP (1996) Immunologic dysfunction in cancer. Hematol Oncol Clin N Am 10:927–951
98. Punglia RS, Morrow M, Winer EP, Harris JR (2007) Local therapy and survival in breast cancer. N Engl J Med 356:2399–2405
99. Visonneau S, Cesano A, Porter DL et al (2000) Phase I trial of TALL-104 cells in patients with refractory metastatic breast cancer. Clin Cancer Res 6:1744–1754
100. Nieto Y, Nawaz S, Jones RB et al (2002) Prognostic model for relapse after high-dose chemotherapy with autologous stem-cell transplantation for stage IV oligometastatic breast cancer. J Clin Oncol 20:707–718
101. Lynch T, Connor S, Clark D (2013) Mapping levels of palliative care development: a global update. J Pain Symptom Manag 45:1094–1106
102. Cleary J, Ddungu H, Distelhorst SR et al (2013) Supportive and palliative care for metastatic breast cancer: resource allocations in low- and middle-income countries. A Breast Health Global Initiative 2013 consensus statement. Breast 22:616–627

Liver Metastases from Kidney Cancer

3

Enrico Pinotti, Francesca Ratti, Federica Cipriani, and Luca Aldrighetti

3.1 Incidence

Kidney cancer is the ninth most frequent cause of malignant tumors in developed countries and accounts for nearly 2 % of all malignancies [1]. The incidence of kidney cancer varies considerably among different populations and regions. Rates are higher in Western and Eastern Europe, North America, and Australia (8–10 cases per 100,000) and lower in Asia, Africa, and the Pacific (1–2 cases per 100,000) [2]. This geographic variation has been ascribed to differences in diagnostic intensity as well as to environmental factors that are likely to play an important role in renal cell carcinogenesis (e.g., smoke and obesity) [2].

Kidney cancer is a tumor of adults occurring primarily after the fifth decade of life, with a mean age of diagnosis of 65 years [3] and a men to women ratio between 1.5:1 and 2.5 [2].

Liver metastases from kidney cancer represent about 5–8 % of secondary noncolorectal nonneuroendocrine liver tumors and are present in 20.3 % of metastatic kidney cancers [4]. Metastases to the liver seem to be associated with a particularly poor prognosis because of their association with widely disseminated disease, and indeed metastases from kidney cancer are confined to the liver in only 10–15 % of cases, while in 85–90 % of cases are associated with extrahepatic disease. In general, the incidence of metastases increases with the size of the primary lesion. Despite this tendency, metastases may occur from very small lesions, and conversely the primary lesion may become quite without identifiable extrarenal disease.

E. Pinotti • F. Ratti • F. Cipriani • L. Aldrighetti (✉)
Hepatobiliary Surgery Unit, IRCCS San Raffaele Hospital,
Via Olgettina 60, Milan, MI 20132, Italy
e-mail: enricopinotti@hotmail.it; ratti.francesca@hsr.it; cipriani.federica@hsr.it; aldrighetti.luca@hsr.it

I. Di Carlo (ed.), *Noncolorectal, Nonneuroendocrine Liver Metastases: Diagnosis and Current Therapies*, DOI 10.1007/978-3-319-09293-5_3

About 10 % of liver metastases from kidney cancer are synchronous and 90 % are metachronous. When liver metastases are present in about 25 % of cases are solitary and in 75 % of cases are multiple [5].

The most important risk factors for liver metastases development in patients with kidney cancer are:

- *Histological subtype*: Approximately 85 % of kidney cancers are renal cell carcinoma (RCC), while others are urothelial cancers of the renal pelvis. Renal cell carcinoma is not a single entity but rather a group of tumors originating from kidney epithelium. The most common histological type is clear cell carcinoma (also called conventional RCC) which represents 75–80 % of RCC. Papillary (10–15 %), chromophobe (5 %), and other more rare forms such as collecting duct carcinoma (<1 %) are other forms of RCC.

  In patients with chromophobe carcinoma, a metastatic spread to the liver is more frequent (39 %) than in patients with clear cell carcinoma (9.2 %) and patients with papillary kidney cancer (18 %) [6].
- *Genetic susceptibility*: Approximately 4–5 % of kidney cancers are hereditary forms and typically occur in younger patients [7]. The most common syndromes associated with renal cell carcinoma are:
  - *Von Hippel–Lindau (VHL) syndrome*. It is a relative rare autosomal dominant disorder with an incidence of 1/35,000. It results from a mutation in VHL gene. About 25–45 % of patients with VHL syndrome develop renal cell carcinoma, typically between 25 and 60 years of age [8]. In these patients, tumor growth is relatively slow, and metastases are infrequent for lesions <3 cm, when tumors are bigger than 3 cm metastases are instead frequent. Liver metastases are present in 20 % of patients with metastatic VHL syndrome [8].
  - Hereditary leiomyomatosis and renal cell carcinoma (HLRCC). This syndrome is caused by mutations in the fumarate hydratase (FH) and usually occurs between 35 and 45 years [9]. When kidney cancer is present, metastatic spread is fast (72 % in 1 year). Liver metastases are present in 20–30 % of cases [9].
  - *Birt–Hogg–Dube (DBH) syndrome*. It is an autosomal dominant disease caused by mutations in *BHD* gene. About 25–35 % of patients with BHD syndrome develop renal tumors. Various histological types of renal cell carcinoma may be present in a single patient affected from BHD syndrome. Chromophobe kidney cancer is frequent in DBH syndrome. Liver metastases are present in 30–40 % of cases.

3.2 Natural History

Liver involvement in patients with renal cell carcinoma may occur with two different patterns: (a) by direct infiltration or (b) by metastatic spread.

(a) Kidney cancer develops as discrete, focal mass lesions and grows in an infiltrating pattern. Local extension through the renal capsule and beyond Gerota fascia may lead to involvement of contiguous retro- or intraperitoneal structures such as psoas, diaphragm, bowel, mesentery, and even liver.

(b) Invasion into segmental branches of the renal vein is not uncommon. Subsequent extension into the inferior vena cava allows hematogenous spread to the lungs, liver, bones, and central nervous system. Metastases have been described in virtually every part of the body. In general, the incidence of metastases increases with the size of the primary lesion [10]. Despite this tendency, metastases may occur from very small lesions, and conversely the primary lesion may become quite large in the absence of visible extrarenal disease.

More than 50 % of the renal cancers are detected incidentally in asymptomatic patients (incidentalomas). At initial presentation, approximately 30 % of patients with renal cell carcinoma have metastatic disease. The most common site of metastatic RCC is the lung (75 % of patients with metastatic RCC [11]). Other frequent sites are the liver and bone. Liver metastases have been reported in 1–7 % of cases and in 20.3 % of metastatic liver cancers. Metastases to the liver seem to be associated with a particularly poor prognosis because of its association with widely disseminated disease. Solitary metastases to the liver are reported to occur in 5.4 % of all cases with metastases [5].

It is well known that metastases in the liver are usually silent. Accordingly, most patients with hepatic metastases are asymptomatic for a long period of time. Laboratory measurements of liver enzymes and tumoral markers have been examined as a method of detecting hepatic metastases and as prognostic determinants. Patients with minute or solitary liver metastases may show a normal biochemical profile. Associated with the progression of metastatic disease, patients may experience cholestatic disease due to neoplastic tissue compression of portobiliary pedicles. When symptoms occur, they may include:

- Loss of appetite
- Weight loss
- Jaundice
- Pain in the upper right abdomen
- Nausea
- Sweats and fever
- Ascites

Symptoms of synchronous liver metastases can be associated with signs and symptoms of primary tumor.

Most frequent symptoms of the primary tumor in the kidney are:

- Classic symptoms of pain, macroscopic hematuria, and palpable mass: less than 10 % of the patients.
- Symptoms due to locally advanced disease including varicocele, or lower extremity edema, which suggests venous involvement: present in advanced renal cell carcinoma.

- Paraneoplastic syndromes: present in 10–40 % of kidney cancers. The most common paraneoplastic syndromes are:
  - Hypercalcemia that occurs in up to 10–20 % of RCC [12] due to the production of parathyroid hormone-related peptide (PTHrP) from the tumor.
  - Hypertension.
  - Polycythemia.
  - Stauffer's syndrome: it is a nonmetastatic hepatic dysfunction characterized by increased alkaline phosphatase, increased transaminases, prolonged prothrombin time (PT), and hepatosplenomegaly in the absence of liver metastases in patients with RCC. The pathophysiology of Stauffer's syndrome is unclear. In most patients the syndrome resolves after nephrectomy and may recur with recurrence of the cancer suggesting involvement of a humoral substance [13]. Anyway in case of increased alkaline phosphatase, increased transaminases, and prolonged prothrombin time, the first step must be the exclusion of liver metastases.

3.3 Diagnosis and Staging

In patient with kidney cancer staging is a fundamental step to determine both prognosis and therapeutical approach.

3.3.1 Transabdominal Ultrasonography (US)

The advantages of ultrasonography are its ready accessibility, low cost, and noninvasive nature. Doppler-enhanced ultrasonography is a potential improvement because it can identify tumor neovascularization even though 20 % of liver metastases from renal cell carcinomas are not hypervascular [14]. On ultrasound (US), liver metastases from RCC are usually hypoechoic but can rarely be even isoechoic or hyperechoic. Doppler ultrasonography also facilitates the assessment of tumor thrombus extension into the renal veins, inferior vena cava, and right side of the heart.

Intraoperative ultrasound (IOUS) is the most accurate imaging technique for detecting liver metastases at the time of primary tumor resection or resection of previously identified hepatic metastases. It is a fundamental tool during resection of liver metastases both for liver anatomy evaluation and for ultrasound-guided resection [15].

3.3.2 Computed Tomography (CT)

CT is the gold standard for detection and characterization of liver masses. CT is associated with ready availability, low cost, and high accuracy for the identification of liver metastases and for staging of renal cell carcinoma. CT accuracy is above 95 % for liver metastases from renal cell carcinoma [16]. On CT liver metastases

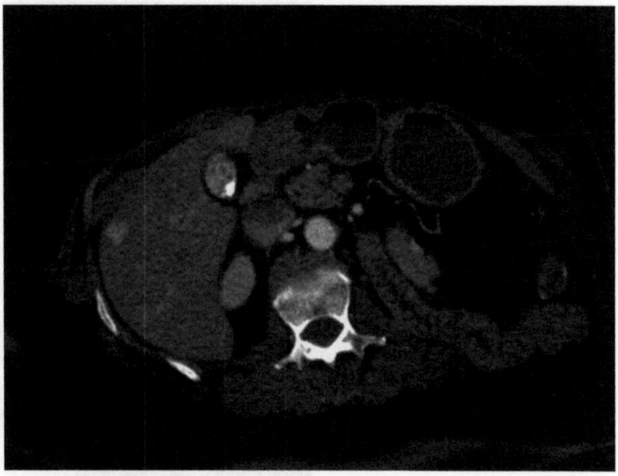

Fig. 3.1 Liver metastases from kidney cancer on CT scan (arterial phase)

are highly vascular, like the primary tumor (Fig. 3.1). Arterial-phase scanning is essential for detecting vascular liver metastases which appear hyperdense. About 10 % of the hepatic lesions are missed in the portal venous phase when smaller than 2 cm [17]. The combination of unenhanced, arterial phase, and portal venous phase should be used in initial evaluation of patients with metastatic RCC for improved lesion detection and characterization. Hepatic metastases may have central necrotic areas which appear hypodense after contrast administration. Occasionally, these lesions are calcified, contain fat, or may present signs of rupture with intraperitoneal hemorrhage.

3.3.3 Magnetic Resonance (MR)

Magnetic resonance imaging is commonly used following CT if there are still issues related to diagnosis or staging of the tumor. In particular it is frequently used to evaluate infiltration of closer organs (e.g., liver involvement in case of right kidney cancer). Liver metastases from RCC are usually hypervascular in gadolinium-enhanced MR imaging such as neuroendocrine tumors, melanoma, and thyroid carcinoma. Liver metastases are hypointense on the T1-weighted image and iso-hyperintense on the T2-weighted image (Figs. 3.2 and 3.3). Morphologic, signal intensity, and contrast enhancement features have been shown to be useful in distinguishing metastatic lesions from common benign lesions such as hemangiomas and cysts.

3.3.4 PET Scan

PET scan is not a recommended technique for the diagnosis and follow-up of liver metastases from kidney cancer due to histopathological characteristics of primary tumor. In low-grade kidney cancer, PET is often negative, and evaluation of primary

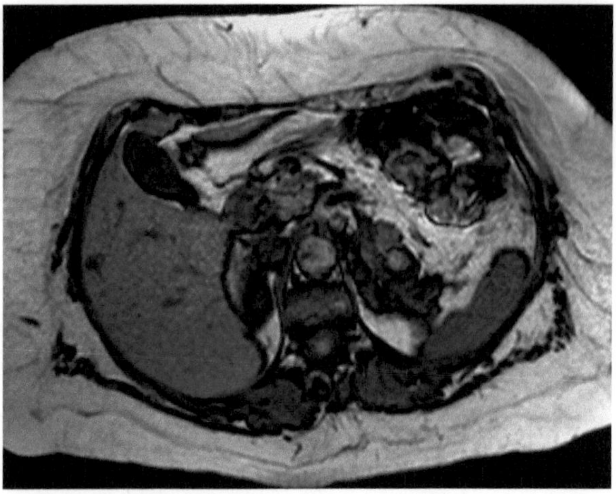

Fig. 3.2 Liver metastases from kidney cancer on RM (T1 weight)

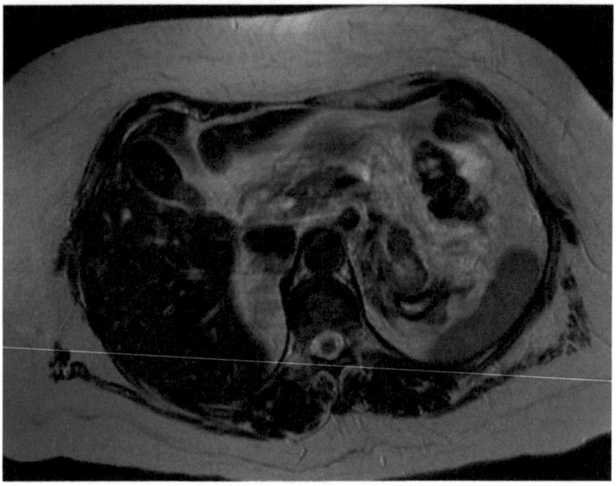

Fig. 3.3 Liver metastases from kidney cancer on RM (T2 weight)

cancer is therefore difficult. Indeed significant uptakes of FDG are normal in kidneys because of the inability of the nephron to reabsorb filtered FDG in the convoluted tubules. That is why PET scan is often falsely positive in kidney cancer, and it is not a recommended technique in diagnosis and follow-up of liver metastases from kidney cancer as well [18].

3.3.5 Staging

The TNM staging system for kidney cancer defines local extension of the primary tumor (T), involvement of regional lymph nodes (N), and presence of distant metastases (M) (Tables 3.1, 3.2 and 3.3). The incidence of liver metastases is associated

Table 3.1 TNM for RCC

		Incidence of synchronous liver metastases [15, 16]	Incidence of metachronous liver metastases after 5 years from primary tumor resection [15, 16]
T0	No evidence of primary tumor	–	–
T1	Tumor ≤7 cm in greatest dimension, limited to the kidney	<1 %	1–2 %
T1a	Tumor ≤4 cm in greatest dimension, limited to the kidney	<0.5 %	1 %
T1b	Tumor >4 cm but not >7 cm in greatest dimension, limited to the kidney	1 %	1–2 %
T2	Tumor >7 cm in greatest dimension, limited to the kidney	2–6 %	4–12 %
T2a	Tumor >7 cm but ≤10 cm in greatest dimension, limited to the kidney	2–3 %	4–6 %
T2b	Tumor >10 cm, limited to the kidney	4–5 %	7–12 %
T3	Tumor extends into major veins or perinephric tissues but not into the ipsilateral adrenal gland and not beyond Gerota fascia	6–14 %	12–27 %
T3a	Tumor grossly extends into the renal vein or its segmental (muscle containing) branches, or tumor invades perirenal and/or renal sinus fat but not beyond Gerota fascia	6–8 %	12–16 %
T3b	Tumor grossly extends into the vena cava below the diaphragm	8–10 %	18–23 %
T3c	Tumor grossly extends into the vena cava above the diaphragm or invades the wall of the vena cava	12–14 %	20–27 %
T4	Tumor invades beyond Gerota fascia (including contiguous extension into the ipsilateral adrenal gland)	12–20 %	>30 %

with local extension of primary tumor (T) (Table 3.1). Synchronous liver metastases are rare in T1a tumors (<4 cm).

In a recent study Kunkle et al. [19] analyzed the incidence of synchronous metastases in 360 patients with kidney cancer and demonstrated that tumors associated with synchronous metastases were significantly larger than those in patients without secondary lesions. In this study there were no patients with tumors <2 cm who presented with confirmed metastatic disease, and less than 5 % of all synchronous metastases occurred in tumors <3.0 cm. In the series of Thompson et al., only 1 patient of 781 with kidney tumor <3 cm had synchronous liver metastases [20].

The incidence of metachronous liver metastases after renal resection is associated with the size of primary tumor. The overall incidence of metastases is, respectively, 3, 13, and 29 % for pT1a, pT1b, and pT2 after 5 years from primary tumor

Table 3.2 TNM for RCC

N	NX	Regional lymph nodes cannot be assessed
	N0	No regional lymph node metastases
	N1	Metastases in a single regional lymph node
	N2	Metastases in more than one regional lymph node
M	MX	Distant metastases cannot be assessed
	M0	No distant metastases
	M1	Distant metastases

Table 3.3 RCC stage

Stage	T	N	M
I	T1	N0	M0
II	T2	N0	M0
III	T1 or T2	N1	M0
	T3	N0 or N1	M0
IV	T4	Any N	M0
	Any T	Any N	M1

resection, and, when metastases are present, liver involvement is observed in 20.3 % of cases (Table 3.1) [20].

When tumor grossly extends into the renal vein or into its segmental branches, invades perirenal and/or renal sinus fat without passing Gerota fascia (pT3a), extends into the vena cava below or above the diaphragm (pT3b, pT3c), or invades beyond Gerota fascia (pT4), the incidence of synchronous and metachronous metastases is higher (30–70 %), and the incidence of liver metastases is 25–50 %.

Risk of metastases according to TNM classification and stage of RCC is shown in Tables 3.1, 3.2, and 3.3.

3.4 Treatment

Options for treatment of liver metastases from renal cancer include surgery, ablative therapies, and chemotherapy. Indications vary depending on the stage of the disease, presence of extrahepatic metastases, and general status of patients and are evaluated on a case-by-case analysis in a multidisciplinary approach with a synergy of surgeons, oncologists, radiologists, and radiotherapists.

3.4.1 Surgery

Liver metastases develop in 30–40 % of patients with metastatic kidney cancer [21] and in most cases coexist with multiple extrahepatic metastases. Prognosis of these patients is generally poor, and without treatment most patients die within 4 months after diagnosis with only 10 % 1-year overall survival. In the series of Suppiah et al., the median survival of 186 untreated patients with hepatic metastases from renal cell carcinoma was 7.8 months [22]. However, in 2–4 % of patients, metastases are limited to the liver, and patients can therefore be candidates to liver resection. Thanks to the development of surgical technique, liver resection is presently a procedure with low mortality (0–2 %) and acceptable morbidity (20–30 %) [23] and represents the only potentially curative treatment for patients with metastases from renal cell carcinoma, offering the chance for long-term survival: indeed renal carcinomas and their metastases rarely respond to traditional systemic chemotherapy, radiotherapy, or hormone modulation therapy.

Synchronous Liver Metastases

Synchronous liver metastases represent about 10 % of liver metastases from kidney cancer. The subset of patients with potentially surgically resectable primary RCC and resectable liver metastases (2–5 %) are candidates to nephrectomy and liver resection. Candidates include patients who initially present with primary RCC and both solitary or multiple resectable liver metastases. Primary tumor and liver metastases may be resected during the same operation or through staged procedures. The most frequent surgical strategy is the second one, while simultaneous nephrectomy and hepatic resection are uncommonly performed during a combined procedure.

Sakaguchi et al. in 1992 demonstrated the feasibility of simultaneous liver resection and nephrectomy for a large RCC with caval thrombus [24]. The main problem to deal with during combined procedure is that liver resection and nephrectomy need conflicting hemodynamic techniques: during nephrectomy, a normovolemic or hypervolemic state is preferred to supply the contralateral kidney with adequate volume, therefore maximizing renal plasma flow to the remnant kidney. By contrast, relative hypovolemia is desired during hepatic resection (low central venous pressure technique) to limit blood loss during parenchymal transection phase of the operation. Anyway, in patients needing caval thrombectomy, hypoperfusion is especially dangerous because of an increased risk of thrombosis [25].

In the most series, the most frequent indication to combined renal and hepatic surgery is instead locally advanced renal cell carcinoma. Outcome of combined procedures is reported only in few limited series from literature [26, 27]; therefore, indications, perioperative management, and postoperative outcomes for simultaneous liver and kidney resection remain poorly defined. In a recent single-center study, Yezhelyev et al. [25] analyzed outcome of 20 patients who underwent synchronous hepatic and renal resection. To optimize perioperative fluid management, hepatectomy was performed before nephrectomy whenever possible. This strategy allowed maintenance of a low central venous pressure (CVP) technique during hepatic parenchymal transection, followed by fluid repletion before and during nephrectomy. Low central venous pressure was maintained as long as adequate urine output of 25 mL/h and systolic blood pressure of 90 mmHg were preserved during transection of liver parenchyma. At the conclusion of the liver resection, crystalloids were administered to achieve a relative hypervolemic state for optimal kidney resection. In this series, 50 % of patients developed major postoperative complications, and postoperative mortality was 5 %. Pulmonary complications were among the most common in the postoperative period (30 %), followed by intra-abdominal (15 %) and surgical site infections (15 %).

Nephrectomy associated with liver resection can therefore be offered to carefully selected patients with synchronous neoplasms of the liver and kidney in centers with high volume of liver and kidney resection. Because of the low number of study about simultaneous hepatic and renal resection, indications of this procedure are still not codificated.

In patients with unresectable synchronous liver metastases, cytoreductive nephrectomy before systemic therapy is recommended. Many randomized clinical studies show that cytoreductive surgery in association with systemic therapy provides a significant survival benefit compared with systemic therapy alone for patients with metastatic RCC [28]. The European Organization for Research and Treatment of Cancer reported a trial where patients with metastatic RCC were randomized to treatment with INF-alpha or INF-alpha plus radical nephrectomy. In the group submitted to radical nephrectomy, the overall survival was 17 months compared to a survival of 7 months reported for patients without nephrectomy [29]. Cytoreductive surgery of primary tumor has been for decades the gold standard treatment for metastatic RCC because spontaneous regression of metastases was expected upon primary cancer removal. Furthermore, surgical resection of large symptomatic cancer may have a significant palliative effect even in terms of quality of life.

Surgical option includes radical nephrectomy and nephron-sparing surgery. A radical nephrectomy requires proximal ligation of the renal artery and vein and removal of the kidney with Gerota fascia, ipsilateral adrenal gland, and regional lymph nodes. Radical nephrectomy is the preferred treatment for tumors extending into the inferior vena cava. Nephron-sparing surgery was originally indicated only if a radical nephrectomy would have rendered patient functionally anephric, necessitating dialysis. It was also indicated in patients with hereditary forms of RCC who may have multiple tumors and in patients with a unilateral tumor and functioning contralateral kidney affected by renal artery stenosis, hydronephrosis, chronic pyelonephritis, reflux, kidney stones, or systemic conditions such as hypertension or diabetes [30]. However, nephron-sparing surgery has been used increasingly in patients with a normal contralateral kidney, with long-term outcomes comparable to radical nephrectomy [31]. The additional benefits of nephrectomy and nephron-sparing surgery include improved performance status, elimination of paraneoplastic syndromes, and eradication of the source of new metastases. Many series in literature showed that survival in patients with metastatic kidney cancer underwent nephron-sparing surgery of the primary tumor and patients underwent radical nephrectomy was comparable [32].

Metachronous Liver Metastases

After surgical excision of the primary tumor from the kidney, 20 to 30 % of patients with localized tumors show disease recurrence. The median time to relapse after surgery ranges between 1 and 2 years, with most recurrences occurring within 3 years. Adjuvant treatment after nephrectomy has no established role in patients who have undergone a complete resection of primary tumor. No systemic therapy has been shown to reduce the risk of recurrence [33], so observation remains standard care after nephrectomy. Follow-up for patients with radical resection includes an abdominal and chest CT scan approximately 4–6 months after surgery, then as clinically indicated considering the stage of the primary tumor. Data about the results of liver resection performed in patients with metachronous liver metastases from renal cell carcinoma are still sparse, and selection criteria for patients suitable for liver resection have not been established yet.

Thelen et al. analyzed the outcome of 31 patients who underwent hepatectomy for metastases from renal cell carcinoma [34]. In this study hepatic resection was considered when resection was likely to be curative in the absence of irresectable extrahepatic metastases. Resectable extrahepatic disease was not considered as a contraindication provided that the overall surgical strategy aimed to be curative. Overall 1-, 3-, and 5-year survival rates were 82.2, 54.3, and 38.9 %, respectively. These long-term results are not inferior to survival rates achieved by liver resection in patients with metastases from colorectal cancer and are comparable to results after resection of pulmonal metastases from renal cell carcinoma, which are presently a generally accepted indication for an aggressive surgical approach in these patients [35]. Tumor recurrence represents the main cause for death after resection of liver metastases from renal cell carcinoma, especially pulmonary recurrences. The survival after hepatectomy with negative margins is superior survival of patients treated by immunotherapy or chemotherapy. Surgical treatment of hepatic metastases from renal cell carcinoma is actually performed in approximately 1 % of patients with liver metastases. Other series from literature suggest that surgical treatment can provide favorable survival rates, with a 5-year survival of 39–60 % [36]. In the multi-institutional analysis of Hatzaras et al. [37], overall 3-year survival after liver resection for metastases from renal cell carcinoma was 62.1 %, 3-year recurrence-free survival was 27.3 %, and the median length of recurrence-free survival was 15.5 months [37].

These data on survival rates after surgery, combined with the unavailability of effective systemic therapies, justify an aggressive surgical approach in patients with hepatic metastases from renal cell carcinoma when a margin-negative resection can be obtained. Prognostic factors predicting long-term survival after resection of liver metastases from renal cell carcinoma included male sex, maximum metastases diameter of 5 cm, disease-free interval of 24 months, and tumor-negative resection margins [34]. Liver resection is considered effective and safe in the treatment of patients with hepatic metastases from renal cell carcinoma and offers the chance of long-term survival and cure. Unfortunately, despite "R0" hepatic resection, many patients will have recurrences both in the liver and at extrahepatic sites. In addition, no reliable serologic marker of recurrence or disease burden exists. As such, the importance of close clinical follow-up after hepatic resection including axial imaging of the thorax and abdomen cannot be understated. Clinical and CT scan follow-up at 3-month intervals for the first 2 years following resection, and subsequent follow-up at 6-month intervals, is recommended [38].

3.4.2 Local Therapies

Ablative therapies, including cryoablation and radiofrequency ablation (RFA) and other local treatment like trans-arterial chemoembolization (TACE), are available for treatment of liver metastases from kidney cancer when surgery is not indicated. Only few studies on this topic are present in literature considering that ablative therapies are relatively recent techniques and that liver metastases from kidney cancer are relatively rare. Radiofrequency ablation and cryoablation can be performed using different approaches: laparoscopic approach (requiring general anesthesia) or percutaneous approach, which can be performed under local anesthesia.

Many studies have demonstrated efficacy of RFA for the treatment of liver metastases from colorectal cancer, but in literature there are no studies about the efficacy of RFA in liver metastases from kidney cancer. In a recent study [39] Bo La Yun et al. analyzed the outcome of 25 patients affected by non-colorectal liver metastases (including metastases from kidney cancer) after percutaneous radiofrequency ablation. They showed that RFA has relatively less therapeutic effectiveness for treatment of non-colorectal origin liver metastases compared with colorectal liver metastases. Survival rate for patients with non-colorectal liver metastases was 86, 39, and 19 % for 1 year, 3 years, and 5 years, respectively. Survival rate for patients with non-colorectal liver metastases was 86, 39, and 19 % for 1 year, 3 years, and 5 years, respectively; studies about RFA in patients with colorectal liver metastases showed that the 1-, 3-, and 5-year estimated survival rates were 87–96 %, 42–57 %, and 24–44 %, respectively [40]. Anyway, the low morbidity and mortality rates and the improved selectivity of candidates for RFA suggest the possible broad application of RFA treatment for liver metastases from kidney cancer when surgical resection cannot be performed [40].

Few studies analyze the topic of trans-arterial chemoembolization treatment for liver metastases from kidney cancer: these metastases are characterized by their hypervascularity, which makes chemoembolization feasible and effective. Nabil et al. [41] analyzed the outcome of 22 patients who underwent TACE for liver metastases from renal cell carcinoma: partial response was achieved in 13.7 %, stable disease in 59 %, and progressive disease was encountered in 27.3 % of the patients. This study demonstrates that TACE can result in a favorable local tumor response in patients with hepatic metastases from kidney cancer, but survival results are still limited.

3.4.3 Medical Treatment

Chemotherapy and immunotherapy can be used in patients with non-resectable synchronous or metachronous liver metastases from kidney cancer. Metastatic renal cell carcinoma has historically been considered resistant to chemotherapy and hormonal therapy. Immunotherapy has been indeed used as a first-line treatment in advanced or metastatic RCC with limited success. However, treatment of metastatic RCC has changed dramatically with the availability of new treatment options.

Molecular research into pathogenesis of RCC has provided valuable information about the altered signaling pathways in RCC. Therapy has changed in metastatic settings with the arrival of targeted agents, with two types of drugs: antiangiogenic agents and mammalian target of rapamycin inhibitors.

Sixty percent of clear cell carcinomas appear to contain an inactivated von Hippel–Lindau (VHL) tumor suppressor gene. Alterations in VHL gene cause elevated protein levels of hypoxiainducible factor-1α (HIF-1α), which upregulates vascular endothelial growth factor (VEGF) and platelet-derived growth factor (PDGF) genes and proteins [42]. Consequently, the overexpression of these growth factors results in tumor angiogenesis and extensive vascularization of primary renal cell carcinoma and metastases. Therefore, tumor angiogenesis has become an important focus of targeted therapy for RCC. This class of agents includes bevacizumab, a monoclonal antibody targeting vascular endothelial growth factor, administered by infusion, and vascular endothelial growth factor receptor tyrosine kinase inhibitors (TKIs) sunitinib, sorafenib, and pazopanib.

Besides inhibition of VEGF signaling, mammalian target of rapamycin (mTOR) is another important therapeutic target in RCC. mTOR pro-survival pathway lies downstream of PI3K/Akt pathway and is regulated by PTEN tumor suppressor gene. mTOR phosphorylation induces translation of messenger RNAs encoding cell cycle regulators and transcription factors that promote proliferation, including HIF. The mTOR inhibition should therefore directly inhibit tumor cell proliferation, as well as it inhibits growth factors regulated by HIF, including VEGF production. Temsirolimus and everolimus as inhibitors of mTOR pathway have demonstrated significant antitumoral activity in metastatic RCC.

Frequently, targeted molecules cause disease stabilization rather than substantial tumor regression in metastatic RCC patients. Currently, several targeted agents have been approved for treatment of metastatic RCC significantly improving long-term perspectives of patients with metastatic RCC. These drugs had distinct mechanisms of action and pathways:

- *Sorafenib* is an oral multikinase inhibitor of several receptor tyrosine kinases, including VEGF receptors (VEGFR)1–3, PDGF receptor-b, Flt-3, and c-KIT. Downstream of these receptor-mediated signaling cascades, sorafenib also blocks serine–threonine kinases of the Raf family. Sorafenib is the only available inhibitor of Raf, a key protein of MAPK pathway. MAPK signals are instrumental in cell proliferation and are overactivated in tumors. Sorafenib, therefore, targets both tumor angiogenesis and tumor proliferation [43].
- *Sunitinib* is a tyrosine kinase inhibitor (TKI) that targets several VEGF and PDGF receptors [44].
- *Pazopanib* is another TKI that targets several VEGF and PDGF receptors with a slightly different kinase profile than sorafenib and sunitinib.
- *Bevacizumab* is the monoclonal antibody that binds to soluble VEGF with great affinity, thus preventing it from reaching its receptor. Bevacizumab was the first agent to prove this principle of angiogenesis inhibition in mRCC, albeit with no significant efficacy as a single agent [45].

- *Temsirolimus* is an intravenously administered inhibitor of mTOR kinase, an enzyme that is a central component of intracellular signal pathways involved in cell growth and proliferation, response to hypoxic stress, and apoptosis. Thus, temsirolimus suppresses both cell cycle and angiogenesis signals.
- *Everolimus* is an oral inhibitor of mTOR kinase.

The availability of approved agents with distinct mechanisms of action (immunotherapy, vascular endothelial growth factor [VEGF] pathway, and mammalian target of rapamycin [mTOR] inhibitors) has complicated treatment decisions for patients with advanced kidney cancer. Identifying the optimal treatment for a particular patient has become an important goal of current investigation. Sunitinib is widely regarded as the preferred first-line and sorafenib as the preferred second-line treatment. Everolimus has demonstrated activity after VEGFR-based therapy in a Phase III study [44].

Nevertheless, they still act as cytotoxic substances in a broader sense and can, therefore, cause side effects that must not be neglected. Fatigue, hypertension, and diarrhea are common side effects of all targeted therapies. Characteristic potential adverse events also include rash, hand/foot/skin reactions, and mucositis, as well as neutropenia and anemia for the kinase inhibitors and gastrointestinal perforation, bleeding, thromboembolic events, anorexia, and proteinuria for the antibody–cytokine combination. In the Phase III trial of sunitinib, 21 % of sunitinib-treated patients developed congestive heart [46]. Sunitinib induces thyroid dysfunction in approximately 30 % of patients [47].

References

1. Parkin DM, Bray F, Ferlay J, Pisani P (2005) Global cancer statistics, 2002. CA Cancer J Clin. 55(2):74–108
2. Mathew A, Devesa SS, Fraumeni JF, Chow WH (2002) Global increases in kidney cancer incidence, 1973–1992. Eur J Cancer Prev 11(2):171–178
3. Siegel R, Naishadham D, Jemal A (2012) Cancer statistic 2012. CA Cancer J Clin 61(1): 10–29
4. Bianchi M, Sun M, Jeldres C, Shariat SF, Trinh QD, Briganti A et al (2012) Distribution of metastatic sites in renal cell carcinoma: a population-based analysis. Annal Oncol 23(4): 973–980
5. Janzen NK, Kim HL, Figlin RA, Belldegrun AS (2013) Surveillance after radical or partial nephrectomy for localized renal cell carcinoma and management of recurrent disease. Urol Clin North Am 30(4):843–852
6. Vera-Badillo FE, Conde E, Duran I (2012) Chromophobe renal cell carcinoma: a review of an uncommon entity. Int J Urol 19(10):894–900
7. García-Donas J, Hernando S, Romero N, Jara C (2011) Knowledge of hereditary renal cancer syndromes: a pending issue for oncologists. Anticancer Drugs 22(Suppl 1):15–20
8. Lonser RR, Glenn GM, Walther M, Chew EY, Libutti SK, Linehan WM et al (2003) Von Hippel-Lindau disease. Lancet 361(9374):2059–2067
9. Toro JR, Wei MH, Glenn GM, Weinreich M, Toure O, Vocke C et al (2008) BHD mutations, clinical and molecular genetic investigations of Birt-Hogg-Dube syndrome: a new series of 50 families and a review of published reports. J Med Genet 45(6):321–331

10. Fowler JE (1987) Nephrectomy in metastatic renal cell carcinoma. Urol Clin N Am 14(4): 749–756
11. Patel NP, Lavengood RW (1978) Renal cell carcinoma: natural history and results of treatment. J Urol 119(6):722–726
12. Gotoh A, Kitazawa S, Mizuno Y, Takenaka A, Arakasawa S, Matsumoto O et al (1993) Common expression of parathyroid hormone-related protein and no correlation of calcium level in renal cell carcinomas. Cancer 71(9):2803–2806
13. Utz D, Warren M, Gregg J, Ludwig J, Kelais PP (1970) Reversible hepatic dysfunction associated with hypernephroma. Mayo Clin Proc 45(3):161–169
14. Warshauer DM, McCarthy SM, Street L, Bookbinder MJ, Glickman MG, Richter J et al (1988) Detection of renal masses: sensitivities and specificities of excretory urography/linear tomography, US, and CT. Radiology 169(2):363–365
15. Jakimowicz JJ (2006) Intraoperative ultrasonography in open and laparoscopic abdominal surgery: an overview. Surg Endosc 20(Suppl 2):425–435
16. Weyman PJ, McClennan BL, Stanley RJ, Levitt RG, Sagel SS (1980) Comparison of computed tomography and angiography in the evaluation of renal cell carcinoma. Radiology 137(2):417–424
17. Mignon F, Mesurolle B (2003) Local recurrence and metastatic dissemination of renal cell carcinoma: clinical and imaging characteristics. J Radiol 84(3):275–284
18. Miyauchi I, Brown RS, Grossman HB, Wojno K, Wahl RL (1996) Correlation between visualization of primary renal cancer by FDG-PET and histopathological findings. J Nucl Med 37(Suppl):64
19. Kunkle DA, Crispen PL, Li T, Uzzo RG (2007) Metastatic renal cell carcinoma: implications for surveillance of small renal masses. J Urol 177(5):1692–1696
20. Thompson H, Hill J, Babayev Y, Cronin A, Kaag M, Kundu S et al (2009) Risk of metastatic renal cancer according to tumor size. J Urol 182(1):41–45
21. Ritchie AWS, Chisholm GD (1983) The natural history of renal carcinoma. Semin Oncol 10:390–400
22. Suppiah R, Shaheen PE, Elson P, Misbah SA, Wood L, Motzer RJ et al (2006) Thrombocytosis as a prognostic factor for survival in patients with metastatic renal cell carcinoma. Cancer 107:1793–1800
23. Hyder O, Pulitano C, Firoozmand A, Dodson R, Wolfgang CL, Choti MA et al (2013) A risk model to predict 90-day mortality among patients undergoing hepatic resection. J Am Coll Surg 216(6):1049–1056
24. Sakaguchi S, Hishiki S, Nakamura S, Koyano K, Kosaka A (1992) Extension incision for renal carcinoma including invaded vena cava and right lobe of liver. Urology 39(3):285–288
25. Yezhelyev M, Master V, Egnatashvili V, Kooby D (2009) Combined nephrectomy and major hepatectomy: indications, outcomes, and recommendations. J Am Coll Surg 208(3):410–418
26. Talarico F, Buli P, Iusco D, Sangiorgi A, Jovine E (2007) Synchronous nephrectomy and right hepatectomy for metastatic chromophobe renal cell carcinoma: report of a case and review of the literature. Chir Ital 59(2):257–261
27. Wong JA, Whelan T, Morse M (2006) Radical nephrectomy with en bloc resection of liver, diaphragm, and lung for locally invasive sarcomatoid renal cell carcinoma. Urology 68(4):890.e1–4
28. Flanigan RC, Mickisch G, Sylvester R, Tangen C, Van Poppel H, Crawford ED (2004) Cytoreductive nephrectomy in patients with metastatic renal cancer: a combined analysis. J Urol 171(3):1071–1076
29. Mickisch GH, Garin A, van Poppel H, de Prijck L, Sylvester R (2001) Radical nephrectomy plus interferon-alfa-based immunotherapy compared with interferon alfa alone in metastatic renal-cell carcinoma: a randomised trial. Lancet 358(9286):966–970
30. Uzo RG, Novick AC (2001) Nephron-saving surgery for renal tumors: indications, techniques and outcomes. J Urol 166(1):6–18
31. Shuch B, Lam JS, Belldegrun AS (2006) Open partial nephrectomy for the treatment of renal cell carcinoma. Curr Urol Rep 7(1):31–38

32. Kranebeck AE, Liebovich BC, Lohse CM, Kwon ED, Zincke H, Blute ML (2006) The role of NSS in metastatic renal cell carcinoma. J Urol 176:1990–1995
33. Kłącz J, Matuszewski M, Michajłowski J, Zachalski W, Markuszewski M, Krajka K (2013) There is no place for targeted therapy neoadjuvant treatment in Polish Health System – an analysis of radical nephrectomies in patients with large kidney tumors. Cent Eur J Urol 66(1):31–35
34. Thelen A, Jonas S, Benckert C, Lopez E, Rudolph B, Neumann U et al (2007) Liver resection for metastases from renal cell carcinoma. World J Surg 31(4):802–807
35. Hofmann HS, Neef H, Krohe K, Andreev P, Silber RE (2005) Prognostic factors and survival after pulmonary resection of metastatic renal cell carcinoma. Eur Urol 48(1):77–81
36. Ruys AT, Tanis PJ, Iris ND, van Duijvendijk P, Verhoef C, Porte RJ et al (2011) Surgical treatment of renal cell cancer liver metastases: a population-based study. Ann Surg Oncol 18(7):1932–1938
37. Hatzaras I, Gleisner AL, Pulitano C, Sandroussi C, Hirose K, Hyder O et al (2012) A multi-institution analysis of outcomes of liver-directed surgery for metastatic renal cell cancer. HPB (Oxford) 14(8):532–538
38. Aloia TA, Adam R, Azoulay D, Bismuth H, Catastaing D (2006) Outcome following hepatic resection of metastatic renal tumors: the Paul Brousse Hospital experience. HPB (Oxford) 8(2):100–105
39. Yun BL, Lee JM, Baek JH, Kim SH, Le JY, Han JK et al (2011) Radiofrequency ablation for treating liver metastases from a non-colorectal origin. Korean J Radiol 12(5):579–587
40. Sorensen SM, Mortensen FV, Nielsen DT (2007) Radiofrequency ablation of colorectal liver metastases: long-term survival. Acta Radiol 48(3):253–258
41. Nabil M, Gruber T, Yakoub D, Ackermann H, Zangos S, Vogl TJ (2008) Repetitive transarterial chemoembolization (TACE) of liver metastases from renal cell carcinoma: local control and survival results. Eur Radiol 18(7):1456–1463
42. Brugarolas J (2007) Renal-cell carcinoma–molecular pathways and therapies. N Engl J Med 356(2):185–187
43. Wilhelm SM, Carter C, Tang L, Wilkie D, McNabola A, Rong H et al (2004) Bay 43-9006 exhibits broad spectrum oral antitumor activity and targets the RAF/MEK/ERK pathway and receptor tyrosine kinases involved in tumor progression and angiogenesis. Cancer Res 64(19):7099–7109
44. Motzer RJ, Escudier B, Oudard S, Hutson TE, Porta C, Bracarda S et al (2008). Efficacy of everolimus in advanced renal cell carcinoma: a double-blind, randomised, placebo-controlled phase III trial. Lancet 372(9637):449–456
45. Yang JC, Haworth L, Sherry RM, Hwu P, Schwartzentruber DJ, Topalin SL et al (2003) A randomized trial of bevacizumab, an antivascular endothelial growth factor antibody, for metastatic renal cancer. N Engl J Med 349(5):427–434
46. Witteles RM, Telli ML, Fisher GA, Srinivas S (2008) Cardiotoxicity associated with the cancer therapeutic agent sunitinib malate. J Clin Oncol 19(9):1613–1618
47. Shinohara N, Takahashi M, Kamishima T, Ikushima H, Otsuka N, Ishizu A et al (2011) The incidence and mechanism of sunitinib-induced thyroid atrophy in patients with metastatic renal cell carcinoma. Br J Cancer 104(2):241–247

Liver Metastases from Larynx Cancer

4

Satyan B. Sreenath, Rupali N. Shah, and Adam M. Zanation

4.1 Epidemiology

4.1.1 Incidence and Risk Factors for Laryngeal Cancer

According to the World Health Organization (WHO) in 2002, there were 600,000 new cases of head and neck cancer with approximately 300,000 deaths worldwide, with larynx cancer being the second most common behind oral cavity cancer [1]. In 2008, larynx, or laryngeal, cancer had the 20th highest incidence in the world amongst all cancers [2] and exhibited a high geographic variability in its disease frequency, with the highest rates seen in southern and eastern Europe [2, 3]. In addition to geographic differences, there are also environmental and gender disparities with regard to laryngeal cancer. In 2008, the International Agency for Research on Cancer (IARC) showed that laryngeal cancer has a higher incidence in more developed than less developed countries [4]. Lastly, in a more recent update by the WHO in 2012, it was noted that the age-adjusted incidence of laryngeal cancer in men worldwide was 3.9 % per 100,000 compared to 0.5 % per 100,000 in women worldwide [5].

S.B. Sreenath • R.N. Shah
Department of Otolaryngology—Head and Neck Surgery,
University of North Carolina at Chapel Hill,
170 Manning Drive, CB #7070, Physician's Office Building Room G-190,
Chapel Hill, NC 27599, USA
e-mail: satyan_sreenath@med.unc.edu; rupali_shah@med.unc.edu

A.M. Zanation (✉)
Department of Otolaryngology—Head and Neck Surgery,
University of North Carolina at Chapel Hill,
170 Manning Drive, CB #7070, Physician's Office Building Room G-190,
Chapel Hill, NC 27599, USA

Department of Neurosurgery, University of North Carolina at Chapel Hill,
Chapel Hill, NC USA
e-mail: adam_zanation@med.unc.edu

I. Di Carlo (ed.), *Noncolorectal, Nonneuroendocrine Liver Metastases: Diagnosis and Current Therapies*, DOI 10.1007/978-3-319-09293-5_4

The major risk factors in the development of head and neck cancer are alcohol and tobacco use, including both smokeless and smoking forms. These two risk factors are associated with approximately 75 % of cases of head and neck cancer worldwide and have been demonstrated to have a multiplicative effect when combined [6]. Regarding laryngeal cancer specifically, smoking has a much greater association with the development of laryngeal cancer when compared to alcohol consumption alone [7, 8]. However, when compared to other common head and neck cancers, laryngeal cancer had the highest association with joint exposure to alcohol and tobacco smoke, demonstrating the promoting effect of alcohol on tobacco smoke as a carcinogen [7]. Other risk factors that are less strongly associated with larynx cancer include a poor diet and occupational exposures to asbestos and diesel exhaust fumes [9, 10]. Also, an association has been demonstrated between laryngeal cancer and a diet low in fresh fruit, vegetables, and vitamins A and C [11, 12].

4.1.2 Incidence of Distant Metastasis

When compared to other major cancers, the incidence of distant metastasis in head and neck squamous cell carcinoma (HNSCC) is relatively low. According to one of the largest published series using the Surveillance Epidemiology and End Results (SEER) database of over 70,000 HNSCC patients recorded from 1988 to 2003, the rate of distant metastasis of HNSCC was 2.82 % at presentation [13]. In other studies reporting on the incidence of distant metastases over the course of disease in patients with HNSCC, the estimated rates range between 10 and 40 % of cases depending on the population, cancer stage, follow-up duration, and locoregional control [14–16]. Additionally, in autopsy reports, the incidence of distant metastases of HNSCC is noted to be even higher from 40 to 50 % of cases [17, 18]. Lastly, amongst the potential sites of distant metastasis, the three most common sites in descending order of frequency have been the lung, bone, and liver, depending on the study population and primary site of disease [19].

In regard to larynx cancer specifically, one of the largest retrospective studies to date reported a 4.4 % rate of distant metastasis over a 20-year period [20]. When analyzed according to laryngeal cancer subsites, the rate of distant metastasis was 14.2 % for subglottic cancer, 4.4 % for glottis cancer, and 3.6 % for supraglottic cancer [20]. In the same study, it was found that advanced tumor stage and regional lymph node metastases significantly predisposed to distant metastasis in glottis cancer.

4.1.3 Incidence of Liver Metastasis

The liver is the third most common site for distant metastasis, behind the bone and lung, respectively [21]. Although the liver is a common site for distant metastasis, a significant difference remains between metastases that are detected clinically and those that are found at autopsy. In studies evaluating the incidence of metastasis found clinically, the rate of liver metastases is close to 1.2 % amongst all cases of HNSCC [21–25]. Notably, in other studies evaluating the incidence of distant metastasis at autopsy in patients with HNSCC, 20–40 % of those patients with distant metastases had evidence of liver metastases [17, 18, 26–28]. Thus, given the discrepancy between the cases detected clinically and those at autopsy, there is a strong indication for the development of a more robust detection method.

With regard to laryngeal cancer specifically, there is a paucity of studies that has specifically investigated the occurrence of liver metastases in cases of laryngeal cancer alone. According to a recent retrospective review, in a total of 202 patients diagnosed with laryngeal cancer, 2.5 % of those patients developed evidence of liver metastases [29].

4.2 Natural History

4.2.1 Anatomy and Staging of Laryngeal Cancer

Laryngeal cancer can be subclassified based on its specific area of origin. The larynx is classically divided into three regions: the supraglottis, the glottis, and the subglottis (Fig. 4.1). The supraglottic region is comprised of the epiglottis, the false vocal cords, the ventricles, the aryepiglottic folds, and the arytenoids. The glottis includes the anterior commissure and the true vocal cords. The subglottic region involves the space below the true vocal cords, extending 5 mm below the free edge of the vocal cord to the inferior border of the cricoid cartilage. Although some controversy exists regarding this anatomic classification system, it is important to attempt to define the anatomic extensions of the tumor, since certain regions demonstrate a higher propensity for metastasis based on proximity of lymphatic and hematogenous channels [30–32]. According to a retrospective analysis of over 2,000 patients with laryngeal and hypopharyngeal cancer, squamous cell carcinomas of the subglottic region had the highest propensity for distant metastasis [20].

Laryngeal cancer is staged clinically, based on the extent of disease at the initial presentation prior to any treatment. The American Joint Committee on Cancer has agreed to designate staging based on the tumor node metastasis (TNM) classification system [33]. Based on this staging system, any laryngeal cancer that demonstrates evidence of distant metastases is automatically classified as a Stage IV(C) tumor. Lastly, since squamous cell carcinomas compose approximately 90–95 % of all laryngeal cancers, the focus on the presentation, diagnosis, and management will be directed toward that form of pathology.

4.2.2 Clinical Presentation and Spread of Primary Laryngeal Cancer

The presenting symptoms of laryngeal cancer depend on the anatomic region that is primarily involved. In glottis cancer, the spectrum of symptoms includes persistent

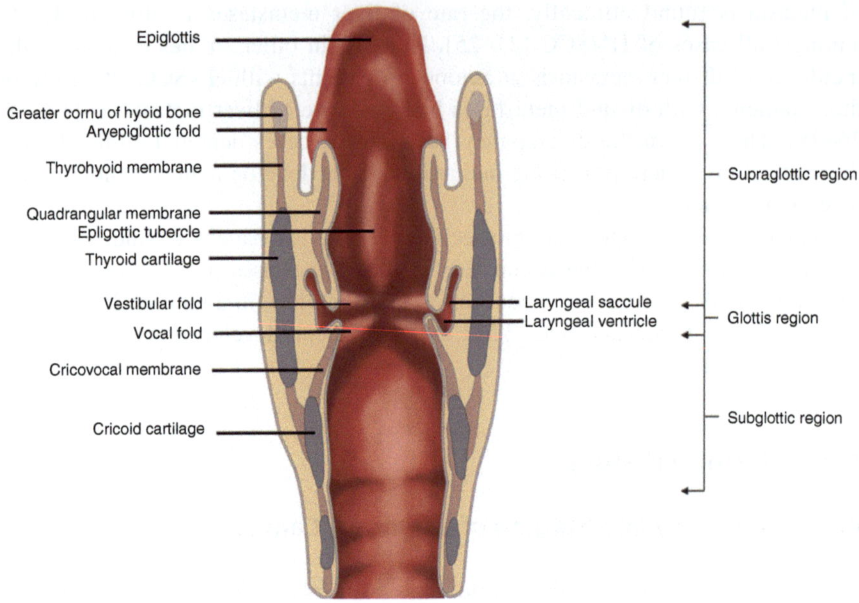

Fig. 4.1 Illustration of the larynx, demonstrating the supraglottic, glottis, and subglottic regions with major anatomic structures

hoarseness, dysphagia, chronic cough, hemoptysis, and referred otalgia. Primary subglottic cancer or extension of disease into the subglottic region can present with stridor or dyspnea on exertion. Lastly, primary supraglottic cancer or extension is often discovered late in the disease process, and patients may present with palpable lymph nodes or airway obstruction.

Locoregionally, laryngeal cancer can spread via lymphatic channels or direct extension. Notably, the supraglottic region has the richest lymphatic supply compared to the glottis, which has little to no lymphatic circulation. From the supraglottic region, local metastasis can proceed to the upper and lower deep cervical lymph nodes. Regarding the subglottic region, although there is very limited lymphatic exposure, metastases can spread to the paratracheal lymph nodes or to the deep cervical lymph nodes as well. Thus, for glottis cancer to metastasize regionally, there must be either direct stromal extension into surrounding tissues or extension of the tumor to the supraglottic and subglottic regions.

Metastases to distant sites, including the liver, occur through hematogenous channels. In laryngeal cancer, tumor cell access to the hematogenous circulation can be achieved through tumor angiogenesis or extension into existing vasculature. Circulatory access can also be achieved indirectly via the lymphatic system, where the deep cervical glands drain to the jugular lymph trunk on the right and the thoracic duct on the left, both of which eventually drain at the junction of the internal jugular vein and subclavian vein.

4.2.3 Risk Factors and Clinical Presentation of Distant Metastases to the Liver

When considering possible sites of distant metastasis, the lungs, liver, and bone are the most common targets for hematogenous tumor spread, and the mediastinum represents the most common site for distant lymphatic tumor spread. To date, there have been no studies evaluating the distinct risk factors for distant metastasis of laryngeal cancer to the liver specifically. In a large retrospective series of over 1,900 patients evaluating the risk factors for distant metastasis in HNSCC, it was found that poor locoregional control, higher N stage, and local extension were significantly associated with a higher risk for distant metastasis, which was consistent with other studies evaluating this property of laryngeal cancer [15, 34]. In other large studies evaluating distant metastasis, delayed regional metastasis, and the role of extracapsular tumor spread for laryngeal and hypopharyngeal cancer, the results confirmed the aforementioned risk factors for distant metastasis and also demonstrated that extracapsular extension in metastatic lymph nodes significantly increased the risk for distant metastases [20, 35]. Additionally, age and site of primary cancer have both been associated with the risk for distant metastases in HNSCC [18]. Lastly, in a smaller series of 650 patients evaluating the factors associated with liver metastases specifically from HNSCC, the same risk factors noted for general distant metastasis were also seen [29].

Although liver metastasis is infrequently associated with advanced laryngeal cancer, its clinical presentation is often indolent during the course of disease. If symptoms are present, they will usually be nonspecific initially including anorexia, weight loss, and vague abdominal pain. Liver-specific symptoms generally will not be present until the disease process has greatly advanced potentially resulting in acute liver failure or cirrhosis. However, during the natural course of the disease, other symptoms can be utilized to alert the physician that either liver metastases are present or a patient is at high risk for liver metastasis. As stated above, advanced locoregional disease including regional lymph node metastasis is strongly associated with the risk for distant metastasis, and thus enlarged deep cervical lymph nodes should be worrisome for distant metastases. Additionally, pulmonary metastases are identified in a significantly greater proportion of patients with liver metastases as compared to those without [29]. Although also nonspecific, symptoms of metastases to the lung include cough, hemoptysis, dyspnea, and chest pain.

4.2.4 Course and Prognosis of Advanced Laryngeal Cancer with Distant Metastasis

Generally speaking, distant metastatic disease from head and neck cancer is incurable, and prognosis is often variable depending on patient comorbidities and tumor pathology. The median time from diagnosis of distant metastases to death ranges from 1 to 12 months, with approximately 88 % of patients dying by 1 year from diagnosis[36–38]. As seen above, advanced locoregional disease often precedes distant metastasis, which can present as worsening dyspnea, airway obstruction, and hoarseness. Progressive nodal disease can result in lymphatic metastasis to the mediastinum, which often presents with similar symptoms as locoregional disease alone, until there is significant involvement of mediastinal structures. As metastases proceed downstream via hematogenous channels to the lungs, liver, and thoracic bones predominately, symptoms remain relatively nonspecific until the disease burden becomes high enough to result in organ failure. The end result of distant metastasis of laryngeal cancer to the liver can either be acute liver failure or decompensated chronic liver failure, which often presents with abdominal pain, ascites, jaundice, confusion, and easy bruising. However, since the majority of patients with laryngeal cancer do not suffer from distant metastatic disease, the end result in the natural course of laryngeal cancer is often related to locoregional disease causing comprise of the airway, requiring immediate and early intervention.

4.3 Diagnosis

4.3.1 Initial Workup of Primary Laryngeal Cancer

When a patient presents with symptoms concerning for laryngeal cancer, he/she undergoes an initial diagnostic evaluation including a thorough physical exam of the head and neck, flexible laryngoscopy to directly visualize the potential lesion, and, under general anesthesia, direct laryngoscopy with biopsy of the lesion for histologic confirmation (Figs. 4.2 and 4.3). Once the diagnosis of laryngeal cancer is confirmed, the patient generally receives further testing for lymphatic and distant metastases at initial presentation. First, computed tomography (CT) or magnetic resonance imaging (MRI) of the neck is generally standard of care for evaluating the extensions of the lesion and detecting locoregional lymphatic spread for staging purposes (Figs. 4.2 and 4.3). Though MRI is superior to CT in providing clearer soft tissue definition for tumor extensions, it is inferior in accurately detecting nodal metastases; thus, MRI and CT be viewed as complementary to one another for evaluation of burden of disease [39]. Although plain chest radiography was historically used to detect pulmonary metastases, it has subsequently been replaced by chest computed tomography (CT) given its higher sensitivity [36, 40]. Other traditional tests for distant metastases include bone scintigraphy and liver function tests for bone and liver metastases, respectively. However, both of these tests lack specificity for metastatic disease processes and thus are relatively unreliable tests for accurately demonstrating distant metastases. Also, given the minimally invasive and inexpensive approach of ultrasonography for detecting liver metastases, it is still generally performed even though it has a lower sensitivity than other imaging modalities [36]. Additionally, abdominal CT may also be used to detect metastases to the liver as well.

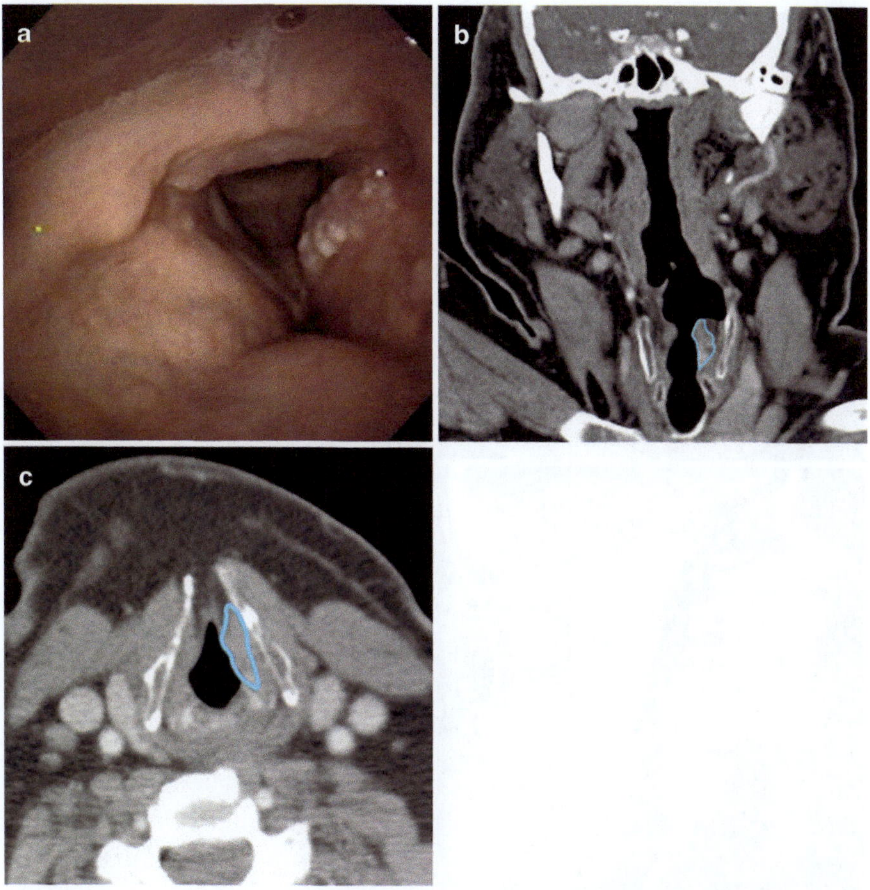

Fig. 4.2 Stage II squamous cell carcinoma of the left true vocal fold and false vocal fold (glottis cancer). (**a**) Laryngoscopic view of the glottis cancer using a flexible, fiberoptic laryngoscope with anterior aspect at the bottom edge of the image and posterior aspect at the *top* edge of the image. (**b**) Computed tomography (*CT*) scan (coronal slice) demonstrating glottis cancer, outlined in *blue*. (**c**) CT scan (axial slice) demonstrating glottis cancer, outline in *blue*

4.3.2 Screening for Liver Metastases

The dogma for an ideal screening modality is that it should be inexpensive, appropriately sensitive, and noninvasive. Although liver function tests (LFTs) are commonly obtained at the initial consultation visit for HNSCC, there is minimal data supporting routine usage of LFTs for metastatic screening. First, given the higher incidence of heavy alcohol use in the head and neck cancer population, elevated LFTs may be unreliable in metastatic surveillance due to concomitant liver disease falsely elevating liver enzymes [38, 41]. In a recent update on the use of LFTs as a screening modality for laryngeal cancer, LFTs were demonstrated to lack adequate sensitivity and specificity in reliably identifying patients with liver metastases from

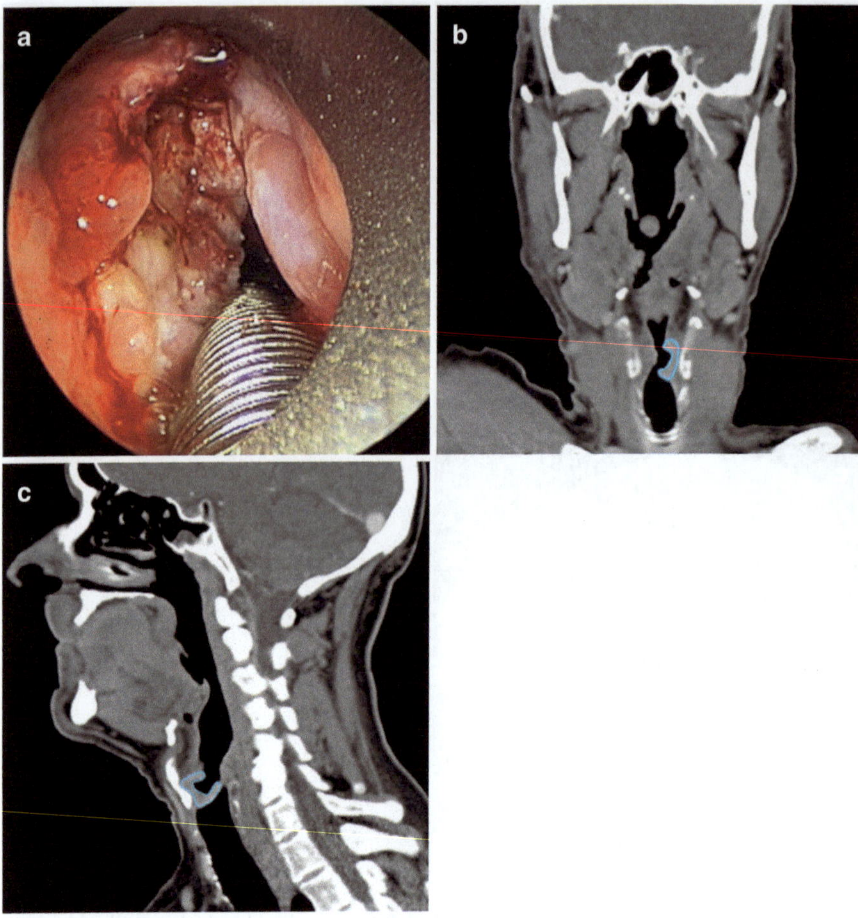

Fig. 4.3 Stage III squamous cell carcinoma of the left transglottic larynx (primary glottis cancer with either supraglottic or subglottic extension or evidence of both). (**a**) Intraoperative view of the transglottic cancer using a rigid laryngoscope with the posterior aspect at the *bottom* edge of the image and anterior aspect at the *top* edge of the image. (**b**) Computed tomography (*CT*) scan (coronal slice) demonstrating transglottic cancer, outline in *blue*. (**c**) CT scan (sagittal slice) demonstrating transglottic cancer, outline in *blue*

HNSCC [29]. Overall sensitivity for all LFTs was found to be very low at 45 %, and specificity was noted to be at 75 % [29] (Table 4.1).

Given these findings, alternative screening modalities have been investigated to determine a more sensitive surveillance method for liver metastases including ultrasound, CT, MRI, and positron emission tomography (PET). Ultrasonography is usually the initial method of choice given that it is relatively inexpensive, generally accurate in detecting liver metastases, and limits unnecessary radiation exposure [25]. Although CT and MRI are more sensitive in detecting metastatic lesions to the liver, they are also comparatively expensive and expose that patient to further

Table 4.1 Sensitivities, specificities, positive predictive values, and negative predictive values of liver function tests

	ALT	AST	LDH	AP	Overall
Sensitivity (95 % CI)	0 (0–16.84)	10.0 (1.23–31.70)	30.0 (11.89–54.28)	20.0 (5.73–43.66)	45.0 (23.06–68.47)
Specificity (95 % CI)	94.33 (92.24–96.0)	89.92 (87.31–92.15)	91.97 (89.58–93.96)	88.03 (85.25–90.45)	74.96 (71.40–78.29)
PPV (95 % CI)	0 (0–9.74)	3.03 (0.37–10.52)	10.53 (3.96–21.52)	5.0 (1.38–12.31)	5.36 (2.48–9.93)
NPV (95 % CI)	96.77 (95.05–98.02)	96.94 (95.21–98.18)	97.65 (96.10–98.71)	97.22 (95.52–98.40)	97.74 (95.99–98.87)

Adapted from, with author's permission: Deal et al. [29]. Sage Publications DOI: 10.1177/0194599811425147

ALT alanine aminotransferase, *AST* aspartate aminotransferase, *LDH* lactate dehydrogenase, *AP* alkaline phosphatase, *CI* confidence interval, *PPV* positive predictive value, *NPV* negative predictive value

radiation [25, 42]. Of note, recent technical advancements have further increased the accuracy of these radiographic methods, including multi-detector row CT and diffusion-weighted MRI, but further studies must be done to evaluate their role as screening tools [43]. Lastly, F-18-fluoro-D-glucose positron emission tomography (FDG-PET) is a functional modality that has been shown to be useful in the initial staging of HNSCC and detection of distant metastases before and after potential therapeutic interventions [44, 45]. Although PET studies are useful in detecting occult metastases, they must be combined with traditional radiographic imaging, such as CT, in order to accurately locate the metastatic lesion. Through analysis of all modalities, it has been seen that screening for distant metastases in advanced HNSCC patients is best performed using FDG-PET combined with CT for high-risk patients [43, 46].

Lastly, the timing of screening for distant metastases is twofold. First, evaluation for distant metastases occurs at the initial consultation visit as part of the initial staging process, which guides providers in forming a treatment plan and providing a prognosis. Depending on availability and cost to the patient, practitioners will employ the imaging modalities described above to determine the presence of distant metastases at presentation. Secondly, regarding metastatic surveillance during the course of disease, routine screening of asymptomatic patients is generally of little clinical value since treatment for distant metastases has no curative intent and palliative interventions are unnecessary when patients remain asymptomatic.

4.4 Treatment

4.4.1 Local Management of Advanced Laryngeal Cancer in the Setting of Distant Metastases

Generally speaking, distant metastatic disease in the setting of laryngeal cancer is incurable. With this notion in mind, principles of oncologic management dictate that interventions with curative intentions should be reserved for those patients with only locoregional disease, whereas palliative interventions and supportive care are intended for patients with evidence of distant, metastatic spread. Given the focus of this chapter, the discussion of treatment will focus on the nuances of palliative interventions for advanced laryngeal cancer in the setting of concomitant liver metastases. Aggressive interventions with curative intent include surgical resection, radiation therapy, or chemoradiotherapy. In regard to the management of locoregional disease from laryngeal cancer, patients with particularly bulky or symptomatic tumors may undergo relatively aggressive interventions with palliative intent including surgical tumor debulking, radiation therapy doses up to 70 Gy, and, very rarely, a total laryngectomy. However, it is important for the patient to be aware that these interventions are not of a curative nature, but instead primarily for improvements in quality of life such as pain control and improvement in dysphagia.

Next, in patients with limited metastatic disease in the liver, palliative interventions can be targeted at hepatic lesions for patients who are symptomatic. Although not studied with specific regard to metastases from laryngeal carcinoma, image-guided radiofrequency ablation is effective in destroying hepatic lesions that are less than 3 cm in the setting of other HNSCC [47, 48]. Recently, it was also observed that larger solitary liver metastases, ranging from 5 to 7 cm, may also be treated with microwave-based ablation, although this approach is more controversial [49]. Additionally, targeted cryotherapy is currently being studied in the treatment of distant metastases in the setting of HNSCC [50]. Lastly, there are no studies to date evaluating the role of partial hepatectomy in managing metastatic disease in the setting of either laryngeal cancer or HNSCC, which may be secondary to the notion that treatment for distant metastases is non-curative by definition.

4.4.2 Systemic Therapy for Liver and Other Distant Sites of Metastases

Palliative systemic therapies generally include palliative chemotherapy and, less frequently, targeted molecular therapies. In the setting of liver metastases, the primary goals of treatment are improving quality of life, cancer-specific symptoms, and overall survival. A broad range of chemotherapeutic agents have been shown to be active against HNSCC, with a response rate of approximately 30–40 % using platinum-based combination regimens albeit with increased incidence of additional toxicities [51, 52]. Unfortunately, evidence of tumor response to multi-agent regimens has not as of yet consistently translated into improved patient survival, with a median survival of 6–9 months [50, 53].

Regarding specific chemotherapy regimens for metastatic laryngeal cancer, cetuximab is generally the chemotherapeutic agent of choice since it has been used in single-agent protocols with modest response rates of approximately 13 % [54]. Notably, when cetuximab is combined with platinum-based chemotherapeutic agents, there has been limited evidence of a moderate survival benefit in the management of metastatic disease in the setting of advanced laryngeal cancer [55]. Aside from chemotherapy protocols, other biologic agents targeted at specific carcinogenic mechanisms are currently under further investigation for their role in palliative treatment for metastatic disease.

References

1. Boyle P, Levin B (eds) (2008) World cancer report. International Agency for Research on Cancer. IARC Press, Lyon
2. Ferlay J, Shin HR, Bray F, Forman D, Mathers C, Parkin DM (2010) Estimates of worldwide burden of cancer in 2008: GLOBOCAN 2008. Int J Cancer 127:2893–2917
3. Parkin DM, Bray F, Ferlay J, Pisani P (2005) Global cancer statistics, 2002. CA Cancer J Clin 55:74–108
4. Jemal A, Bray F, Center MM, Ferlay J, Ward E, Forman D (2011) Global cancer statistics. CA Cancer J Clin 61:69–90
5. Siegel R, Naishadham D, Jemal A (2013) Cancer statistics, 2013. CA Cancer J Clin 63:11–30

6. Conway DI, Hashibe M, Boffetta P, Wunsch-Filho V, Muscat J, La Vecchia C, Winn DM (2009) Enhancing epidemiologic research on head and neck cancer: INHANCE – the international head and neck cancer epidemiology consortium. Oral Oncol 45:743–746
7. Anantharaman D, Marron M, Lagiou P, Samoli E, Ahrens W, Pohlabeln H, Slamova A, Schejbalova M, Merletti F, Richiardi L, Kjaerheim K, Castellsague X, Agudo A, Talamini R, Barzan L, Macfarlane TV, Tickle M, Simonato L, Canova C, Conway DI, Mckinney PA, Thomson P, Znaor A, Healy CM, Mccartan BE, Hashibe M, Brennan P, Macfarlane GJ (2011) Population attributable risk of tobacco and alcohol for upper aerodigestive tract cancer. Oral Oncol 47:725–731
8. Tuyns AJ, Esteve J, Raymond L, Berrino F, Benhamou E, Blanchet F, Boffetta P, Crosignani P, del Moral A, Lehmann W et al (1988) Cancer of the larynx/hypopharynx, tobacco and alcohol: IARC international case-control study in Turin and Varese (Italy), Zaragoza and Navarra (Spain), Geneva (Switzerland) and Calvados (France). Int J Cancer 41:483–491
9. Boyle P, Macfarlane GJ, Zheng T, Maisonneuve P, Evstifeeva T, Scully C (1992) Recent advances in epidemiology of head and neck cancer. Curr Opin Oncol 4:471–477
10. Graham S, Mettlin C, Marshall J, Priore R, Rzepka T, Shedd D (1981) Dietary factors in the epidemiology of cancer of the larynx. Am J Epidemiol 113:675–680
11. de Stefani E, Correa P, Oreggia F, Leiva J, Rivero S, Fernandez G, Deneo-Pellegrini H, Zavala D, Fontham E (1987) Risk factors for laryngeal cancer. Cancer 60:3087–3091
12. LA Vecchia C, Negri E, D'avanzo B, Franceschi S, Decarli A, Boyle P (1990) Dietary indicators of laryngeal cancer risk. Cancer Res 50:4497–4500
13. Kuperman DI, Auethavekiat V, Adkins DR, Nussenbaum B, Collins S, Boonchalermvichian C, Trinkaus K, Chen L, Morgensztern D (2011) Squamous cell cancer of the head and neck with distant metastasis at presentation. Head Neck 33:714–718
14. Alvi A, Johnson JT (1997) Development of distant metastasis after treatment of advanced-stage head and neck cancer. Head Neck 19:500–505
15. Garavello W, Ciardo A, Spreafico R, Gaini RM (2006) Risk factors for distant metastases in head and neck squamous cell carcinoma. Arch Otolaryngol Head Neck Surg 132:762–766
16. Leibel SA, Scott CB, Mohiuddin M, Marcial VA, Coia LR, Davis LW, Fuks Z (1991) The effect of local-regional control on distant metastatic dissemination in carcinoma of the head and neck: results of an analysis from the RTOG head and neck database. Int J Radiat Oncol Biol Phys 21:549–556
17. Nishijima W, Takooda S, Tokita N, Takayama S, Sakura M (1993) Analyses of distant metastases in squamous cell carcinoma of the head and neck and lesions above the clavicle at autopsy. Arch Otolaryngol Head Neck Surg 119:65–68
18. Zbaren P, Lehmann W (1987) Frequency and sites of distant metastases in head and neck squamous cell carcinoma. An analysis of 101 cases at autopsy. Arch Otolaryngol Head Neck Surg 113:762–764
19. Takes RP, Rinaldo A, Silver CE, Haigentz M Jr, Woolgar JA, Triantafyllou A, Mondin V, Paccagnella D, de Bree R, Shaha AR, Hartl DM, Ferlito A (2012) Distant metastases from head and neck squamous cell carcinoma. Part I. Basic aspects. Oral Oncol 48:775–779
20. Spector JG, Sessions DG, Haughey BH, Chao KS, Simpson J, el Mofty S, Perez CA (2001) Delayed regional metastases, distant metastases, and second primary malignancies in squamous cell carcinomas of the larynx and hypopharynx. Laryngoscope 111:1079–1087
21. Ferlito A, Shaha AR, Silver CE, Rinaldo A, Mondin V (2001) Incidence and sites of distant metastases from head and neck cancer. ORL J Otorhinolaryngol Relat Spec 63:202–207
22. de Bree R, Haigentz M Jr, Silver CE, Paccagnella D, Hamoir M, Hartl DM, Machiels JP, Paleri V, Rinaldo A, Shaha AR, Takes RP, Leemans CR, Ferlito A (2012) Distant metastases from head and neck squamous cell carcinoma. Part II. Diagnosis. Oral Oncol 48:780–786
23. Jackel MC, Rausch H (1999) Distant metastasis of squamous epithelial carcinomas of the upper aerodigestive tract. The effect of clinical tumor parameters and course of illness. HNO 47:38–44
24. Papac RJ (1984) Distant metastases from head and neck cancer. Cancer 53:342–345
25. Troell RJ, Terris DJ (1995) Detection of metastases from head and neck cancers. Laryngoscope 105:247–250

26. Dennington ML, Carter DR, Meyers AD (1980) Distant metastases in head and neck epidermoid carcinoma. Laryngoscope 90:196–201
27. Kotwall C, Sako K, Razack MS, Rao U, Bakamjian V, Shedd DP (1987) Metastatic patterns in squamous cell cancer of the head and neck. Am J Surg 154:439–442
28. O'brien PH, Carlson R, Steubner EA Jr, Staley CT (1971) Distant metastases in epidermoid cell carcinoma of the head and neck. Cancer 27:304–307
29. Deal AM, Patel MR, Thorp BD, Cannon TY, Shores CG, Zanation AM (2012) Liver function tests: inadequate screening modality for detection of liver metastasis in head and neck carcinoma. Otolaryngol Head Neck Surg 146:88–91
30. Harrison DF (1971) The pathology and management of subglottic cancer. Ann Otol Rhinol Laryngol 80:6–12
31. Reidenbach MM (1998) Subglottic region: normal topography and possible clinical implications. Clin Anat 11:9–21
32. Stell PM, Tobin KE (1975) The behavior of cancer affecting the subglottic space. Can J Otolaryngol 4:612–617
33. AJCC (2010) Larynx. In: Edge S, Byrd DR, Compton CC et al (eds) AJCC cancer staging manual, 7th edn. Springer, New York
34. Leon X, Quer M, Orus C, del Prado Venegas M, Lopez M (2000) Distant metastases in head and neck cancer patients who achieved loco-regional control. Head Neck 22:680–686
35. Oosterkamp S, dE Jong JM, Van den Ende PL, Mmanni JJ, dehing-Oberije C, Kremer B (2006) Predictive value of lymph node metastases and extracapsular extension for the risk of distant metastases in laryngeal carcinoma. Laryngoscope 116:2067–2070
36. de Bree R, Deurloo EE, Snow GB, Leemans CR (2000) Screening for distant metastases in patients with head and neck cancer. Laryngoscope 110:397–401
37. Ferlito A, Rinaldo A (2000) The pathology and management of subglottic cancer. Eur Arch Otorhinolaryngol 257:168–173
38. Probert JC, Thompson RW, Bagshaw MA (1974) Patterns of spread of distant metastases in head and neck cancer. Cancer 33:127–133
39. Sakata K, Hareyama M, Tamakawa M, Oouchi A, Sido M, Nagakura H, Akiba H, Koito K, Himi T, Asakura K (1999) Prognostic factors of nasopharynx tumors investigated by MR imaging and the value of MR imaging in the newly published TNM staging. Int J Radiat Oncol Biol Phys 43:273–278
40. Leong SC, Javed F, Elliot S, Mortimore S (2008) Effectiveness of X-ray and computed tomography screening for assessing pulmonary involvement in patients with head and neck squamous cell carcinoma. J Laryngol Otol 122:961–966
41. Korver KD, Graham SM, Hoffman HT, Mcculloch T, Funk GF (1995) Liver function studies in the assessment of head and neck cancer patients. Head Neck 17:531–534
42. Scherer U, Rothe R, Eisenburg J, Schildberg F, Meister P, Lissner J (1978) Diagnostic accuracy of CT in circumscript liver disease. AJR Am J Roentgenol 130:711–714
43. de Bree R, Castelijns JA, Hoekstra OS, Leemans CR (2009) Advances in imaging in the work-up of head and neck cancer patients. Oral Oncol 45:930–935
44. Brouwer J, Senft A, de Bree R, Comans EF, Golding RP, Castelijns JA, Hoekstra OS, Leemans CR (2006) Screening for distant metastases in patients with head and neck cancer: is there a role for (18)FDG-PET? Oral Oncol 42:275–280
45. Jeong HS, Baek CH, Son YI, Ki Chung M, Kyung Lee D, Young Choi J, Kim BT, Kim HJ (2007) Use of integrated 18F-FDG PET/CT to improve the accuracy of initial cervical nodal evaluation in patients with head and neck squamous cell carcinoma. Head Neck 29:203–210
46. Gourin CG, Watts TL, Williams HT, Patel VS, Bilodeau PA, Coleman TA (2008) Identification of distant metastases with positron-emission tomography-computed tomography in patients with previously untreated head and neck cancer. Laryngoscope 118:671–675
47. Karatzas A, Katsanos K, Maroulis I, Kalogeropoulou C, Tzorakoleftherakis E, Karnabatidis D (2011) Multi-modality curative treatment of salivary gland cancer liver metastases with drug-eluting bead chemoembolization, radiofrequency ablation, and surgical resection: a case report. J Med Case Rep 5:416

48. Palussiere J, Italiano A, Descat E, Ferron S, Cornelis F, Avril A, Brouste V, Bui BN (2011) Sarcoma lung metastases treated with percutaneous radiofrequency ablation: results from 29 patients. Ann Surg Oncol 18:3771–3777
49. Livraghi T, Meloni F, Solbiati L, Zanus G (2012) Complications of microwave ablation for liver tumors: results of a multicenter study. Cardiovasc Intervent Radiol 35:868–874
50. Haigentz M Jr, Hartl DM, Silver CE, Langendijk JA, Strojan P, Paleri V, de Bree R, Machiels JP, Hamoir M, Rinaldo A, Paccagnella D, Shaha AR, Takes RP, Ferlito A (2012) Distant metastases from head and neck squamous cell carcinoma. Part III. Treatment. Oral Oncol 48:787–793
51. Forastiere AA, Metch B, Schuller DE, Ensley JF, Hutchins LF, Triozzi P, Kish JA, Mcclure S, Vonfeldt E, Williamson SK et al (1992) Randomized comparison of cisplatin plus fluorouracil and carboplatin plus fluorouracil versus methotrexate in advanced squamous-cell carcinoma of the head and neck: a Southwest Oncology Group study. J Clin Oncol 10:1245–1251
52. Liverpool Head and Neck Oncology Group (1990) A phase III randomised trial of cisplatinum, methotrextate, cisplatinum + methotrexate and cisplatinum + 5-FU in end stage squamous carcinoma of the head and neck. Liverpool Head and Neck Oncology Group. Br J Cancer 61:311–315
53. Haigentz M, Silver CE, Hartl DM, Takes RP, Rodrigo JP, Robbins KT, Rinaldo A, Ferlito A (2010) Chemotherapy regimens and treatment protocols for laryngeal cancer. Expert Opin Pharmacother 11:1305–1316
54. Vermorken JB, Trigo J, Hitt R, Koralewski P, Diaz-Rubio E, Rolland F, Knecht R, Amellal N, Schueler A, Baselga J (2007) Open-label, uncontrolled, multicenter phase II study to evaluate the efficacy and toxicity of cetuximab as a single agent in patients with recurrent and/or metastatic squamous cell carcinoma of the head and neck who failed to respond to platinum-based therapy. J Clin Oncol 25:2171–2177
55. Vermorken JB, Mesia R, Rivera F, Remenar E, Kawecki A, Rottey S, Erfan J, Zabolotnyy D, Kienzer HR, Cupissol D, Peyrade F, Benasso M, Vynnychenko I, de Raucourt D, Bokemeyer C, Schueler A, Amellal N, Hitt R (2008) Platinum-based chemotherapy plus cetuximab in head and neck cancer. N Engl J Med 359:1116–1127

Liver Metastases from Lung Cancer

5

Giorgio Ercolani, Flavia Neri, Matteo Ravaioli, Matteo Cescon, and Antonio Daniele Pinna

5.1 Incidence

Lung cancer is the most common cancer worldwide, with an estimated 1,600,000 new cases and 1,380,000 deaths in 2008, which makes it the leading cause of cancer-related mortality [1].

The majority of lung malignancies can be described either as small cell lung cancer (SCLC) (13 %) or as non-small cell lung cancer (NSCLC) (81 %), which can be further classified into adenocarcinoma (38 %), squamous cell carcinoma (20 %), large cell carcinoma (5 %), and other non-small cell carcinomas (18 %) [2].

Lung cancer can spread to any organ and present with either synchronous or metachronous metastases. The most frequent sites of extrathoracic metastatic lesions are brain (10 %), bone (7 %), liver (5 %), and adrenal glands (3 %) [3].

Hepatic metastases are quite uncommon at an early stage, while their incidence rises later in the course of the disease as showed by some autopsy studies conducted on patients affected by NSCLC and SCLC; the incidence of hepatic disease in deceased patients after treated lung cancer is almost 50 % [4, 5].

5.2 Natural History

The TNM stage at presentation has the major impact on prognosis for patients affected by lung cancer.

While patients in stage I have a prognosis of almost 60 months, those in stage IV, equivalent to metastatic disease, have a median survival time of 4–9 months

G. Ercolani (✉) • F. Neri • M. Ravaioli • M. Cescon • A.D. Pinna
General Surgery and Transplantation, S. Orsola – Malpighi Hospital,
University of Bologna, V. Massarenti 9, Bologna 40138, Italy
e-mail: giorgio.ercolani@aosp.bo.it; flavia.neri84@gmail.com;
mraval@hotmail.com; matteo.cescon@aosp.bo.it; antoniodaniele.pinna@unibo.it

I. Di Carlo (ed.), *Noncolorectal, Nonneuroendocrine Liver Metastases: Diagnosis and Current Therapies*, DOI 10.1007/978-3-319-09293-5_5

[6]. However when the metastatic disease is solitary and a resective treatment is feasible, the survival benefit is considerable compared to palliative therapies [7]. A metachronous interval between the primary pulmonary lesion and the appearance of metastases seems to be a favorable prognostic factor.

5.3 Diagnosis

Contrast-enhanced thorax computed tomography (CT) completed by total-body CT scan is the gold standard diagnostic imaging technique for patients with suspected lung cancer. It allows not only a detailed characterization of the primary tumor but also the identification of possible intra- or extrathoracic lesions.

PET scan can be a useful integrative tool as it can sometimes identify unexpected liver metastases in about 20 % of patients [8, 9].

Tumor sampling can be required if synchronous diffuse lesions are detected by imaging techniques. In these cases the histopathological diagnosis is necessary in order to identify the primitive tumor and to assess the stage of the disease.

If the metastatic lesion is metachronous, then the detection of a positivity at the PET scan is generally sufficient to establish the diagnosis of metastases unless there is a high suspicion for a new primitive tumor. Anyway, a CT scan or MR is useful to evaluate the precise localization of the metastatic nodule and its relation to vascular structures.

5.4 Treatment

Although resection of solitary metastases from lung cancer is suggested for treatment of advanced disease, few cases are reported in literature related to the outcome of hepatic resection when single or multiple liver lesions are detected [10].

Fifteen English-written papers describing a total of 25 resected patients for hepatic metastases from lung tumor have been reported in terms of case-report or small series [11–24]. However, the period span is considerable as the first report was in 1978 and the latest in 2014. Patients' characteristics and outcome are summarized in Table 5.1.

Papers published up to the 2000s report outcome of these patients together with other cases of non-colorectal and non-neuroendocrine liver metastases, and therefore there is a lack of sufficient details for correct analysis. However it seems that before the 1990s, a surgical operation for such cases was not considered worthwhile because of the dismal short-term outcome related to postoperative complications. With the improvements in surgical techniques and perioperative management, the resectability rate for hepatobiliary tumors has been greatly increased [25]; in particular non-colorectal, non-neuroendocrine liver metastases have been considered unresectable disease anymore. The primary site and the extension of the metastatic disease seem to be strictly related to the outcome. While the prognosis is poor for metastases from gastrointestinal carcinoma (survival of 24.6 % at 5 years), a better outcome has been reported for genitourinary metastatic tumors (survival of 37.8 %

Table 5.1 Patients' characteristics and outcome of the reported case series

Author	Year	No. of cases	Primary tumor	Time of occurrence	Diameter (mm) of hepatic lesion	Disease-free interval (mo)	Type of resection	Mean survival (months)
Foster et al. [11]	1978	2	NR	NR	NR	NR	NR	NR
Thomas-de La Vega et al. [13]	1984	1	NR	NR	NR	NR	NR	NR
Cobourn et al. [12]	1987	1	NR	NR	NR	NR	NR	NR
Stehlin et al. [14]	1988	1	NR	NR	NR	NR	major	9
Schwartz et al. [15]	1995	2	NR	NR	NR	NR	NR	NR
Berney et al. [16]	1998	3	NR	NR	NR	NR	NR	NR
Lindell et al. [17]	1998	1	Adenocarcinoma	NR	NR	NR	NR	185
Hamy et al. [18]	2000	1	Epidermoid tumor	NR	NR	NR	Minor	13
Di Carlo et al. [19]	2003	1	Adenocarcinoma	Metachronous	50	48	Minor	36
Nagashima et al. [20]	2004	1	Adenocarcinoma	Metachronous	NR	6	Minor	>60
Ercolani et al. [21]	2006	3	Adenocarcinoma	Synchronous	20	–	Minor	24
				Metachronous	50	24	Major	
				Metachronous	60	18	Minor	
O'Rourke et al. [22]	2008	2	Squamous carcinoma	NR	NR	NR	NR	NR
Ileana et al. [23]	2010	2	Adenocarcinoma	Metachronous	NR	16	Major	21
				Synchronous		–		
Ueda et al. [24]	2012	2	Large cell tumor/ adenocarcinoma	Metachronous	50	8	Minor	20
					20	20		
Slotta et al. [25]	2014	2	NR	NR	NR	NR	NR	16

NR not reported

at 5 years) [26]. A metastatic lung tumor shows an extremely variable range of survival rate, and an assessment of the outcome for the resection of this tumor is extremely difficult.

From available data of the literature, it seems that resected liver metastases were metachronous in most of the patients, without presence of extrahepatic lesions.

The timing of metastatic diagnosis ranged from 6 months to 4 years after resection of the primary tumor, and in all cases the hepatic metastases appeared after adjuvant chemoradiotherapy treatments. The diagnosis was generally obtained by abdominal CT and PET scan to exclude extrahepatic disease. When metastases were detected a long period after the primary tumor resection (more than 16 months), colonoscopy and gastroscopy were performed in order to rule out the presence of new primary gastrointestinal tumors of which the hepatic lesion could be synchronous metastases. All authors describe perioperative chemo- and radiotherapy, which were mostly performed after the hepatic surgery unless liver metastases appeared synchronously to the pulmonary primitive tumor; in these cases chemoradiotherapy was performed with neoadjuvant intent. Most of the papers reported minor resections for single or two lesions. Although it was not always specified what the authors intended for major resection, only three patients underwent such procedures, two of them were right hepatectomies. According to data reported in the literature, neither perioperative mortality (within 30 days from the surgical operation) nor major complications related to the liver resection occurred. The postoperative median survival time was 21 months, ranging from 9 months to more than 10 years; when death occurred it was related to disease recurrence.

It is difficult to identify common features among the cases that had the worse outcome, not only because little information is available but also because they are spread in a large period and among different hepatobiliary centers. Several strategies are described for the treatment of liver metastases from lung tumors since no common consensus has yet been established about this topic.

From the data obtained from these papers, it seems that patients with single or few lesions (under 3) are the best candidates for resective surgery even when a major hepatectomy is needed, since generally liver function is preserved in these patients. The best prognosis seems to be obtained in those who present with metachronous oligometastases limited to the liver appearing after a disease-free interval longer than 1 year.

The general condition of the single patient is also taken into account as much as the entity of the metastatic disease and the function of the remnant liver.

Although initial studies showed poor prognosis for this type of patients, the surgical advances have allowed good postoperative outcome and the assessment of the real benefit of hepatic surgery even for this indication. It appears that if the primary pulmonary malignancy has been removed, liver oligometastases are present and can be totally resected and no extrahepatic disease is detected at PET/CT scan, then hepatic surgery has a considerable role in increasing the survival benefit of these patients. In all these borderline cases where there are no clear guidelines, the management of this pathology relies on a multidisciplinary team in which various factors are considered in order to decide the better strategy.

References

1. Jemal A et al (2011) Global cancer statistics. CA Cancer J Clin 61(2):69
2. Travis WD et al (2004) Pathology and genetics of tumours of the lung, pleura, thymus and heart. In: World Health Organization classification of tumours. IARC Press, Lyon
3. Quint LE et al (1996) Distribution of distant metastases from newly-diagnosed non-small cell lung cancer. Ann Thorac Surg 62:246–250
4. Jereczek B et al (1996) Autopsy findings in small cell lung cancer. Neoplasma 43(2):133
5. Hillers TK et al (1994) Analysis of published studies on the detection of extrathoracic metastases in patients presumed to have operable non-small cell lung cancer. Thorax 49(1):14
6. Groome PA et al (2007) The IASLC Lung Cancer Staging Project: validation of the proposals for revision of the T, N, and M descriptors and consequent stage groupings in the forthcoming (seventh) edition of the TNM classification of malignant tumours. J Thorac Oncol 2(8):694–705
7. Albain KS et al (1991) Survival determinants in extensive-stage non-small cell lung cancer: the Southwest Oncology Group experience. J Clin Oncol 9:1618–1626
8. Van Tinteren H et al (2002) Effectiveness of positron emission tomography in the preoperative assessment of patients with suspected non-small-cell lung cancer: the PLUS multicentre randomised trial. Lancet 359(9315):1388
9. De Wever W et al (2007) Detection of extrapulmonary lesions with integrated PET/CT in the staging of lung cancer. Eur Respir J 29(5):955
10. Pfannschmidt J et al (2010) Surgical treatment of oligometastatic non-small cell lung cancer. Lung Cancer 69:251–258
11. Foster JH et al (1978) Survival after liver resection for secondary tumors. Am J Surg 135:389–394
12. Cobourn CS et al (1987) Examination of patient selection and outcome for hepatic resection for metastatic disease. Surg Gynecol Obstet 165:239–246
13. Thomas-de la Vega JE et al (1984) A ten year experience of with hepatic resection. Surg Gynecol Obstet 159:223–228
14. Stehlin JS Jr et al (1988) Treatment of cancer of the liver. Twenty years' experience with infusion and resection in 414 patients. Ann Surg 208:23–35
15. Schwartz SI et al (1995) Hepatic resection for noncolorectal non neuroendocrine metastases. World J Surg 19:72–75
16. Berney T et al (1998) Results of surgical resection of liver metastases from non-colorectal primaries. Br J Surg 85:1423–1427
17. Lindell G et al (1998) Liver resection of noncolorectal secondaries. J Surg Oncol 69:66–70
18. Hamy A et al (2000) Liver resection for noncolorectal, nonneuroendocrine metastases. Results of 32 hepatectomies in 27 patients. Ann Chir 125:124–130
19. Di Carlo I et al (2003) Liver metastases from lung cancer: is surgical resection justified? Ann Thorac Surg 76:293–295
20. Nagashima A et al (2004) Long-term survival after surgical resection of liver metastasis from lung cancer. Jpn J Thorac Cardiovasc Surg 52(6):311–313
21. Ercolani G et al (2006) The role of liver resection for metastases from lung carcinoma. HPB 8:114–115
22. O'Rourke TR et al (2008) Long-term results of liver resection for non-colorectal, non neuroendocrine metastases. Ann Surg Oncol 15:207–218
23. Ileana C et al (2010) Surgical resection of liver non-small cell lung cancer metastases: a dual weapon? Lung Cancer 70:221–222
24. Ueda J et al (2012) Surgical resection of solitary metastatic liver tumor arising from lung cancer: a case series. Hepato-Gastroenterology 59:2307–2309
25. Slotta JE et al (2014) Hepatic resection of non-colorectal and non-neuroendocrine liver metastases – survival benefit for patients with non gastrointestinal primary cancers – a case-controlled study. Int J Surg 12:163–168
26. Ercolani G et al (2005) The role of liver resections for noncolorectal, nonneuroendocrine metastases: experience with 142 observed cases. Ann Surg Oncol 12(6):1–8

Liver Metastases from Melanoma Cancer 6

Charbel Sandroussi

6.1 Introduction

Melanocytes are found in the epidermis and hair follicles where they are involved in the production of melanin, the iris and choroid of the eye where they provide pigment behind the retina, and the inner cochlear where they are involved in hearing. Melanocyte pigments are important in the prevention of damage by ultraviolet radiation by scattering the incoming rays thereby preventing DNA changes and cellular damage. Frequent intense ultraviolet exposure particularly in childhood increases the risk of melanoma developing. One quarter of new cutaneous melanoma arises from preexisting nevi, and the remainder is due to transformation of melanocytes.

The transformation of melanocytes into malignant melanoma involves a complex series of genetic mutations, involving BRAF, n-RAS, KIT genes, as well other genes involved in cell cycle regulation. These genetic mutations are not uniform and differ depending on the body site and the degree of sun exposure where a melanoma has occurred. Personal risk factors for melanoma include skin type (fair skin, easily burnt, multiple freckles), repeated episodes of burning sun exposure especially in childhood, family history of melanoma, and a large number of nevi. Patients who have a large congenital nevus, or who have had a melanoma in the past, have a much higher rate of development of melanoma.

Over several decades the incidence of melanoma has increased across all age groups. This increase in the incidence rate has plateaued over the past 10 years. Melanoma is the third most common malignancy in both males and females, representing approximately 10 % of all new cancers. The incidence increases up to the sixth and seventh decades, and it accounts for 5 % of skin cancers and 70–80 % of

C. Sandroussi
Hepatobiliary and Upper Gastrointestinal Surgery, Royal Prince Alfred Hospital, Camperdown, NSW 2050, Australia
e-mail: charbel.sandroussi@sydney.edu.au

I. Di Carlo (ed.), *Noncolorectal, Nonneuroendocrine Liver Metastases: Diagnosis and Current Therapies*, DOI 10.1007/978-3-319-09293-5_6

cancer deaths. The age standardized rate of melanoma is approximately 60 per 100,000 in males and 40 per 100,000 in females. The increased incidence has led to a 2 % increase in mortality each year for the past 40 years [1].

6.2 Melanoma Staging

Primary melanomas are staged according to the thickness of the tumor. The depth of invasion can be classified according to Breslow's depth, Table 6.1, and Clark's levels, Table 6.2, more recently the AJCC guidelines for TNM stage [2], have become more widely used Table 6.3. Depth of invasion is important because it correlates with the survival, presence of lymph node metastases at the time of diagnosis, and occurrence of both locoregional and distant recurrence. The 5-year survival rates for patients with stage 0 or I melanoma are 95–100 %, stage II melanoma are 45–80 %, stage III melanoma are 25–70 %, and stage IV melanoma are 7–20 %. Half of all initial metastases are to locoregional lymph nodes, whereas distant metastatic disease represents a quarter of the initial metastasis from the primary melanoma and in transit metastases represent approximately 20 % of all metastasis. The site of the primary melanoma is strongly associated with the location of the first metastasis, with melanomas situated on the limbs more likely to metastasize to regional lymph nodes or to be discovered in transit sites. Melanomas that arise on the trunk, and on the head and neck, are more likely to have direct distant metastatic disease.

Intra-abdominal metastases are common in patients with melanoma. In the vast majority of patients, the disease is disseminated, and of those patients undergoing surgery, two thirds are treatable with intention for complete extirpation of the tumor

Table 6.1 Breslow's depth

Stage	Depth
I	Less or equal to 0.75 mm
II	0.75–1.5 mm
III	1.51–2.25 mm
IV	2.26–3.0 mm
V	Greater than 3.0 mm

Table 6.2 Clark's levels

Level	Depth
I	Melanoma confined to the epidermis
2	Invasion into the papillary dermis
3	Invasion into the junction of the papillary and reticular dermis
4	Invasion into the reticular dermis
5	Invasion into the subcutaneous fat

Table 6.3 AJCC staging

Primary tumor	
Tx	Primary cannot be assessed
T0	No evidence of primary tumor
Tis	Melanoma in situ
T1	≤1 mm thick
T2	1.01–2.0 mm thick
T3	2.01–4.0 mm thick
T4	>4.0 mm thick

Regional lymph nodes		
Nx	Regional nodes cannot be assessed	
N0	No regional metastases detected	
N1	Single regional node	a – micrometastasis
		b – macrometastasis
N2	2–3 nodes	a – micrometastasis
		b – macrometastasis
		c – in transit metastasis without lymph nodes
N3	4 or more metastatic nodes or matted nodes or in transit metastasis with metastatic nodes	

Distant metastasis	Site of metastasis	LDH
M0	No detectable evidence of distant metastasis	
M1a	Skin, subcutaneous, or nodal metastasis	Normal
M1b	Lung	Normal
M1c	All other visceral metastases	Normal
	Any distant metastasis	Elevated

Clinical staging			
Stage 0	T1s	N0	M0
Stage IA	T1a	N0	M0
Stage IB	T1b	N0	M0
	T2a	N0	M0
Stage IIA	T2b	N0	M0
	T3a	N0	M0
Stage IIB	T3b	N0	M0
	T4a	N0	M0
Stage IIC	T4b	N0	M0
Stage III	Any T	≥N1	M0
Stage IV	Any T	Any N	Any M

a without ulceration, *b* with ulcerations

[3]. The liver is a very common site for metastases from melanoma. Approximately 3 % of all patients have metastases to the liver. Cutaneous melanomas metastasized to the liver in up to 20 % of those patients with metastatic disease. The incidence of hepatic metastases is much more common in patients with ocular melanomas, with up to 40 % of patients having liver metastases at the time of diagnosis [4]. The liver is involved with metastasis from ocular melanoma in over 90 % of cases. Despite the high frequency of metastatic disease, the pattern of disease and associated extra-hepatic disease means that only a very small proportion of patients are suitable for surgical treatment [5].

6.3 Surveillance for Metastatic Disease

Follow-up of patients after resection of primary melanomas is related to the depth of invasion of the lesion. For patients with lesions that are less than 1 mm, the risk of recurrence is quite small, and as such if they do not have specific risk factors for the development of a second melanoma, then close follow-up is not necessary. They should have yearly skin checks for 2–3 years, and then review as necessary depending on clinical symptoms. For patients with melanomas thicker than 1 mm, clinical examination of the locoregional lymph nodes, and a complete skin examination, is necessary. As the thickness of the melanoma increases, the frequency of recurrence increases, and more extensive investigations may be required.

In patients with melanomas greater than 4 mm thick serum LDH, staging investigations looking for metastatic disease are required at presentation. There is no evidence that routine surveillance imaging confers a survival benefit, even if metastases are detected earlier, then clinical symptoms arise. In patients where symptoms are present, axial CT scanning and magnetic resonance imaging are appropriate initial investigations. Where there is a high suspicion of recurrence, 18 fluorodeoxyglucose positron emission tomography scan is the most appropriate investigation.

6.4 Staging of Recurrence

When metastatic liver disease is detected, all appropriate clinical and pathological staging investigation should be undertaken. The patients require a serum lactate dehydrogenase level, as well as an axial CT scan of their head, neck, chest, and abdomen. Patients affected by metastases should also undergo an 18 FDG PET scan.

6.5 LDH

Lactate dehydrogenase is secreted when melanoma cells outgrow their vascular supply. It is the strongest independent prognostic factor in metastatic melanoma, and it predicts a poorer survival and a reduction in response to treatment. This is independent of the volume of metastatic disease present. Due to the potential false-positive values for lactate dehydrogenase, it is advised that more than one sample is obtained when using it as a prognostic marker [6].

6.6 Other Serum Markers

Other serum markers have also been identified, which may have a role in predicting prognosis in patients with metastatic disease. S-100, melanoma-inhibiting activity, and vascular endothelial growth factor have all been shown in small studies to predict survival and response to treatment. Given the heterogeneity of the studies, the small sample size, and the cost of these markers, none of these have come into routine clinical practice.

6.7 Computed Tomography

CT scanning of patients with higher risk primary melanomas has not been shown to improve survival and has a very low yield in the absence of symptoms, without significant survival advantage compared with clinically detected metastasis. CT scans undertaken at 6 monthly intervals for patients with stage II and III melanomas were able to detect treatable recurrence in 20 and 30 % of patients, respectively. Less frequent surveillance intervals reduce this detection rate, and there was a very high rate of false positives, and the test had very low positive predictive values [7]. There is a role for its use in the protection of false negatives, and it may function as baseline, when surgery is undertaken for metastatic disease.

6.8 Positron Emission Tomography (PET and PET/CT)

Locoregional and distant metastases from melanoma are highly glucose avid, and as such PET scanning is a useful adjunct in the surveillance for and diagnosis of metastases. PET scanning has a very high sensitivity, and specificity for the identification of metastatic melanoma, when compared with other imaging modalities [8]. PET scanning has a 10 % false-positive rate [9], and although metastatic lesions are able to be detected, the influence on survival is limited [7]. Within the hepatic parenchyma, many factors influence the uptake of glucose, into normal hepatic parenchyma as well as metastatic lesions. PET scans are accurate in the detection of metastases to the liver, but the spatial resolution is inferior to other imaging modalities, even when combined with CT scanning with and without contrast [10]. PET scanning should be undertaken as a routine, in patients undergoing staging prior to resection of visceral metastases, including hepatic metastasis. This would identify the majority of patients who have extrahepatic disease, and either deem them unresectable, or alter the nature of their resection to include the extrahepatic disease.

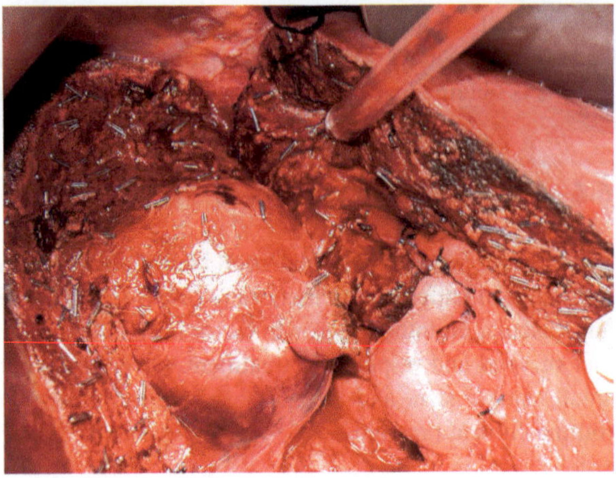

Fig. 6.1 Extended right hepatectomy for metastasis from cutaneous melanoma

6.9 Therapy for Melanoma Metastasis to the Liver

Three percent of all patients with melanoma will develop liver metastases [5]. Of these only a small proportion are treatable with attempt to cure the metastases, by complete surgical resection. Patients who are found to have isolated liver disease, which is resectable, or liver disease that occurs in association with low-volume and resectable extrahepatic disease are candidates for surgical treatment. When considering patients for surgical treatment of liver metastases from melanoma, the standard perioperative considerations are made. Patients will need to have preservation of two contiguous segments of the liver, with appropriate inflow and outflow as well as biliary drainage. It is unusual for the metastases to occur in the context of liver disease, and as such extensive resections can be undertaken where necessary for patients leaving a 25–30 % functional liver remnant. The presence of vascular invasion, and the need for major vascular resection, and reconstruction is not a contraindication to undertaking surgical resection for metastases (Fig. 6.1).

There are limited data on the outcome of patients following liver resection for metastases, and all of the studies are small cohort studies [4, 5, 11–14] from single centers or multiple centers with pooled data. Liver resection for patients with isolated hepatic metastases from ocular melanoma occurred in isolation in up to 90 % of patients, and this is significantly different from patients who have liver metastases from cutaneous melanoma where 40 % of patients have extrahepatic disease at the time of diagnosis of the liver metastases [5, 11–14]. As a consequence of a high proportion of people having localized liver disease, patients with metastasis from ocular melanomas more commonly undergo major hepatic resections. This has been a consistent finding across all of the studies reporting on the outcomes of patients with either ocular or cutaneous melanoma metastasis. Similarly patients with ocular melanomas have a longer disease-free interval from the time of treatment of the primary melanoma, until the development of metastases.

There are limited data available on the long-term survival, following resection of melanoma metastasis to the liver. In the series where long-term survival is reported, it ranges from 0 to 42 % [5, 11, 14]. Similarly median survival across this cohort of patients ranges from 14 to 30 months. More favorable survival has been seen where there is a longer disease-free interval from the time of initial melanoma, complete resection of all liver metastases, and a lower number of liver metastases. In patients where microscopically clear margins can be obtained following liver resection, survival has been reported to be up to 50 % at 5 years. It has been reported that metastases from ocular melanomas have a more favorable prognosis than those from cutaneous melanomas [11], but this finding has been inconsistent across various studies, and with very small numbers of patients in the cohort undergoing resection for metastases from cutaneous melanoma, it is still advisable to offer these patients surgical resection if the liver disease is isolated or occurs in association with low-volume resectable extrahepatic disease. In this cohort up to 40 % 5-year survival can be achieved with appropriate patient selection [4, 5, 12].

Extrahepatic disease is not a contraindication to liver resection, although it does lead to a worse overall survival and an increased recurrence rate. Where present an attempt should be made to resect all extrahepatic disease, with a microscopically clear margin. Even with complete extirpation of the tumor, recurrence rates have been reported up to 92 % [4]. Recurrence tends to be lower in patients with unilateral metastases and tumors less than 5 cm; however, given the small numbers in this group of patients, recommendations about the cutoff surgical resection are difficult to make given that even patients with more advanced disease have prolongation of the survival even if recurrence does occur.

It needs to be remembered that in all series reporting outcomes of patients following resection of metastatic melanoma that the cohort of patients undergoing resection come from a highly selected group of patients and represent only 3 % of all patients with liver metastases from melanoma. Appropriate investigations to identify those patients who have unresectable hepatic and extrahepatic disease are central to the selection of those patients undergoing resection and also lead to improved long-term postoperative outcomes.

6.10 Intrahepatic Chemotherapy

Intrahepatic chemotherapy has been used in the treatment of patients with hepatic metastases, that are unresectable, or in the presence of significant extrahepatic disease, in order to prolong survival. It has been shown to lead to a partial response in two thirds of patients and a complete response in approximately 10 % of patients [15]. The reported median survival for patients treated with intrahepatic chemotherapy is up to 24 months, and as a result arterially based treatment should be considered for those who are unsuitable for systemic chemotherapy. The regimes reported in the literature are heterogeneous, and it is not possible to define what represents the best regime for treating metastatic disease.

6.11 Chemotherapy

There has been rapid progression in the available systemic therapies for patients with metastatic melanoma over the past few years. Agents targeting specific part of the cell cycle, such as anti-PD1 antibodies, selective B-RAF inhibitors, c-kit inhibitors, and MEK inhibitors, have all been shown in vitro to have antitumor effects.

Activating mutations of the B-RAF genes are found in half of patients with metastatic melanoma. In patients with the V600 mutation, treatment with trametinib, a selective B-RAF inhibitor, leads to an improvement in progression-free (HR 0.45, $P<0.001$) and overall survival compared with standard chemotherapy (81 % versus 67 % at 6 months) [16].

Inhibition of the CTLA-4 antigen on the cytotoxic T cell with ipilimumab increases the immune response to metastatic melanoma and leads to an improvement in median survival, for those patients with unresectable disease. Other immunomodulators can be used, in addition, to improve the antitumor effects and lead to an improvement in median survival [17].

The c-kit mutation is commonly found in patients with metastatic melanoma, and selective inhibition using imatinib mesylate allows the disease to be controlled in half of the patients treated, with an overall response rate of 23 % [18]. More recently the various targeted agents have been used in combination in an attempt to improve response rates and prolong overall survival. Combination therapy with a B-RAF inhibitor, and a selective MAPK kinase inhibitor, has been shown to improve median progression-free survival by 4 months (9.4 months versus 5.8 months) compared with monotherapy alone. The response rates were also higher in the group treated with combination therapy (76 % versus 54 %) [19].

Where targeted agents, or clinical trials for these targeted agents, are unavailable, standard cytotoxic medications can be used. Dacarbazine (DTIC), taxanes, platinum derivatives, or cytokines such as interferon or interleukin-2 can be used either alone or in combination to treat metastatic disease. Multiple drug regimes can lead to better initial response rate, but they do not prolong overall survival.

In summary, complete surgical resection of liver metastasis in appropriately selected patients can lead to long-term survival. The presence of low-volume resectable extrahepatic disease is not a contraindication to surgical resection of liver metastasis. Where patients are unsuitable for or unable to have complete resection of tumors, it is appropriate that they undergo treatment with one of the newer agents which are cell cycle specific either alone or in combination as part of a controlled clinical trial.

References

1. Rigel DS (2010) Epidemiology of melanoma. Semin Cutan Med Surg 29(4):204–209
2. Balch CM et al (2009) Final version of 2009 AJCC melanoma staging and classification. J Clin Oncol 27(36):6199–6206
3. Sanki A, Scolyer RA, Thompson JF (2009) Surgery for melanoma metastases of the gastrointestinal tract: indications and results. Eur J Surg Oncol 35(3):313–319

4. Caralt M et al (2011) Outcome of patients following hepatic resection for metastatic cutaneous and ocular melanoma. J Hepatobiliary Pancreat Sci 18(2):268–275
5. Ryu SW et al (2013) Liver resection for metastatic melanoma: equivalent survival for cutaneous and ocular primaries. J Surg Oncol 108(2):129–135
6. Yi JH et al (2011) Dacarbazine-based chemotherapy as first-line treatment in noncutaneous metastatic melanoma: multicenter, retrospective analysis in Asia. Melanoma Res 21(3): 223–227
7. Rueth NM et al (2014) Is surveillance imaging effective for detecting surgically treatable recurrences in patients with melanoma? A comparative analysis of stage-specific surveillance strategies. Ann Surg 259(6):1215–1222
8. Holder WD Jr et al (1998) Effectiveness of positron emission tomography for the detection of melanoma metastases. Ann Surg 227(5):764–769; discussion 769–71
9. Xing Y et al (2011) Contemporary diagnostic imaging modalities for the staging and surveillance of melanoma patients: a meta-analysis. J Natl Cancer Inst 103(2):129–142
10. Orcurto V et al (2012) (18)F-fluorodeoxyglucose positron emission tomography/computed tomography and magnetic resonance imaging in patients with liver metastases from uveal melanoma: results from a pilot study. Melanoma Res 22(1):63–69
11. Pawlik TM et al (2006) Hepatic resection for metastatic melanoma: distinct patterns of recurrence and prognosis for ocular versus cutaneous disease. Ann Surg Oncol 13(5):712–720
12. Frenkel S et al (2009) Long-term survival of uveal melanoma patients after surgery for liver metastases. Br J Ophthalmol 93(8):1042–1046
13. Mariani P, Servois V, Piperno-Neumann S (2012) Therapeutic options in metastatic uveal melanoma. Dev Ophthalmol 49:166–181
14. Rivoire M et al (2005) Treatment of liver metastases from uveal melanoma. Ann Surg Oncol 12(6):422–428
15. Sharma KV et al (2008) Hepatic arterial chemoembolization for management of metastatic melanoma. AJR Am J Roentgenol 190(1):99–104
16. Flaherty KT et al (2012) Improved survival with MEK inhibition in BRAF-mutated melanoma. N Engl J Med 367(2):107–114
17. Hodi FS et al (2010) Improved survival with ipilimumab in patients with metastatic melanoma. N Engl J Med 363(8):711–723
18. Guo J et al (2011) Phase II, open-label, single-arm trial of imatinib mesylate in patients with metastatic melanoma harboring c-Kit mutation or amplification. J Clin Oncol 29(21): 2904–2909
19. Flaherty KT et al (2012) Combined BRAF and MEK inhibition in melanoma with BRAF V600 mutations. N Engl J Med 367(18):1694–1703

4. Caralt M et al (2011) Outcome of patients following hepatic resection for metastatic cutaneous and ocular melanoma. J Hepatobiliary Pancreat Sci 18(2):268–275
5. Ryu SW et al (2013) Liver resection for metastatic melanoma: equivalent survival for cutaneous and ocular primaries. J Surg Oncol 108(2):129–135
6. Yi JH et al (2011) Dacarbazine-based chemotherapy as first-line treatment in noncutaneous metastatic melanoma: multicenter, retrospective analysis in Asia. Melanoma Res 21(3):223–227
[illegible]

7 Liver Metastases from Ovarian and Uterus Cancer

Anya Adair and Stephen J. Wigmore

7.1 Introduction

Almost any solid organ malignancy can spread to the liver. Those cancers originating from the gastrointestinal tract spread directly via the portal circulation. Other tumors travel to the liver via systemic hematogenous spread or via peritoneal seeding, as can be the case in ovarian malignancy.

Until the 1990s, development of liver metastasis was regarded as a preterminal event with palliation the only treatment option. During the same time period, liver resection for malignant disease carried mortality rates of up to 29 % [1].

Improvements in preoperative imaging, anesthesia, perioperative care, operative techniques, and improved understanding of segmental anatomy have all contributed to the reduction in mortality rates for liver resection to <5 % [2]. In addition the proportion of patients now eligible for liver resection has greatly increased due to the introduction of staged hepatic resection and techniques such as portal vein embolization [3–5].

Hepatic resection is now considered the treatment of choice for many patients with colorectal and neuroendocrine tumor metastases resulting in 5-year survival rates of 50 and 75 %, respectively [3, 4, 6]. Long-term survival has also been reported following hepatic resection of non-colorectal metastases from Wilms' tumors, carcinoid, adrenal carcinoma, and other malignancies [7, 8].

As a consequence of these successful outcomes and the accompanying low mortality rates, hepatic resection for non-colorectal primary tumors is now being considered as a possibility. There does however still remain a lack of prospective

A. Adair • S.J. Wigmore (✉)
Department of Surgery, Royal Infirmary of Edinburgh,
51 Little France Crescent, Edinburgh EH16 4SA, UK
e-mail: anyadair@hotmail.com; s.wigmore@ed.ac.uk

I. Di Carlo (ed.), *Noncolorectal, Nonneuroendocrine Liver Metastases: Diagnosis and Current Therapies*, DOI 10.1007/978-3-319-09293-5_7

evidence and therefore no clear consensus related to liver resection for metastases from many solid organ tumors.

The role of hepatic resection for gynecological tumors still remains undecided, possibly due to the fact that liver metastases of these tumors tend to occur in the setting of regional dissemination making hepatic resection inappropriate [9].

In this chapter we consider the role of hepatic resection in the management of gynecological malignancy.

7.2 Ovarian Cancer

7.2.1 Introduction

Ovarian cancer is the second most common gynecological malignancy and the fifth most commonly diagnosed cancer in women worldwide [10, 11].

The incidence of ovarian cancer increases with age becoming most prevalent in the eighth decade with a median age at presentation of 63 years [12].

Increased risks identified for the development of ovarian cancer include being nulliparous or being of more advanced age at first pregnancy [13]. In addition family history accounts for a small proportion of ovarian malignancies, approximately 5 %, with an increased risk linked to BRCA1 and two genotypes and HNPCC [14].

Epithelial ovarian cancer is responsible for approximately 90 % of ovarian cancers. Tumors arising from germ cells or the sex cords and stroma of the ovary account for the remaining 10 %. Approximately 80 % of epithelial ovarian cancers are of serous histological type, and less common are mucinous, endometrioid, clear cell, Brenner, and undifferentiated cancers [14].

Most ovarian cancers are not diagnosed at an early stage due to the location of the ovaries and the nonspecific symptoms with which patients present including bloating, pelvic and abdominal pain, early satiety, and urinary symptoms [15].

Due to this indolent presentation, greater than 70 % of patients are diagnosed with advanced stage disease [16], with over 50 % of patients diagnosed with peritoneal seeding from the pelvis to the upper abdomen [17].

Fewer than 40 % of women with ovarian cancer are cured, and the 5-year survival for patients with advanced disease is between 5 and 20 % [11, 12].

Stage of disease is highly significant in determining prognosis and treatment options in ovarian malignancy. Ovarian cancer is classified as stages I–IV. Since 1997 no significant changes have been made in the TNM and FIGO (International Federation of Gynecology and Obstetric) staging systems for ovarian cancer [12, 18] (Table 7.1).

Ovarian cancer spreads by direct extension and intraperitoneal seeding, via lymphatic pathways or hematogenous spread. The most common route of spread is via intraperitoneal seeding as the tumor cells shed and circulate in the peritoneal fluid. Approximately 70 % of patients are found to have peritoneal metastases at the time of staging laparotomy.

Table 7.1 FIGO staging system for ovarian cancer

Stage I disease confined to the ovary
Stage II disease confined to the pelvis
Stage III peritoneal seeding in the abdominal cavity including pancreatic, diaphragmatic, and bowel invasion
Stage IV hepatic parenchymal metastasis

UK website, FIGO Cancer Committee staging announcement [64]

In contrast hematogenous spread is the least common form of ovarian metastasis and is rarely present at the time of diagnosis. The most common sites for this form of dissemination are the colon, liver, intestine, and lung in 50, 48, 44, and 34 % of patients, respectively [19].

Initial investigations include physical examination, ultrasound scan of the pelvis, and CT chest abdomen pelvis [12]. MRI has been used more recently in the detection of early peritoneal carcinomatosis and PET CT when investigating recurrent disease [16].

7.2.2 Treatment

Cytoreductive surgery to minimize residual tumor followed by platinum- and taxane-based chemotherapy is the standard treatment for advanced epithelial ovarian cancer [18].

Management first requires surgical staging in the form of staging laparotomy, and at this time approximately 30 % of patients are upstaged [20].

Total abdominal hysterectomy and bilateral oophorectomy alone are performed for stage I disease. Cytoreductive surgery is carried out for patients with stage II–IV disease [20–22, 23]. This is followed by systemic platinum-based chemotherapy [12].

For patients with bulky stage III/IV disease who are not surgical candidates, neoadjuvant chemotherapy followed by primary cytoreduction can be considered [16, 24–27].

7.2.3 Cytoreductive Surgery

As early as 1935 Meigs recognized the importance of cytoreduction and removing as much tumor as possible to improve the effects of postoperative radiation in the management of ovarian cancer [28]. Forty years later Griffiths published a study that demonstrated conclusively an inverse relationship between the maximal residual tumor diameter and patient survival [29].

Cytoreductive surgery or debulking is the standard treatment recommendation for patients with clinical stage II–IV disease [20–23]. Cytoreductive surgery can be performed at the time of index surgery termed primary cytoreduction, following neoadjuvant chemotherapy, or for recurrent disease termed secondary cytoreduction.

The aim of cytoreduction is to fully stage the disease and achieve maximal clearance to less than 1 cm residual disease, or resection of all visible disease in appropriate circumstances.

Procedures that may be considered for optimal surgical cytoreduction include radical pelvic dissection, omentectomy, bowel resection, diaphragm stripping, splenectomy, partial hepatectomy, and distal pancreatectomy [30].

Chi et al. studied the impact of extensive upper abdominal primary cytoreduction including splenectomy, distal pancreatectomy, hepatic resection, and resection of porta hepatis tumors (Group 2) compared to earlier more conservative cytoreduction which involved only TAH, BSO ± omentectomy, and bowel resection (Group 1). Optimal cytoreduction rates defined as <1 cm residual disease (total disease less than 1 cm left behind) increased from 50 to 70 % between groups 1 and 2.

Operative time and estimated blood loss were greater in group 2 than group 1, $P<0.001$ for both; however, complication rates and length of hospitalization were not significantly different between the two groups [31].

For patients with bulky stage III/IV disease who are not surgical candidates, neoadjuvant chemotherapy followed by primary interval cytoreduction can be considered [16, 24, 26, 27, 32].

Secondary cytoreductive surgery can be considered for patients who experience recurrence after a long disease-free interval (>6 months) [33].

7.2.4 Liver Metastases from the Ovary

Ovarian malignancy can disseminate to the liver via intraperitoneal seeding or hematogenous spread.

With peritoneal seeding, initially the cells move downward into the pelvis due to the pull of gravity, and they then travel cranially in the circulating peritoneal fluid, moving through the right paracolic gutter to the pouch of Morrison and the right subdiaphragmatic space. The peritoneal fluid from the posterior subphrenic space travels along the right coronary ligament to the hepatic bare area and spreads throughout the perihepatic space.

The tumor cells initially seed to the liver capsule producing peritoneal lesion on the liver surface – stage III disease. The tumor can then advance to involve the liver parenchyma – stage IV disease [16, 18].

Hematogenous spread is generally seen in advanced disease the liver being affected in 48 % of cases.

Liver involvement can be present at the initial diagnosis of ovarian cancer usually due to peritoneal seeding, and the presence of adhesions resembling those seen in Fitz-Hugh-Curtis disease may be an early indicator of carcinomatosis [16].

Alternatively metachronous liver metastasis diagnosed during follow-up following initial cytoreduction and chemotherapy can occur. These can be either due to peritoneal seeding or hematogenous spread.

As stated liver involvement can therefore occur in both stage III and IV disease. Sixteen percent of ovarian cancer cases are stage IV at the time of diagnosis. Both stages of ovarian cancer have a poor prognosis with 5-year survival for stage III and IV disease approximately 37 and 25 %, respectively [34–36].

When considering liver resection in ovarian cancer metastasis, consideration needs to be given to the stage of disease and whether the tumor is synchronous or metachronous.

Liver resection has been considered in the setting of:

1. Primary cytoreduction pre-chemotherapy treatment
2. Primary cytoreduction following neoadjuvant chemotherapy
3. Secondary cytoreduction for recurrent disease following primary cytoreduction and adjuvant chemotherapy
4. Secondary cytoreduction for recurrent disease following neoadjuvant chemotherapy for bulky disease

7.2.5 Liver Resection for Ovarian Cancer

The literature surrounding liver resection for ovarian malignancy is limited and mainly restricted to retrospective reviews.

The majority of papers have reviewed the role of hepatic resection in secondary cytoreduction for recurrent disease following chemotherapy.

Liver resection has been carried out in the context of both stage III and IV disease, with and without the presence of extrahepatic disease. Resection was performed for both single and multiple metastases [37–43].

Median survival ranged from 11 to 62 months combining stage III and IV disease. Two studies looking at only stage IV had wide variation in median survival, 11 and 40 months [40]. Similar survival rates are seen with and without the presence of extrahepatic disease [38, 39, 41, 43].

There was no perioperative mortality reported, and complication rates are reported between 11 and 21 %. All studies had a long median disease-free interval ranged between primary cytoreduction and the development of liver metastasis ranging 32–68.5 months.

Both univariate and multivariate analysis demonstrated the importance of length of disease free interval to the development of liver metastases as a good prognostic factor. This possibly indicates favorable tumor biology. Other prognostic factors include optimal cytoreduction of residual disease to <1 cm and clear surgical margins, survival of 52 months with R0 resection compared to 22 months R1 [38]. Nui et al. found that the number of liver lesions affected prognosis [38], and this was however not found by others [37]. Abood et al. demonstrated improved prognosis if the size of the largest metastatic tumor was >5 cm, and speculating this may be due to overall less tumor burden due to smaller number of tumors [42].

Liver resection can be considered for both single and multiple liver lesions. The presence of extrahepatic disease should not exclude liver resection as long as adequate debulking is possible. Neoadjuvant chemotherapy can be performed in the presence of bulky stage IIIc/IV disease in an attempt to downstage the tumor and improve the chance of tumor clearance and achieving an R0 resection. In addition it may reduce the extent of resection required and therefore the possible surgical morbidity.

Table 7.2 Prognostic factors in liver resection as secondary cytoreduction for ovarian cancer

Disease-free interval from primary cytoreduction to liver metastases
R0 resection
Cytoreduction to <1 cm of residual disease
Number of liver lesions
Size of the largest liver lesion

The patients considered for liver resection, as with other hepatic metastases, should have good performance status. Many of the patients undergoing secondary cytoreduction and liver resection subsequently completed a further course of adjuvant chemotherapy (Table 7.2).

Liver Resection as a Component of Primary Cytoreduction

Less has been written about liver resection as part of primary cytoreduction. Lim and Bristow independently looked at the effect of hepatic resection as part of primary cytoreduction both before and after chemotherapy for synchronous liver metastases.

Bristow et al. retrospectively reviewed the results of primary cytoreduction for stage IV disease. In this population of patients, the median survival for those with synchronous parenchymal liver metastasis was 18 months. This was comparable to survival rates seen with pulmonary or other extrahepatic synchronous disease.

There was a significant relationship between performance status and survival following primary cytoreduction. In addition prognosis was significantly impacted on by the success of debulking. Those with <1 cm residual tumor experienced a 38.4-month median survival compared with 10.3 months for those with suboptimal debulking. The survival of those patients with parenchymal hepatic disease also correlated with the number of liver lesions, 1–2 hepatic lesions median survival 20.9 months compared with 6.4 months for patients with three or more lesions ($P=0.0012$).

Lim et al. retrospectively reviewed hepatic resection as part of primary cytoreduction for hepatic parenchymal metastases from peritoneal seeding for both stage IIIc and IV disease and found 5-year progression-free survival rates of 25 and 23 %, respectively, and overall 5-year survival rate of 55 and 51 %, respectively [18].

In summary liver resection in the context of stage III/IV disease is a viable option with acceptable morbidity and mortality, which should be considered as part of cytoreduction in a selected patient population at the time of both primary and secondary cytoreduction.

7.3 Endometrial Cancer

7.3.1 Introduction

Endometrial cancer is the most frequent malignant disease of the female reproductive tract [44, 45] accounting for 6 % of all cancers in women. The mean age at diagnosis is 68 years.

Table 7.3 FIGO staging of endometrial cancer

Stage I confined to the uterus
Stage II involvement of the uterine cervix
Stage III direct invasion to involve surface of the uterus, fallopian tubes, or vagina
Stage IV distant metastases
IVa to bowel, bladder
IVb to the liver, lungs, bone

This malignancy, as a rule, has a good prognosis with postmenopausal bleeding allowing for early diagnosis. At the time of diagnosis, 75 % of patients have stage 1 disease with 5-year survival rates of up to 88.9 % [45, 46]. Stage IV disease is seen in only 3.7 % of patients at initial diagnosis but is responsible for 23 % of cancer-related deaths in the first year following diagnosis and has an overall 5-year survival rate of 10–25 % [46–49].

Most patients who die from their disease have metastases beyond the pelvis at the time of death. Studies suggest that death from endometrial cancer is largely due to abdominal and distant metastases with a high proportion demonstrating liver and lung involvement [45, 49]. Approximately 50 % of patients dying as a result of endometrial cancer will demonstrate hepatic metastases at autopsy [43].

In cases of endometrial cancer, the tumor markers CA 15-3, CA72-4, and CA125 have been correlated with the disease stage, depth of myometrial invasion, and nodal status [50, 51]. There is however no difference in tumor marker levels in patients with or without distant metastases. Endometrial cancer cells are also known to express CEA, and significant differences in the level of this marker have only been seen when both hepatic and pulmonary metastases are present [49].

As with ovarian cancer the FIGO (International Federation of Gynecology and Obstetrics) system is also used in the staging of endometrial cancer (Table 7.3).

Endometrial carcinoma has four histological subtypes (endometrioid, papillary serous, clear cell, carcinosarcoma) of which endometrioid subtype is the most common affecting 75–80 % of patients [45, 46, 52]. Unlike ovarian carcinoma it is an important independent variable for prognosis and potential treatment. Endometrioid endometrial adenocarcinoma has a better prognosis than the other subtypes.

After surgical treatment of primary endometrial carcinoma, both local and distant recurrences are a serious concern in high-risk patients [53].

Recurrence is defined as "local tumor regrowth or the development of distant metastasis discovered 6 months or more after complete regression of the treated tumor." Approximately 60 % of recurrences are seen within 2 years following primary treatment [54].

Local or pelvic recurrence in endometrial carcinoma is frequently seen in patients treated with adjuvant chemotherapy alone and involves the vagina, pelvic nodes, cervix, adnexa, and peritoneum [55]. Adjuvant pelvic radiotherapy has been associated with decreased risk of local recurrence [56]. Peritoneal carcinomatosis is one of the most classical sites of recurrent endometrial carcinoma [57].

Endometrial cancer usually spreads by lymphatic dissemination. Hematogenous metastases are uncommon. The most common sites of distant metastases are the bone, lung, and liver [54]. Pulmonary metastases from gynecological malignancies are seen most commonly with endometrial carcinoma [54, 57]. Recurrent endometrial carcinoma is less commonly seen in intra-abdominal organs; however, the liver is the most common intra-abdominal organ to become involved. Liver metastases are seen as single or multiple liver lesions with peripheral enhancement [52].

PET/CT is a highly sensitive and specific modality in the diagnosis of recurrent endometrial carcinoma. It provides good anatomical and functional localization of sites of recurrence and distant metastases before it becomes symptomatic or detectable by other imaging modalities [52].

7.3.2 Liver Metastases from Endometrial Cancer

Published data on hepatic resection for metastatic endometrial carcinoma is sparse with all cases being of endometrioid histology [11].

In two case reports the patients underwent resection of isolated lesions followed by chemotherapy. One patient survived, and the second patient developed secondary recurrence at 8 months and died 2 months after this diagnosis [32, 43].

Chi had two patients with endometrial carcinoma in his series of gynecological malignancies and hepatic resection. Both were endometrioid, both had undergone TAH and BSO as primary treatment, both had single liver deposits, and both underwent postoperative pelvic irradiation. One patient had synchronous pulmonary metastases also resected.

One patient had synchronous pulmonary metastases also resected. One patient developed secondary recurrence in the brain which was resected with postoperative irradiation, and there was no evidence of disease 19 months after completing her radiotherapy [43].

Harrison published a series of 96 cases undergoing hepatic resection for non-colorectal non-neuroendocrine metastases including genitourinary, gastrointestinal, and soft tissue; this series included four endometrial carcinomas. There was no postoperative mortality, and there were some long-time survivors, but none of the endometrial metastases reached 5-year survival [2].

Knowles et al. retrospectively reviewed hepatic resection for endometrioid carcinoma of both ovarian and endometrial origin over a 20-year period. This made up only 0.8 % of the total liver resections performed in a tertiary referral hepatobiliary unit over this time period. Two were endometrial in origin with follow-up at 48 and 66 months showing both patients alive and disease-free [9] (Fig. 7.1).

Bristow et al. undertook a retrospective study of the role of primary cytoreductive surgery in the clinical management of patients with stage IVb endometrial carcinoma. An optimal surgical result was defined as no residual tumor nodule <1 cm in maximal diameter. Only one patient 1.5 % underwent liver resection as part of primary cytoreduction.

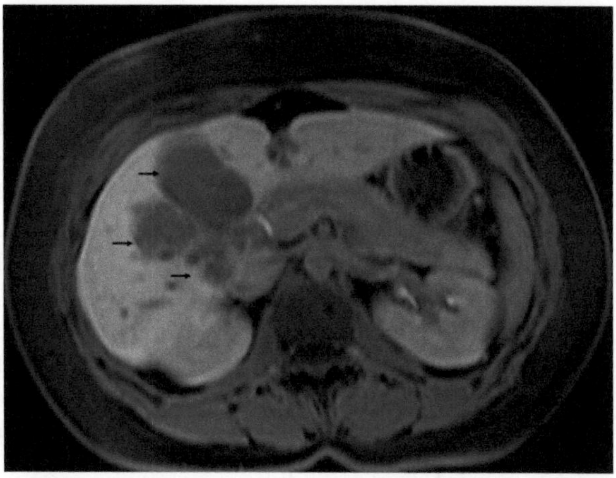

Fig. 7.1 MRI scan showing endometrial carcinoma metastasis in the right lobe of liver (*black arrows*). The lesion was resected by a right trisegmentectomy

Table 7.4 Similarities and differences in presentation, prognosis and management of ovarian and endometrial cancer

	Ovarian epithelial carcinoma	Endometrial carcinoma
Prognosis	Poor	Good
Diagnosis	Late	Early
Symptoms	Specific	Vague
Metastases	Common	Not common
Prognosis dependent on histological type	No	Yes
Chemotherapy	Standard	Controversial
Present with stage III/IV disease	High	Low
Stage IV disease at presentation	16 %	3.7 %
Most common histological type	Serous	Endometrioid

The median survival for the entire patient population was 14.8 months (range 0.4–102.7 months, mean survival 22.1 months). After a median follow-up of 14.7 months, 15 patients were alive without evidence of disease (23.1 %).

When evaluating adjuvant therapy modalities, no association between survival outcome and either chemotherapy or radiation therapy, when administered alone, was seen. In contrast, the 14 patients who received treatment with chemotherapy followed by radiation therapy had a median survival rate of 40.0 months, compared with only 14.0 months for patients not receiving this combination ($P=0.004$).

Patients with a performance status of 0 demonstrated a statistically significant survival advantage (median survival 20.1 months) compared with patients with a performance status of ≥1 (median survival 10.5 months, $P=0.0005$). Multivariate analysis only was presented which demonstrated that age <58 years ($P=0.023$), performance status = 0 ($P=0.043$), and residual disease <1 cm ($P=0.0001$) maintained significance as predictors of survival. Residual disease showed the strongest independent effect. These findings are consistent with those seen with ovarian cancer (Table 7.4).

7.3.3 Carcinoma of the Uterine Cervix

Cervical cancer is generally a local problem, and when recurrent or metastatic disease is present, this is difficult to treat. In these situations surgery is usually confined to pelvic exenteration or debulking with palliative chemotherapy being the mainstay of treatment for advanced disease. Liver resection for cervical carcinoma is therefore rare (Fig. 7.2). Patients who receive palliative chemotherapy for metastatic cervical cancer have a median survival of 12 months [58], and this is reduced to 10 months in those who have liver metastases as part of their pattern of spread [59].

There are a number of case reports that have described liver resection of cervical carcinoma metastases. In general cases were unusual in that they had single or small numbers of hepatic metastases with low volume of disease. The survival of patients who underwent resection of liver metastases from cervical cancer varied between 5 and 50 months [8, 43, 60–63].

Strong recommendations cannot be made regarding the appropriateness of resection of liver metastases arising from cervical cancer although there is case evidence that selected patients with limited disease may derive survival benefit.

Conclusions

The role of liver resection in the management of gynecological malignancy remains undefined. However with the excellent results seen in the management of colorectal metastasis and the improved surgical results of liver resection, interest in its role in the management of advanced gynecological malignancy has now been stimulated.

When considering the role of liver resection for metastatic disease, thought has to be given to the biological differences existing between solid organ tumors and the nonsurgical treatment options available to each cancer.

There does appear to be a role for liver resection in the setting of metastatic ovarian and endometrial metastases.

Ovarian cancer commonly presents late with distant metastases and liver involvement a common finding. Overall prognosis is poor; however, there are effective chemotherapy options available, and both primary and secondary cytoreduction do seem to improve survival. Liver resection in this context does appear to be advantageous if the patient population is chosen well.

Liver resection can be considered for both stage IV and IV disease as part of primary or secondary cytoreduction although most experience centers around resection in the setting of secondary cytoreduction.

Resection is not appropriate for all patients with liver metastases and should be limited to a selective population of patients who possess good performance status and long time interval between primary resection and recurrence of disease. The best median survival is seen when cytoreduction has achieved <1 cm of residual disease and an R0 liver resection. The presence of extrahepatic disease is not a contraindication.

Endometrial cancer in contrast is often diagnosed at an early stage, and metastases to the liver are less common. There are less studies exploring the role

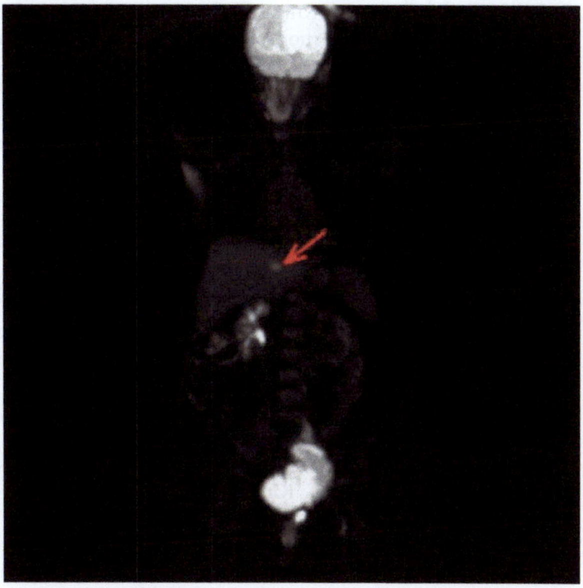

Fig. 7.2 Fluorodeoxyglucose positron emission tomography (FDG PET) showing cervical carcinoma metastasis in the left lateral section of the liver (*red arrow*)

of liver resection in this setting; however, as with ovarian cancer results are best in younger patients with good performance status and when able to achieve clearance with <1 cm residual disease.

Cervical cancer rarely metastasizes but when this occurs is difficult to manage with treatment options generally palliative.

References

1. Brunschwig A (1963) Hepatic lobectomy for metastatic cancer. Cancer 16:277–282
2. Harrison LE, Brennan MF, Newman E, Fortner JG, Picardo A, Blumgart LH, Fong Y (1997) Hepatic resection for noncolorectal, nonneuroendocrine metastases: a fifteen-year experience with ninety-six patients. Surgery 121(6):625–632
3. Shah SA, Bromberg R, Coates A, Rempel E, Simunovic M, Gallinger S (2007) Survival after liver resection for metastatic colorectal carcinoma in a large population. J Am Coll Surg 205(5):676–683
4. Fong Y, Fortner J, Sun RL, Brennan MF, Blumgart LH (1999) Clinical score for predicting recurrence after hepatic resection for metastatic colorectal cancer: analysis of 1,001 consecutive cases. Ann Surg 230(3):309–318; discussion 318–321
5. Abad A, Figueras J, Valls C, Carrato A, Pardo F, Diaz-Rubio E, Aranda E (2007) Guidelines for the detection and treatment of liver metastases of colorectal cancer. Clin Transl Oncol 9(11):723–730
6. Madoff DC, Gupta S, Ahrar K, Murthy R, Yao JC (2006) Update on the management of neuroendocrine hepatic metastases. J Vasc Interv Radiol 17(8):1235–1249; quiz 1250
7. Cobourn CS, Makowka L, Langer B, Taylor BR, Falk RE (1987) Examination of patient selection and outcome for hepatic resection for metastatic disease. Surg Gynecol Obstet 165(3):239–246

8. Wolf RF, Goodnight JE, Krag DE, Schneider PD (1991) Results of resection and proposed guidelines for patient selection in instances of non-colorectal hepatic metastases. Surg Gynecol Obstet 173(6):454–460
9. Knowles B, Bellamy CO, Oniscu A, Wigmore SJ (2010) Hepatic resection for metastatic endometrioid carcinoma. HPB (Oxford) 12(6):412–417
10. Permuth-Wey J, Sellers TA (2009) Epidemiology of ovarian cancer. Methods Mol Biol 472:413–437
11. Tangjitgamol S, Levenback CF, Beller U, Kavanagh JJ (2004) Role of surgical resection for lung, liver, and central nervous system metastases in patients with gynecological cancer: a literature review. Int J Gynecol Cancer 14(3):399–422
12. Morgan RJ Jr, Alvarez RD, Armstrong DK, Boston B, Burger RA, Chen LM, Copeland L, Crispens MA, Gershenson D, Gray HJ, Grigsby PW, Hakam A, Havrilesky LJ, Johnston C, Lele S, Matulonis UA, O'Malley DM, Penson RT, Remmenga SW, Sabbatini P, Schilder RJ, Schink JC, Teng N, Werner TL, National Comprehensive Cancer Network (2011) Epithelial ovarian cancer. J Natl Compr Canc Netw 9(1):82–113
13. Morch LS, Lokkegaard E, Andreasen AH, Kruger-Kjaer S, Lidegaard O (2009) Hormone therapy and ovarian cancer. JAMA 302(3):298–305
14. Finch A, Beiner M, Lubinski J, Lynch HT, Moller P, Rosen B, Murphy J, Ghadirian P, Friedman E, Foulkes WD, Kim-Sing C, Wagner T, Tung N, Couch F, Stoppa-Lyonnet D, Ainsworth P, Daly M, Pasini B, Gershoni-Baruch R, Eng C, Olopade OI, McLennan J, Karlan B, Weitzel J, Sun P, Narod SA (2006) Hereditary ovarian cancer clinical study G. Salpingo-oophorectomy and the risk of ovarian, fallopian tube, and peritoneal cancers in women with a BRCA1 or BRCA2 mutation. JAMA 296(2):185–192
15. Goff BA, Mandel LS, Drescher CW, Urban N, Gough S, Schurman KM, Patras J, Mahony BS, Andersen MR (2007) Development of an ovarian cancer symptom index: possibilities for earlier detection. Cancer 109(2):221–227
16. Nougaret S, Addley HC, Colombo PE, Fujii S, Al Sharif SS, Tirumani SH, Jardon K, Sala E, Reinhold C (2012) Ovarian carcinomatosis: how the radiologist can help plan the surgical approach. Radiographics 32(6):1775–1800; discussion 1800–1773
17. Zivanovic O, Eisenhauer EL, Zhou Q, Iasonos A, Sabbatini P, Sonoda Y, Abu-Rustum NR, Barakat RR, Chi DS (2008) The impact of bulky upper abdominal disease cephalad to the greater omentum on surgical outcome for stage IIIC epithelial ovarian, fallopian tube, and primary peritoneal cancer. Gynecol Oncol 108(2):287–292
18. Lim MC, Kang S, Lee KS, Han SS, Park SJ, Seo SS, Park SY (2009) The clinical significance of hepatic parenchymal metastasis in patients with primary epithelial ovarian cancer. Gynecol Oncol 112(1):28–34
19. Rose PG, Piver MS, Tsukada Y, Lau TS (1989) Metastatic patterns in histologic variants of ovarian cancer. An autopsy study. Cancer 64(7):1508–1513
20. Stier EA, Barakat RR, Curtin JP, Brown CL, Jones WB, Hoskins WJ (1996) Laparotomy to complete staging of presumed early ovarian cancer. Obstet Gynecol 87(5 Pt 1):737–740
21. du Bois A, Quinn M, Thigpen T, Vermorken J, Avall-Lundqvist E, Bookman M, Bowtell D, Brady M, Casado A, Cervantes A, Eisenhauer E, Friedlaender M, Fujiwara K, Grenman S, Guastalla JP, Harper P, Hogberg T, Kaye S, Kitchener H, Kristensen G, Mannel R, Meier W, Miller B, Neijt JP, Oza A, Ozols R, Parmar M, Pecorelli S, Pfisterer J, Poveda A, Provencher D, Pujade-Lauraine E, Randall M, Rochon J, Rustin G, Sagae S, Stehman F, Stuart G, Trimble E, Vasey P, Vergote I, Verheijen R, Wagner U, Gynecologic Cancer Intergroup, Ago Ovar, Anzgog, Eortc, Geico, Gineco, Gog, Jgog, Mrc/Ncri, Ncic CTG, Nci US, Nsgo, Rtog, Sgctg, Igcs, Organizational team of the two prior International OCCC (2005) 2004 consensus statements on the management of ovarian cancer: final document of the 3rd International Gynecologic Cancer Intergroup Ovarian Cancer Consensus Conference (GCIG OCCC 2004). Ann Oncol 16(Suppl 8):viii7–viii12
22. Eisenhauer EL, Abu-Rustum NR, Sonoda Y, Levine DA, Poynor EA, Aghajanian C, Jarnagin WR, DeMatteo RP, D'Angelica MI, Barakat RR, Chi DS (2006) The addition of extensive

upper abdominal surgery to achieve optimal cytoreduction improves survival in patients with stages IIIC-IV epithelial ovarian cancer. Gynecol Oncol 103(3):1083–1090
23. du Bois A, Reuss A, Pujade-Lauraine E, Harter P, Ray-Coquard I, Pfisterer J (2009) Role of surgical outcome as prognostic factor in advanced epithelial ovarian cancer: a combined exploratory analysis of 3 prospectively randomized phase 3 multicenter trials: by the Arbeitsgemeinschaft Gynaekologische Onkologie Studiengruppe Ovarialkarzinom (AGO-OVAR) and the Groupe d'Investigateurs Nationaux Pour les Etudes des Cancers de l'Ovaire (GINECO). Cancer 115(6):1234–1244
24. Steed H, Oza AM, Murphy J, Laframboise S, Lockwood G, DEP D, Sturgeon J, Rosen B (2006) A retrospective analysis of neoadjuvant platinum-based chemotherapy versus up-front surgery in advanced ovarian cancer. Int J Gynecol Cancer 16(Suppl 1):47–53
25. Tangjitgamol S, Manusirivithaya S, Laopaiboon M, Lumbiganon P (2009) Interval debulking surgery for advanced epithelial ovarian cancer: a Cochrane systematic review. Gynecol Oncol 112(1):257–264
26. Vandenput I, Van Calster B, Capoen A, Leunen K, Berteloot P, Neven P, Moerman P, Vergote I, Amant F (2009) Neoadjuvant chemotherapy followed by interval debulking surgery in patients with serous endometrial cancer with transperitoneal spread (stage IV): a new preferred treatment? Br J Cancer 101(2):244–249
27. Tiersten AD, Liu PY, Smith HO, Wilczynski SP, Robinson WR 3rd, Markman M, Alberts DS (2009) Phase II evaluation of neoadjuvant chemotherapy and debulking followed by intraperitoneal chemotherapy in women with stage III and IV epithelial ovarian, fallopian tube or primary peritoneal cancer: Southwest Oncology Group Study S0009. Gynecol Oncol 112(3):444–449
28. Meigs JV (1935) Ovarian tumors with endocrine significance. Ann Surg 102(5):834–848
29. Griffiths CT (1975) Surgical resection of tumor bulk in the primary treatment of ovarian carcinoma. Natl Cancer Inst Monogr 42:101–104
30. Wimberger P, Lehmann N, Kimmig R, Burges A, Meier W, Du Bois A, Arbeitsgemeinschaft Gynaekologische Onkologie Ovarian Cancer Study Group (2007) Prognostic factors for complete debulking in advanced ovarian cancer and its impact on survival. An exploratory analysis of a prospectively randomized phase III study of the Arbeitsgemeinschaft Gynaekologische Onkologie Ovarian Cancer Study Group (AGO-OVAR). Gynecol Oncol 106(1):69–74
31. Chi DS, Eisenhauer EL, Lang J, Huh J, Haddad L, Abu-Rustum NR, Sonoda Y, Levine DA, Hensley M, Barakat RR (2006) What is the optimal goal of primary cytoreductive surgery for bulky stage IIIC epithelial ovarian carcinoma (EOC)? Gynecol Oncol 103(2):559–564
32. Tangjitgamol S, Manusirivithaya S, Laopaiboon M, Lumbiganon P (2013) Interval debulking surgery for advanced epithelial ovarian cancer. Cochrane Database Syst Rev 2:CD006014
33. Eisenkop SM, Friedman RL, Spirtos NM (2000) The role of secondary cytoreductive surgery in the treatment of patients with recurrent epithelial ovarian carcinoma. Cancer 88(1):144–153
34. Jemal A, Siegel R, Ward E, Hao Y, Xu J, Thun MJ (2009) Cancer statistics. CA Cancer J Clin 59(4):225–249
35. Averette HE, Donato DM (1990) Ovarian carcinoma. Advances in diagnosis, staging, and treatment. Cancer 65(3 Suppl):703–708
36. Wagner BJ, Buck JL, Seidman JD, McCabe KM (1994) From the archives of the AFIP. Ovarian epithelial neoplasms: radiologic-pathologic correlation. Radiographics 14(6):1351–1374; quiz 1375–1356
37. Kolev V, Pereira EB, Schwartz M, Sarpel U, Roayaie S, Labow D, Momeni M, Chuang L, Dottino P, Rahaman J, Zakashansky K (2014) The role of liver resection at the time of secondary cytoreduction in patients with recurrent ovarian cancer. Int J Gynecol Cancer 24(1):70–74
38. Niu GC, Shen CM, Cui W, Li Q (2012) Hepatic resection is safe for metachronous hepatic metastases from ovarian cancer. Cancer Biol Med 9(3):182–187

39. Pekmezci S, Saribeyoglu K, Aytac E, Arvas M, Demirkiran F, Ozguroglu M (2010) Surgery for isolated liver metastasis of ovarian cancer. Asian J Surg 33(2):83–88
40. Naik R, Nordin A, Cross PA, Hemming D, de Barros LA, Monaghan JM (2000) Optimal cytoreductive surgery is an independent prognostic indicator in stage IV epithelial ovarian cancer with hepatic metastases. Gynecol Oncol 78(2):171–175
41. Yoon SS, Jarnagin WR, Fong Y, DeMatteo RP, Barakat RR, Blumgart LH, Chi DS (2003) Resection of recurrent ovarian or fallopian tube carcinoma involving the liver. Gynecol Oncol 91(2):383–388
42. Abood G, Bowen M, Potkul R, Aranha G, Shoup M (2008) Hepatic resection for recurrent metastatic ovarian cancer. Am J Surg 195(3):370–373; discussion 373
43. Chi DS, Fong Y, Venkatraman ES, Barakat RR (1997) Hepatic resection for metastatic gynecologic carcinomas. Gynecol Oncol 66(1):45–51
44. Prat J (2004) Prognostic parameters of endometrial carcinoma. Hum Pathol 35(6):649–662
45. Barlin JN, Wysham WZ, Ferda AM, Khoury-Collado F, Cassella DK, Alektiar KM, Hensley ML, Chi DS, Barakat RR, Abu-Rustum NR (2012) Location of disease in patients who die from endometrial cancer: a study of 414 patients from a single institution. Int J Gynecol Cancer 22(9):1527–1531
46. Creasman WT, Kohler MF, Odicino F, Maisonneuve P, Boyle P (2004) Prognosis of papillary serous, clear cell, and grade 3 stage I carcinoma of the endometrium. Gynecol Oncol 95(3): 593–596
47. Hacker NF, Berek JS, Lagasse LD, Nieberg RK, Elashoff RM (1983) Primary cytoreductive surgery for epithelial ovarian cancer. Obstet Gynecol 61(4):413–420
48. Hoskins WJ, Rubin SC (1991) Surgery in the treatment of patients with advanced ovarian cancer. Semin Oncol 18(3):213–221
49. Heyer H, Grunwald S, Kohler G, Ohlinger R (2007) Significance of laboratory studies for ruling out metastases in primary endometrial carcinoma. Anticancer Res 27(3B):1673–1677
50. Yamazawa K, Hirashiki K, Usui H, Mitsuhashi A, Matsui H, Sekiya S (2005) Discordance between serum level and tissue immunohistochemical staining of CA125 in endometrioid adenocarcinoma of the uterine corpus. Int J Gynecol Pathol 24(3):254–259
51. Santala M, Talvensaari-Mattila A, Kauppila A (2003) Peritoneal cytology and preoperative serum CA 125 level are important prognostic indicators of overall survival in advanced endometrial cancer. Anticancer Res 23(3C):3097–3103
52. Kurra V, Krajewski KM, Jagannathan J, Giardino A, Berlin S, Ramaiya N (2013) Typical and atypical metastatic sites of recurrent endometrial carcinoma. Cancer Imaging 13:113–122
53. Grigsby PW, Perez CA, Kuten A, Simpson JR, Garcia DM, Camel HM, Kao MS, Galakatos AE (1992) Clinical stage I endometrial cancer: prognostic factors for local control and distant metastasis and implications of the new FIGO surgical staging system. Int J Radiat Oncol Biol Phys 22(5):905–911
54. Aalders JG, Abeler V, Kolstad P (1984) Recurrent adenocarcinoma of the endometrium: a clinical and histopathological study of 379 patients. Gynecol Oncol 17(1):85–103
55. Mundt AJ, McBride R, Rotmensch J, Waggoner SE, Yamada SD, Connell PP (2001) Significant pelvic recurrence in high-risk pathologic stage I–IV endometrial carcinoma patients after adjuvant chemotherapy alone: implications for adjuvant radiation therapy. Int J Radiat Oncol Biol Phys 50(5):1145–1153
56. Elliott P, Green D, Coates A, Krieger M, Russell P, Coppleson M, Solomon J, Tattersall M (1994) The efficacy of postoperative vaginal irradiation in preventing vaginal recurrence in endometrial cancer. Int J Gynecol Cancer 4(2):84–93
57. Sohaib SA, Houghton SL, Meroni R, Rockall AG, Blake P, Reznek RH (2007) Recurrent endometrial cancer: patterns of recurrent disease and assessment of prognosis. Clin Radiol 62(1):28–34; discussion 35–26
58. Monk BJ, Sill MW, McMeekin DS, Cohn DE, Ramondetta LM, Boardman CH, Benda J, Cella D (2009) Phase III trial of four cisplatin-containing doublet combinations in stage IVB,

recurrent, or persistent cervical carcinoma: a Gynecologic Oncology Group study. J Clin Oncol 27(28):4649–4655

59. Kim GE, Lee SW, Suh CO, Park TK, Kim JW, Park JT, Shim JU (1998) Hepatic metastases from carcinoma of the uterine cervix. Gynecol Oncol 70(1):56–60
60. Kaseki H, Yasui K, Niwa K, Mizuno K, Inoue T, Ota M (1992) Hepatic resection for metastatic squamous cell carcinoma from the uterine cervix. Gynecol Oncol 44(3):284–287
61. Papadia A, Moya Y, Rodgers SE, Lucci JA 3rd, Diaz JP (2011) Surgical resection of recurrent upper abdominal cervical cancer: a case report and review of the literature. Gynecol Oncol Case Rep 1(1):8–9
62. Foster JH (1978) Survival after liver resection for secondary tumors. Am J Surg 135(3): 389–394
63. La Fianza A, Alberici E, Biasina AM, Preda L, Tateo S, Campani R (1999) Spontaneous hemorrhage of a liver metastasis from squamous cell cervical carcinoma: case report and review of the literature. Tumori 85(4):290–293
64. FIGO Cancer Committee staging announcement (1968) Gynecol Oncol 25:383–385

Liver Metastases from Pancreatic Adenocarcinoma

8

Jin He, David Cosgrove, Joseph M. Herman, and Timothy M. Pawlik

8.1 Introduction

Pancreatic cancer is the fourth leading cause of cancer-related death in Europe and the United States [1]. At the time of diagnosis, approximately half of patients with pancreatic adenocarcinoma will have synchronous metastasis. Patients with metastatic pancreatic cancer generally have a median survival of 6 months and a 5-year survival of about 2–5 %. The liver is a frequent site of metastasis as pancreatic adenocarcinoma can metastasize to the liver through portal venous or intra-abdominal lymphatic drainage. For example, in a study from Johns Hopkins Hospital, among 838 patients with pancreatic adenocarcinoma who underwent a pancreatectomy, 46 % subsequently developed metachronous liver metastasis. Of note, among those patients with pancreatic cancer metastatic to the liver, 60 % had isolated liver metastasis without extrahepatic recurrence at the time of last follow-up.

Although surgery is an accepted treatment modality for liver metastases from colorectal cancer [2] or gastrointestinal neuroendocrine tumors [3], the role of resection for pancreatic adenocarcinoma metastatic to the liver is less defined and certainly controversial. Several topics of ongoing debate include whether concomitant hepatic resection is ever justifiable for synchronous metastasis, when (if ever) should

J. He, MD, PhD
Department of Surgery, Johns Hopkins Hospital, Baltimore, MD, USA

D. Cosgrove, MD
Department of Medical Oncology, Johns Hopkins Hospital, Baltimore, MD, USA

J.M. Herman, MD, MSc
Department of Radiation Oncology, Johns Hopkins Hospital, Baltimore, MD, USA

T.M. Pawlik, MD, MPH, PhD (✉)
Division of Surgical Oncology, Department of Surgery, Johns Hopkins Hospital, Harvey 611, 600 North Wolfe Street, Blalock 688, Baltimore, MD 21287, USA
e-mail: tpawlik1@jhmi.ed

I. Di Carlo (ed.), *Noncolorectal, Nonneuroendocrine Liver Metastases: Diagnosis and Current Therapies*, DOI 10.1007/978-3-319-09293-5_8

resection be considered in patients with metachronous disease, and whether surgery provides a better chance at long-term survival versus chemotherapy alone. The data on the surgical management of pancreatic adenocarcinoma metastatic to the liver are relatively limited. In fact, most data are derived from retrospective data, and many studies are single institution. Notwithstanding these limitations, we herein review the role of surgical management of pancreatic adenocarcinoma metastatic to the liver.

8.2 Natural History

Less than 20 % of patients diagnosed with pancreatic cancer are candidates for curative surgical resection. Advanced pancreatic cancer can invade local major vascular structures such as the celiac axis, hepatic artery, superior mesenteric artery, portal vein, and/or superior mesenteric vein. Pancreatic cancer can often also metastasize hematogenously to distant organs. Iacobuzio et al. profiled the patterns of failure in 76 autopsies of patients who died of pancreatic cancer; 30 % of patients died with locally advanced pancreatic cancer, while 70 % of patients died with widespread metastatic disease [4]. The liver was noted to be the most common site of metastatic disease (70 %), followed by the peritoneum and lung [4]. Multi-organ metastasis is also common. In this same study, 57 (88 %) of 65 patients with distant metastases had metastatic disease in multiple organ sites, most commonly involving the liver in combination with peritoneal and/or lung metastases [4].

Without treatment, the survival of patients with pancreatic adenocarcinoma liver metastasis is dismal. Lavu et al. noted that the median survival of patients with synchronous pancreatic cancer and liver metastasis after palliative bypass or celiac plexus neurolysis was about 6 months [5]. In a separate study, Kneuertz et al. noted a comparable median survival of 5 months among a group of 130 patients with pancreatic adenocarcinoma liver metastasis who underwent palliative bypass only [6]. Interestingly, in a study examining patients with metachronous pancreatic adenocarcinoma liver metastasis, Sperti et al. also noted an abysmal survival of only 4–6 months from the time liver metastasis was diagnosed [7].

8.3 Diagnosis

Liver protocol (3-phase) computed tomography (CT) is probably the most common imaging modality used to evaluate patients with pancreatic adenocarcinoma. Accurate definition of the number and distribution of pancreatic adenocarcinoma liver metastasis is obviously critical to help determine the therapeutic plan. On an unenhanced CT scan, pancreatic adenocarcinoma liver metastasis usually appears as a hypoattenuating lesion compared with the surrounding hepatic parenchyma. In general, the metastases are often more clearly seen on the venous phase of the CT scan. Other features of pancreatic liver metastasis can vary depending on the size and vascularity of the metastasis as well as the characteristics of the adjacent non-tumorous liver. In addition, the imaging characteristics of the metastasis may change in response to treatment, highlighting the importance of comparing pre- and posttreatment images.

MRI is another commonly used technique that can be particularly helpful in characterizing liver lesions. A liver protocol MRI may be an even more effective approach than CT scan in the evaluation of patients with possible pancreatic adenocarcinoma liver metastasis and in the assessment of the candidacy for surgery [8, 9]. Motosuqi et al. reported on 15 patients with pancreatic ductal adenocarcinoma who had 62 liver metastases [10]. Three radiologists who were blinded to the final diagnosis interpreted all MR (precontrast T1- and T2-weighted and contrast-enhanced dynamic and hepatocyte phase MR images) and tetraphasic dynamic contrast-enhanced CT images and assessed the presence or absence of liver metastasis on patient-by-patient and lesion-by-lesion basis. MRI had greater sensitivity in detecting liver metastases versus multi-detector row CT (MDCT) on the lesion-by-lesion analysis (92–94 % vs. 74–76 %, $p=0.03$–0.04) [10]. In a separate study, Holzapfel et al. compared the performance of diffusion-weighted MRI (DWI) with MDCT in the detection of pancreatic adenocarcinoma liver metastasis among 31 patients with newly diagnosed pancreatic cancer. The sensitivity and specificity in detecting liver metastases were 86.7 and 97.5 % for DWI versus 53.3 and 77.8 % for MDCT, respectively. Of note, DWI would have changed the therapeutic management in 4 out of 31 patients (12.9 %) [11].

Contrast agents such as Gd-DTPA may improve the detection of liver lesions [9]. Gd-DTPA can be injected as a bolus and is taken up selectively by functioning hepatocytes 20 min after injection. Thus, liver metastases are spared from contrast and are characterized by a hypointense signal relative the surrounding bright liver [8]. On contrast-enhanced dynamic MRI, pancreatic adenocarcinoma liver metastases usually have low signal intensity on T1-weighted images and are hyperintense on T2-weighted images. Unlike benign lesions that tend to have well-defined borders, the shape and borders of liver metastases may be less well circumscribed. Liver metastases may enhance irregularly, predominantly in the periphery of the lesion with the central portion not demonstrating as much contrast enhancement due to inherent necrosis. In most metastatic lesions, the peripheral rim typically washes out and appears hypointense on delayed images. Together, these characteristic enhancement patterns can help differentiate pancreatic adenocarcinoma liver metastasis from other benign liver lesions.

PET may also play an important role in the diagnosis and staging of pancreatic cancer (Fig. 8.1) [12]. The value of PET in detecting pancreatic adenocarcinoma liver metastasis is not well defined, however [13]. A recent meta-analysis by Wang et al. noted that the pooled sensitivity of PET in diagnosing pancreatic adenocarcinoma liver metastasis (7 studies, 316 patients) was 67 % (95 % CI: 52–79 %), and the corresponding specificity was 96 % (95 % CI: 89–98 %). Subgroup analysis showed that PET/CT was more sensitive than PEt alone in evaluating pancreatic adenocarcinoma liver metastasis [82 % (95 % CI: 48–98 %) and 67 % (95 % CI: 52–79 %), respectively [14]. As such, PET/CT may be a valuable tool to identify new metastases and help differentiate malignant from benign lesions in some patients with pancreatic adenocarcinoma.

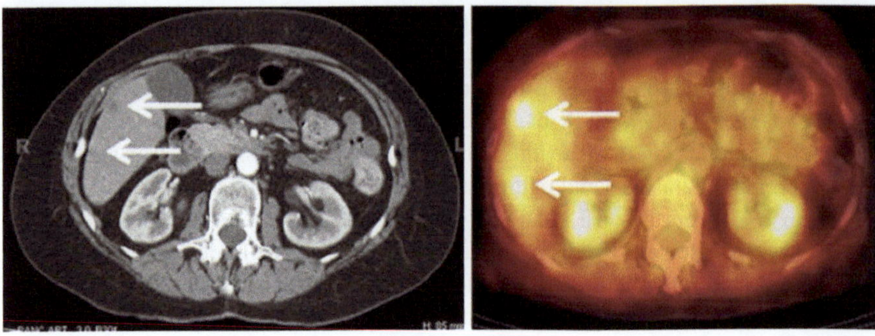

Fig. 8.1 PET/CT confirmation of CT findings. CT and PET/CT scan in a 59-year-old female with an adenocarcinoma in the head of the pancreas with suspicious hypodensities in the right lobe of the liver. PET/CT demonstrated these lesions to be hypermetabolic. *Arrows* point to liver metastases (Reproduced with permission from Farma et al. [52])

8.4 Treatment

8.4.1 Resection of Liver Metastases

Synchronous liver metastasis from pancreatic cancer, regardless of the number or size, has long been considered a marker of systemic disease and poor tumor biology. In turn, synchronous liver metastasis is generally considered a strong absolute contraindication to resection of the pancreatic primary tumor. In a number of small series, patients who underwent an aggressive simultaneous resection of both the primary pancreatic tumor and the metastatic hepatic lesions were noted to do poorly with very limited survival. Takada et al. reported on 11 patients with pancreatic adenocarcinoma who had synchronous liver metastasis and underwent concomitant pancreaticoduodenectomy and partial liver resection [15]. The authors noted no difference in the overall survival of patients who underwent palliative bypass alone versus patients who underwent resection of both the primary and metastatic pancreatic cancer (6 vs. 4 months, respectively). In fact, all patients who underwent pancreaticoduodenectomy with resection of synchronous liver metastasis died from multiple recurrent liver metastases within 1 year [15]. In a separate study, Gleisner and colleagues reported on a small group of patients with synchronous liver metastasis who underwent surgical resection [16]. In this series, the extent of hepatic disease in the liver was minimal (median tumor size 0.6 cm, 91 % patients with 1 liver metastasis), yet simultaneous resection of the pancreas primary adenocarcinoma and the liver metastasis yield a median survival of only 5.9 month, which was no different than the control group who underwent palliative bypass only (Fig. 8.2). In fact, simultaneous resection of the pancreas primary and the liver metastasis resulted in increased morbidity, length of stay, and mortality [16]. In a follow-up study from the group, de Jong et al. reported similar morbidity and mortality between simultaneous and stage hepatic resections for liver metastasis from periampullary malignancies [17]. In another study by Shrikhande et al. of 11 patients who

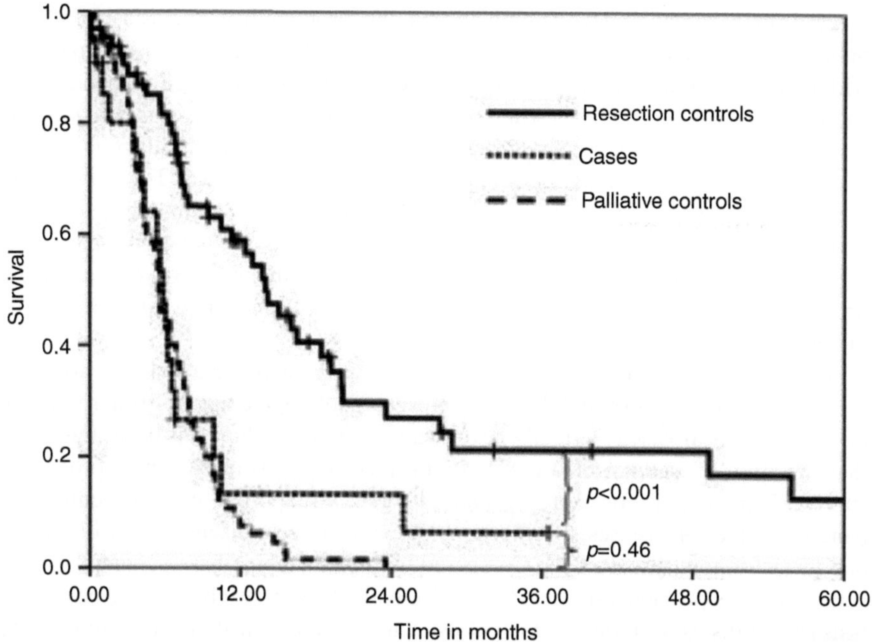

Fig. 8.2 Results of matched survival analysis. Patients ($n = 22$) who underwent simultaneous resection for primary adenocarcinoma and for liver metastasis had a similar overall survival (median, 5.9 months) compared with patients ($n = 66$) who underwent palliative bypass alone (5.6 months; $p = 0.46$), but they had a significantly shorter survival compared with patients who had no liver metastasis and, thus, underwent resection of the primary tumor alone (median, 14.1 months; $p < 0.001$) (Reproduced with permission from Gleisner et al. [16])

underwent combined pancreatic and liver resection for metastatic pancreatic cancer, the authors reported a median survival of 11.4 months [18]. Klein et al. reported on 22 patients with pancreatic adenocarcinoma metastatic to the liver who underwent simultaneous liver resection and pancreatectomy. In this small cohort of patients, the postoperative morbidity and mortality were no higher among patients who underwent pancreatectomy alone; however, the overall survival among patients who underwent resection in the setting of synchronous liver metastasis was very poor [19]. In contrast, Yamada et al. reported somewhat better results among six patients who underwent simultaneously resection of pancreatic cancer and liver metastasis [20]. Specifically, the authors noted an overall 1-, 3-, and 5-year survival after combined hepatectomy and pancreatic resection of 66.7, 33.3, and 16.7 %. In fact, one patient with liver metastasis was alive at 65.4 months following surgery; however, it is important to note that this patient had metastasis from a pancreatic cystadenocarcinoma, which may have a different biologic behavior compared with pancreatic ductal adenocarcinoma [20].

In aggregate, resection of synchronous liver metastasis from pancreatic adenocarcinoma should be avoided. While the level of data is poor, being based on small retrospective cohort studies, findings are generally consistent. Patients offered surgery for pancreatic adenocarcinoma and synchronous liver metastasis do very poorly. Overall survival is short and recurrence is nearly universal. As such, patients with pancreas adenocarcinoma who have liver metastasis diagnosed preoperatively should not be offered surgery. When unsuspected synchronous liver metastases are discovered at the time of surgery, resection of the primary tumor with concomitant resection of the liver lesions should also be strongly discouraged. The data would suggest that even when the burden of disease in the liver is small that these patients derive little benefit from surgery [18]. Rather patients should undergo a palliative procedure if warranted and then be referred for chemotherapy. Avoiding a bypass procedure (unless indicated) may decrease recovery time and allow earlier initiation of chemotherapy.

The possible role of resection for metachronous pancreatic adenocarcinoma to the liver is more controversial. Whereas most surgeons agree that up-front resection of synchronous disease is virtually never warranted, some clinicians have suggested that resection of well-selected patients with metachronous disease may provide a survival benefit [21]. For example, Dünschede et al. reported on 23 patients with pancreatic liver metastases, 14 of whom had synchronous disease and 9 of whom had metachronous disease [21]. Compared with gemcitabine-based chemotherapy, surgery did not provide a survival benefit for patients with synchronous liver metastasis (8 months vs. 11 months). In contrast, among patients with metachronous liver metastases, surgical resection was associated with a median survival of 31 months compared with only 11 months for those patients treated with chemotherapy alone. Klempnauer et al. have shown a median survival of 8.3 months after curative resection of synchronous PCLM ($n=16$) and 5.8 months after resection of metachronous PCLM ($n=7$) (Fig. 8.3; Table 8.1) [22]. In a separate study, Adam et al. reported on liver resection for metachronous liver metastases among 40 patients with primary pancreatic exocrine cancer [23]. In this subset of 40 patients with metachronous pancreatic adenocarcinoma liver metastasis, the estimated 5-year survival following liver resection was 20 % – better than anticipated for patients with stage IV disease. Patients with metastases from pancreatic adenocarcinoma who underwent hepatic resection had, however, a lower survival than those with metastases from ampullary primary tumors [23]. In a separate study, Gleisner and colleagues reported a small group of patients with periampullary cancer with synchronous liver metastasis who underwent surgical resection [16]. Patients with nonpancreatic primary cancer (duodenal or ampullary) had longer median survival compared with those who underwent resection of pancreatic cancer liver metastasis [16]. This was confirmed by study from de Jong et al. who showed median survival following resection of liver metastases from intestinal-type tumors ($n=15$) was 23 months compared with 13 months for patients with pancreaticobiliary tumors ($n=25$) ($p=0.05$) [17]. In a systematic review of data from 103 patients with liver metastases from pancreatic adenocarcinoma, Michalski and colleagues reported that resection of metachronous lesions was safe and associated with a median survival of 5.8–11.4 months [24].

While patient selection clearly plays a very important part in explaining the survival benefit associated with surgery, these data suggest that liver resection may be warranted in a select subset of patients with metachronous disease. Selection of

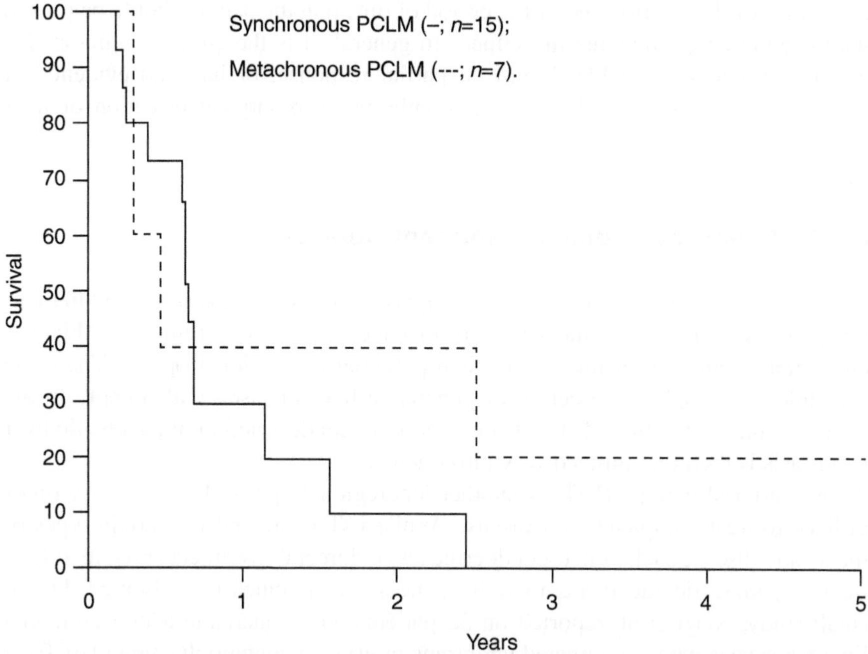

Fig. 8.3 Survival after synchronous resection of the pancreatic primary tumor and the liver metastasis (—; $n=15$) and after metachronous resection of liver metastases of pancreatic cancer (– – – –; $n=7$) (Reproduced with permission from Klempnauer et al. [27])

Table 8.1 Summary of studies on resection of PCLM

Author (year)	# patients with pancreatic cancer liver metastasis	Median survival	1- and 5-year actuarial survival
Klempnauer et al. (1996) [22]	15 synchronous	8.3 months	41 and 0 %
Takada et al. (1997) [15]	11 synchronous	4 months	0 and 0 %
Yamada et al. (2006) [20]	6 synchronous	n/a	67 and 17 %
Gleisner et al. (2007) [16]	17 synchronous	5.9 months	13 and 0 %
Shrikhande et al. (2007) [18]	11 synchronous	11.4 months	42 and 0 %
Klein et al. (2012) [19]	22 synchronous	7.6 months	30 and 0 %
Dünschede et al. (2010) [21]	9 metachronous	31 months	n/a
Adam et al. (2006) [23]	40 metachronous	20 months	n/a and 25 %

patients for resection of metachronous liver metastasis from pancreatic cancer needs to be very stringent. In addition, candidates for surgery should have a good performance status, adequate future liver remnant, and have disease that is amenable to a complete R0 resection. Typically, only patients who have been treated and who have responded to systemic chemotherapy and those patients with a long disease-free interval should even be considered for possible surgical resection [25]. The duration of the disease-free period and/or the period of time that the patient should be treated with chemotherapy remains ill defined. In general, it is the authors' opinion that patients should have stable disease, a partial response, or have no evidence of progressive disease for at least 6–12 months prior to surgical resection of liver metastases.

8.4.2 Other Locoregional Treatment Options

In addition to surgery, other locoregional options are sometimes considered in treating patients with hepatic metastasis from pancreatic adenocarcinoma. Ablation, either radiofrequency or microwave, is a potential locoregional option. The same principles that apply to resection of pancreatic liver metastasis also apply to the local thermal destruction of such liver disease. Local destruction of pancreatic liver metastasis is therefore utilized very infrequently.

Intra-arterial therapy (IAT) is another locoregional approach that is sometimes utilized to treat malignant liver disease. While IAT is utilized for certain types of metastatic disease such as neuroendocrine and colorectal liver metastasis, its role in treating pancreatic adenocarcinoma liver metastasis is much more limited. In one small study, Azizi et al. reported on 32 patients with pancreatic adenocarcinoma liver metastasis who were treated with trans-arterial chemoembolization (TACE) at 4–8-week intervals [26]. Following TACE, 71.9 and 9.4 % of patients had either stable disease or a partial response, whereas 18.8 % of patients had progressive disease. The 1-, 3-, and 5-year survival from the time of the first TACE was 60, 25, and 11 %, respectively. Furthermore, survival was better among patients with oligonodular disease (<5 lesions) versus multinodular disease (≥5 lesions) (1-year survival: oligonodular, 84 % vs. multinodular, 50 %) [26]. As such, the authors postulated that TACE might control liver metastases from pancreatic cancer in a certain subset of patients. In a separate study, Tajima et al. investigated hepatic arterial infusion chemotherapy with gemcitabine (GEM) plus 5-fluorouracil or oral S-1 in seven patients with metachronous liver metastases from pancreatic cancer. Three of the seven cases showed a partial response, and stable disease was achieved in another three of the seven cases (response rate, 85.7 %). While no life-threatening toxicities arose, six patients (85.7 %) developed catheter-related complications [27].

In addition to the biologic and oncologic issues that make thermal ablation and IAT of generally not applicable for pancreatic hepatic metastasis, the risk of infectious complications can also make this therapeutic approach undesirable. Specifically, following pancreaticoduodenectomy and the creation of a bilioenteric anastomosis, the biliary tree can become colonized with enteric flora. In turn, liver abscess can be much more common after any liver-directed intervention in the presence of a biliary-enteric anastomosis. Elias et al. reported on percutaneous liver RFA among 11 patients with an enterobiliary anastomosis or biliary stenting [28]. The incidence of liver abscess rate was about 40–50 % after RFA [28]. In another study, De Jong and colleagues reviewed liver-directed therapy in 126 patients with pancreatic liver metastases including 42 patients with pancreatic adenocarcinoma hepatic metastases [29]. Following liver-directed therapy (RFA or IAT), the overall morbidity rate was 34 %, and most complications were major (Clavien grade >3) requiring an invasive intervention [29].

Another locoregional option involves the use of radiation therapy. Traditionally, the liver had been considered to be very radiosensitive, and therefore radiation therapy was utilized somewhat sparingly. More recently, however, radiation therapy has been increasingly used to treat liver tumors. Wiley et al. reported on the results of a prospective study of 17 patients with pancreatic ductal adenocarcinoma liver metastasis who underwent a 2-week hepatic artery infusion of 5-fluorouracil and irradiation of the liver with 20 Gy. The authors noted that the combination of 5-fluorouracil infusion and hepatic irradiation may suppress subclinical (microscopic) liver metastases without significant hepatic toxicity [30]. The efficacy of prophylactic low-dose whole irradiation to the liver was, however, marginal. In a separate study, De Jong et al. reported on the use of adjuvant "prophylactic" whole-liver irradiation (5-fluorouracil plus 30 Gy external beam) in 28 patients with primary pancreatic adenocarcinoma with no clinical evidence of liver metastasis. The treatment was well tolerated, and only one patient developed radiation hepatitis and a liver abscess [29]. Low-dose whole-liver radiotherapy can benefit patients with symptomatic liver metastases with few side effects [31]. Bydder et al. treated 28 patients who had symptomatic liver metastases with liver irradiation consisting of 10 Gy in two fractions over 2 days. Individual symptom response rates were 53–66 % at 2 weeks. Partial or complete global symptomatic improvement was noted in 15 patients (54 %) overall. The treatment was well tolerated with two patients (7 %) experiencing grade 3 toxicity (one vomiting and one diarrhea).

More recently, the use of conformal/stereotactic radiation therapy to ablate liver metastases has emerged with the development of 3D imaging. Conformal radiation therapy uses a multi-leaf collimator (3–4 Fields) to deliver higher doses of radiation to the targeted tumor area. With better imaging guidance, many modulated fields (5–100 s fields) can be precisely focused on the tumor using stereotactic body radiation therapy (SBRT). Goodman et al. reported their experience using SBRT in 19 patients with liver metastases from 2004 to 2008. There were three patients with pancreatic cancer liver metastasis. The prescribed radiation dose was escalated from 18 to 30 Gy at 4-Gy increments with a planned maximum dose of 30 Gy. All patients tolerated the single-fraction SBRT well without developing dose-limiting toxicity. After a median of 17 months follow-up (range, 2–55 months), the cumulative risk of local failure at 12 months was 23 %. Median survival was 28.6 months, and the 2-year actuarial overall survival was 50.4 % [32]. Ideal candidates for SBRT should have good performance status (ECOG 0–1), adequate liver function, no extrahepatic disease, and uninvolved liver volume of 700 ml or greater [33]. There is no current phase III trial showing survival benefit of SBRT for patients with liver metastasis. However, an international survey of radiation therapy (RT) of liver metastases done by the Liver Cancer Workgroup of the Third International Consensus on Metastases Workshop at the 2010 American Society for Radiation Oncology (ASTRO) meeting showed a 36 % increase in the average annual number of referrals for liver radiation therapy (RT) over the past 5 years. The majority of experience in liver metastases is with SBRT for focal metastases rather than low-dose palliative whole-liver RT for symptom control [34].

8.4.3 Systemic Chemotherapy Options

The overwhelming majority of patients with pancreatic adenocarcinoma liver metastases will not be candidates for surgery. Liver metastasis almost universally signifies additional systemic disease, and, as noted, the results with surgery are largely poor. As such, systemic chemotherapy constitutes the backbone of therapy for patients with liver metastasis and pancreatic adenocarcinoma. Gemcitabine (Gemzar™; 2′,2′-difluorodeoxycytidine) is a pyrimidine antimetabolite and a specific analogue of deoxycytidine. Since 1997, gemcitabine monotherapy has been the standard first-line treatment for patients with metastatic pancreatic ductal adenocarcinoma [35]. While there have been numerous attempts to identify a suitable companion drug for gemcitabine as doublet therapy, many phase 3 trials had failed to establish the superiority of any doublet regimen over monotherapy with gemcitabine alone. Recently, the MPACT (Metastatic Pancreatic Adenocarcinoma Clinical Trial) trial demonstrated in a randomized phase 3 trial that gemcitabine combined with nab-paclitaxel led to an improvement in survival among patients with metastatic pancreatic ductal adenocarcinoma, including patients with liver metastases. Specifically, for patient with pancreatic adenocarcinoma liver metastasis, overall survival and progression-free survival was better in the gemcitabine plus nab-paclitaxel group versus the gemcitabine-only group (Hazard ratio for death 0.69, 95 % CI 0.59–0.81; hazard ratio for progression 0.65, 95 % CI 0.54–0.78) [36]. Gemcitabine plus nab-paclitaxel is now the standard of care for this patient group.

The combination of 5-fluorouracil, irinotecan, and oxaliplatin (FOLFIRINOX) has also recently been demonstrated in a randomized clinical trial to produce an overall survival benefit among patients with advanced pancreatic adenocarcinoma [37]. In the PRODIGE study, patients with metastatic pancreatic ductal adenocarcinoma were randomized to receive FOLFIRINOX or gemcitabine monotherapy (Table 8.2). The median overall survival was 11.1 months in the FOLFIRINOX group compared with 6.8 months in the gemcitabine group (HR for death, 0.57;

Table 8.2 Summary of trials of chemotherapy in patients with pancreatic cancer liver metastasis

Trial name	Chemotherapy drugs investigated	# patients with pancreatic liver metastasis in each arm	Median overall survival	*p* value
MPACT	Gem ± nab-paclitaxel	309 vs. 290	8.5 vs. 6.7 months	<0.001
PRODIGE	Gem vs. FOLFIRINOX	130 vs. 113	6.8 vs. 11.1 months	<0.001
Van Cutsem et al. [51]	Gem ± tipifarnib	60 vs. 63	193 vs. 182 days	0.75

MPACT metastatic pancreatic adenocarcinoma clinical trial, *PRODIGE* Partenariat de Recherche en Oncologie Digestive, *FOLFIRINOX* oxaliplatin, irinotecan, leucovorin, and fluorouracil, *tipifarnib* farnesyltransferase inhibitor 15084616

95 % CI 0.45–0.73; $p<0.001$). Of note, the majority of patients (62 %) had distal pancreatic lesions, while a smaller subset had pancreatic ductal adenocarcinoma in the head of the pancreas. In addition, most patients had advanced disease with 71 % having liver metastasis. The median survival for patients with pancreatic cancer liver metastasis treated with FOLFIRINOX was significantly better compared survival among patients treated with gemcitabine (HR for death, 0.61; 95 % CI 0.48–0.79; $p<0.001$). Grade 3 or 4 toxicity was, however, higher in the FOLFIRINOX. Specifically, more patients developed neutropenia, diarrhea, sensory neuropathy, and elevated level of alanine aminotransferase in the FOLFIRINOX group. As such, FOLFIRINOX is typically only offered to younger patients (<75 years) and those with good ECOG performance status (<2). Of interest, while toxicity was higher in the FOLFIRINOX group, there was an improvement in global health status and emotional functioning among patients treated with FOLFIRINOX compared with patients treated with gemcitabine. Specifically, patients experienced a decrease in pain, insomnia, anorexia, and constipation when treated with FOLFIRINOX [37]. In light of these data, FOLFIRINOX should be considered as a first-line treatment option for patients with metastatic pancreatic ductal adenocarcinoma to the liver.

In addition to cytotoxic chemotherapy, there are emerging data on targeted therapy for patients with advanced pancreatic adenocarcinoma. Human epidermal growth factor receptor (EGFR) is overexpressed in many pancreatic tumors and is associated with liver metastasis and disease progression [38]. Blocking EGFR tyrosine kinase signaling has been shown to decrease the growth and metastasis of human pancreatic tumor xenografts [39]. Erlotinib is an oral tyrosine kinase inhibitor targeting EGFR and is currently approved for patients with non-small cell lung cancer. Moore et al. conducted a phase 3 randomized controlled trial investigating the effect of erlotinib in combination with gemcitabine on survival in patients with advanced pancreatic cancer. Five hundred sixty-nine patients were randomly assigned to receive gemcitabine either with or without erlotinib. Patients treated with the combination of gemcitabine and erlotinib had an improved overall survival with a decreased hazard of death ($HR=0.82$, $p=0.038$). Risk of progression was also lower among patients treated with erlotinib and gemcitabine ($HR=0.77$, $p=0.004$) [40]. Although the VEGF-targeting agent bevacizumab initially showed promise in a phase 2 trial in patients with advanced pancreatic ductal adenocarcinoma [41], the addition of bevacizumab to gemcitabine-erlotinib [42] or gemcitabine [43] has not led to a significant improvement in overall survival. The hedgehog signaling pathway also plays a role in pancreatic cancer metastasis and resistance to chemotherapy. In preclinical studies, blocking hedgehog signaling not only inhibited pancreatic cancer metastases but also enhanced the delivery of gemcitabine to pancreatic cancer cells [44, 45]. Several oral hedgehog pathway inhibitors are being tested in advanced and metastatic pancreatic adenocarcinoma in early phase clinical trials, but initial results have not been promising [46].

8.5 Palliative Care

Palliation plays an important role in the care of patients with pancreatic adenocarcinoma metastatic to the liver. Palliative care should include social, psychological, as well as physical considerations. Many patients with advanced pancreatic cancer may experience pain, and adequate control of symptoms is critical. Pain control may necessitate a celiac plexus block and/or pain medications administered through other routes (e.g., oral, transdermal, etc.). Patients with pancreatic adenocarcinoma and synchronous liver metastasis can sometimes present with impending biliary or gastric obstruction. In general, nonoperative options such as endoscopic biliary and duodenal stents are preferable compared with surgical options. Self-expanding metal stents have been shown to be a safe and durable option. Specifically, the median patency time of self-expanding metal stents is longer than that of plastic stents (3.6 vs. 1.8 months, respectively, $p=0.02$) [47, 48]. For patients who are discovered to have the incidental findings of synchronous pancreatic adenocarcinoma liver metastasis during laparotomy, the approach should be tailored to the individual situation. For patients who have biliary obstruction that has not been addressed by endoscopic or percutaneous biliary stents, surgical choledochojejunostomy or hepaticojejunostomy can provide durable palliation [49]. Similarly, for patients with gastric outlet obstruction, a palliative gastrojejunostomy can provide relief. "Prophylactic" biliary and gastric decompression may be reasonable in patients with locally advanced pancreatic adenocarcinoma in the absence of liver metastasis [50]. In contrast, the performance of surgical palliative procedures is probably unwarranted in patients who have liver metastasis and who are otherwise asymptomatic or already adequately decompressed via stenting.

Conclusion

Patients with pancreatic adenocarcinoma metastatic to the liver have a poor prognosis. Liver metastasis almost universally denotes incurable systemic disease. As such, surgical resection and other locoregional therapies to treat pancreatic adenocarcinoma liver metastasis are generally not indicated. Patients with synchronous disease have a particularly grim prognosis, and therefore surgical resection should not be considered – whether found preoperatively or incidentally at the time of surgery. While patients with metachronous liver metastasis have a similarly poor long-term survival, surgical resection or locoregional therapy may be considered in very highly selected situations after thorough multidisciplinary review. In general, resection should only be considered in patients with limited disease, a long disease-free period, and in those patients who have not progressed following preoperative systemic chemotherapy. Ultimately, systemic chemotherapy is the standard of care for patients with pancreatic adenocarcinoma liver metastasis. Similar to the advances made in treating metastatic colorectal cancer to the liver, advances in systemic chemotherapy for pancreatic adenocarcinoma will be critical to expanding the indication for liver-directed therapies and surgical resection, as well as prolonging the life of patients with this disease.

References

1. Malvezzi M, Bertuccio P, Levi F, La Vecchia C, Negri E (2013) European cancer mortality predictions for the year 2013. Ann Oncol 24(3):792–800
2. Ito K, Govindarajan A, Ito H, Fong Y (2010) Surgical treatment of hepatic colorectal metastasis: evolving role in the setting of improving systemic therapies and ablative treatments in the 21st century. Cancer J 16(2):103–110
3. Mayo SC, Herman JM, Cosgrove D, Bhagat N, Kamel I, Geschwind JF et al (2013) Emerging approaches in the management of patients with neuroendocrine liver metastasis: role of liver-directed and systemic therapies. J Am Coll Surg 216(1):123–134
4. Iacobuzio-Donahue CA, Fu B, Yachida S, Luo M, Abe H, Henderson CM et al (2009) DPC4 gene status of the primary carcinoma correlates with patterns of failure in patients with pancreatic cancer. J Clin Oncol 27(11):1806–1813
5. Lavu H, Mascaro AA, Grenda DR, Sauter PK, Leiby BE, Croker SP et al (2009) Margin positive pancreaticoduodenectomy is superior to palliative bypass in locally advanced pancreatic ductal adenocarcinoma. J Gastrointest Surg 13(11):1937–1946; discussion 46–7
6. Kneuertz PJ, Cunningham SC, Cameron JL, Torrez S, Tapazoglou N, Herman JM et al (2011) Palliative surgical management of patients with unresectable pancreatic adenocarcinoma: trends and lessons learned from a large, single institution experience. J Gastrointest Surg 15(11):1917–1927
7. Sperti C, Pasquali C, Piccoli A, Pedrazzoli S (1997) Recurrence after resection for ductal adenocarcinoma of the pancreas. World J Surg 21(2):195–200
8. Zech CJ, Herrmann KA, Reiser MF, Schoenberg SO (2007) MR imaging in patients with suspected liver metastases: value of liver-specific contrast agent Gd-EOB-DTPA. Magn Reson Med Sci 6(1):43–52
9. Imam K, Bluemke DA (2000) MR imaging in the evaluation of hepatic metastases. Magn Reson Imaging Clin N Am 8(4):741–756
10. Motosugi U, Ichikawa T, Morisaka H, Sou H, Muhi A, Kimura K et al (2011) Detection of pancreatic carcinoma and liver metastases with gadoxetic acid-enhanced MR imaging: comparison with contrast-enhanced multi-detector row CT. Radiology 260(2):446–453
11. Holzapfel K, Reiser-Erkan C, Fingerle AA, Erkan M, Eiber MJ, Rummeny EJ et al (2011) Comparison of diffusion-weighted MR imaging and multidetector-row CT in the detection of liver metastases in patients operated for pancreatic cancer. Abdom Imaging 36(2):179–184
12. Grassetto G, Rubello D (2011) Role of FDG-PET/CT in diagnosis, staging, response to treatment, and prognosis of pancreatic cancer. Am J Clin Oncol 34(2):111–114
13. Mansour JC, Schwartz L, Pandit-Taskar N, D'Angelica M, Fong Y, Larson SM et al (2006) The utility of F-18 fluorodeoxyglucose whole body PET imaging for determining malignancy in cystic lesions of the pancreas. J Gastrointest Surg 10(10):1354–1360
14. Wang Z, Chen JQ, Liu JL, Qin XG, Huang Y (2013) FDG-PET in diagnosis, staging and prognosis of pancreatic carcinoma: a meta-analysis. World J Gastroenterol 19(29):4808–4817
15. Takada T, Yasuda H, Amano H, Yoshida M, Uchida T (1997) Simultaneous hepatic resection with pancreato-duodenectomy for metastatic pancreatic head carcinoma: does it improve survival? Hepatogastroenterology 44(14):567–573
16. Gleisner AL, Assumpcao L, Cameron JL, Wolfgang CL, Choti MA, Herman JM et al (2007) Is resection of periampullary or pancreatic adenocarcinoma with synchronous hepatic metastasis justified? Cancer 110(11):2484–2492
17. de Jong MC, Tsai S, Cameron JL, Wolfgang CL, Hirose K, van Vledder MG et al (2010) Safety and efficacy of curative intent surgery for peri-ampullary liver metastasis. J Surg Oncol 102(3):256–263
18. Shrikhande SV, Kleeff J, Reiser C, Weitz J, Hinz U, Esposito I et al (2007) Pancreatic resection for M1 pancreatic ductal adenocarcinoma. Ann Surg Oncol 14(1):118–127
19. Klein F, Puhl G, Guckelberger O, Pelzer U, Pullankavumkal JR, Guel S et al (2012) The impact of simultaneous liver resection for occult liver metastases of pancreatic adenocarcinoma. Gastroenterol Res Pract 2012:939350

20. Yamada H, Hirano S, Tanaka E, Shichinohe T, Kondo S (2006) Surgical treatment of liver metastases from pancreatic cancer. HPB (Oxford) 8(2):85–88
21. Dunschede F, Will L, von Langsdorf C, Mohler M, Galle PR, Otto G et al (2010) Treatment of metachronous and simultaneous liver metastases of pancreatic cancer. Eur Surg Res Europaische Chir Forsch Rech Chir Europeennes 44(3–4):209–213
22. Klempnauer J, Ridder GJ, Piso P, Pichlmayr R (1996) Is liver resection in metastases of exocrine pancreatic carcinoma justified? Der Chirurg Zeitschrift Alle Gebiete Operativen Medizen 67(4):366–370
23. Adam R, Chiche L, Aloia T, Elias D, Salmon R, Rivoire M et al (2006) Hepatic resection for noncolorectal nonendocrine liver metastases: analysis of 1,452 patients and development of a prognostic model. Ann Surg 244(4):524–535
24. Michalski CW, Erkan M, Huser N, Muller MW, Hartel M, Friess H et al (2008) Resection of primary pancreatic cancer and liver metastasis: a systematic review. Dig Surg 25(6):473–480
25. Fong Y (1999) Surgical therapy of hepatic colorectal metastasis. CA Cancer J Clin 49(4): 231–255
26. Azizi A, Naguib NN, Mbalisike E, Farshid P, Emami AH, Vogl TJ (2011) Liver metastases of pancreatic cancer: role of repetitive transarterial chemoembolization (TACE) on tumor response and survival. Pancreas 40(8):1271–1275
27. Tajima H, Ohta T, Kitagawa H, Sakai S, Makino I, Hayashi H et al (2011) Pilot study of hepatic arterial infusion chemotherapy with gemcitabine and 5-fluorouracil for patients with postoperative liver metastases from pancreatic cancer. Exp Ther Med 2(2):265–269
28. Elias D, Di Pietroantonio D, Gachot B, Menegon P, Hakime A, De Baere T (2006) Liver abscess after radiofrequency ablation of tumors in patients with a biliary tract procedure. Gastroenterol Clin Biol 30(6–7):823–827
29. De Jong MC, Farnell MB, Sclabas G, Cunningham SC, Cameron JL, Geschwind JF et al (2010) Liver-directed therapy for hepatic metastases in patients undergoing pancreaticoduodenectomy: a dual-center analysis. Ann Surg 252(1):142–148
30. Wiley AL Jr, Wirtanen GW, Mehta MP, Ramirez G, Shahabi S (1988) Treatment of probable subclinical liver metastases and gross pancreatic carcinoma with hepatic artery 5-fluorouracil infusion and radiation therapy. Acta Oncol 27(4):377–381
31. Bydder S, Spry NA, Christie DR, Roos D, Burmeister BH, Krawitz H et al (2003) A prospective trial of short-fractionation radiotherapy for the palliation of liver metastases. Australas Radiol 47(3):284–288
32. Goodman KA, Wiegner EA, Maturen KE, Zhang Z, Mo Q, Yang G et al (2010) Dose-escalation study of single-fraction stereotactic body radiotherapy for liver malignancies. Int J Radiat Oncol Biol Phys 78(2):486–493
33. Hoyer M, Swaminath A, Bydder S, Lock M, Mendez Romero A, Kavanagh B et al (2012) Radiotherapy for liver metastases: a review of evidence. Int J Radiat Oncol Biol Phys 82(3):1047–1057
34. Lock MI, Hoyer M, Bydder SA, Okunieff P, Hahn CA, Vichare A et al (2012) An international survey on liver metastases radiotherapy. Acta Oncol 51(5):568–574
35. Burris HA 3rd, Moore MJ, Andersen J, Green MR, Rothenberg ML, Modiano MR et al (1997) Improvements in survival and clinical benefit with gemcitabine as first-line therapy for patients with advanced pancreas cancer: a randomized trial. J Clin Oncol 15(6):2403–2413
36. Von Hoff DD, Ervin T, Arena FP, Chiorean EG, Infante J, Moore M et al (2013) Increased survival in pancreatic cancer with nab-paclitaxel plus gemcitabine. N Engl J Med 369(18): 1691–1703
37. Gourgou-Bourgade S, Bascoul-Mollevi C, Desseigne F, Ychou M, Bouche O, Guimbaud R et al (2013) Impact of FOLFIRINOX compared with gemcitabine on quality of life in patients with metastatic pancreatic cancer: results from the PRODIGE 4/ACCORD 11 randomized trial. J Clin Oncol 31(1):23–29
38. Tobita K, Kijima H, Dowaki S, Kashiwagi H, Ohtani Y, Oida Y et al (2003) Epidermal growth factor receptor expression in human pancreatic cancer: significance for liver metastasis. Int J Mol Med 11(3):305–309

39. Bruns CJ, Solorzano CC, Harbison MT, Ozawa S, Tsan R, Fan D et al (2000) Blockade of the epidermal growth factor receptor signaling by a novel tyrosine kinase inhibitor leads to apoptosis of endothelial cells and therapy of human pancreatic carcinoma. Cancer Res 60(11):2926–2935
40. Moore MJ, Goldstein D, Hamm J, Figer A, Hecht JR, Gallinger S et al (2007) Erlotinib plus gemcitabine compared with gemcitabine alone in patients with advanced pancreatic cancer: a phase III trial of the National Cancer Institute of Canada Clinical Trials Group. J Clin Oncol 25(15):1960–1966
41. Kindler HL, Friberg G, Singh DA, Locker G, Nattam S, Kozloff M et al (2005) Phase II trial of bevacizumab plus gemcitabine in patients with advanced pancreatic cancer. J Clin Oncol 23(31):8033–8040
42. Van Cutsem E, Vervenne WL, Bennouna J, Humblet Y, Gill S, Van Laethem JL et al (2009) Phase III trial of bevacizumab in combination with gemcitabine and erlotinib in patients with metastatic pancreatic cancer. J Clin Oncol 27(13):2231–2237
43. Kindler HL, Niedzwiecki D, Hollis D, Sutherland S, Schrag D, Hurwitz H et al (2010) Gemcitabine plus bevacizumab compared with gemcitabine plus placebo in patients with advanced pancreatic cancer: phase III trial of the Cancer and Leukemia Group B (CALGB 80303). J Clin Oncol 28(22):3617–3622
44. Feldmann G, Dhara S, Fendrich V, Bedja D, Beaty R, Mullendore M et al (2007) Blockade of hedgehog signaling inhibits pancreatic cancer invasion and metastases: a new paradigm for combination therapy in solid cancers. Cancer Res 67(5):2187–2196
45. Olive KP, Jacobetz MA, Davidson CJ, Gopinathan A, McIntyre D, Honess D et al (2009) Inhibition of Hedgehog signaling enhances delivery of chemotherapy in a mouse model of pancreatic cancer. Science 324(5933):1457–1461
46. Bisht S, Brossart P, Maitra A, Feldmann G (2010) Agents targeting the Hedgehog pathway for pancreatic cancer treatment. Curr Opin Investig Drugs 11(12):1387–1398
47. Moss AC, Morris E, Mac Mathuna P (2006) Palliative biliary stents for obstructing pancreatic carcinoma. Cochrane Database Syst Rev 2:CD004200
48. Maire F, Hammel P, Ponsot P, Aubert A, O'Toole D, Hentic O et al (2006) Long-term outcome of biliary and duodenal stents in palliative treatment of patients with unresectable adenocarcinoma of the head of pancreas. Am J Gastroenterol 101(4):735–742
49. Lillemoe KD, Cameron JL, Hardacre JM, Sohn TA, Sauter PK, Coleman J et al (1999) Is prophylactic gastrojejunostomy indicated for unresectable periampullary cancer? A prospective randomized trial. Ann Surg 230(3):322–328; discussion 8–30
50. Gurusamy KS, Kumar S, Davidson BR (2013) Prophylactic gastrojejunostomy for unresectable periampullary carcinoma. Cochrane Database Syst Rev 2:CD008533
51. Van Cutsem E, van de Velde H, Karasek P, Oettle H, Vervenne WL, Szawlowski A et al (2004) Phase III trial of gemcitabine plus tipifarnib compared with gemcitabine plus placebo in advanced pancreatic cancer. J Clin Oncol 22(8):1430–1438
52. Farma T et al (2008) PET/CT fusion scan enhances CT staging in patients with pancreatic neoplasms. Ann Surg Oncol 15(9):2465–2471

Liver Metastasis from Salivary Gland Tumors

9

Parul J. Shukla and Chetan Merchant

9.1 Introduction

Salivary gland cancer is rare with a worldwide incidence of 0.3–3 per 100,000 [1]. Over the last four decades, there has been an increase in the incidence of these tumors in the USA, from 6.3 % of all head and neck cancers in 1974–1976 to 8.1 % in 1998–1999 [2]. The majority of salivary gland tumors are benign in nature, and only 20 % turn out to be malignant. The malignant salivary gland tumors tend to have both local and distant metastases, with the liver being an infrequent organ for metastasis. In this chapter we intend to review the literature and discuss the management of hepatic metastasis from the malignant salivary gland tumors.

9.2 Epidemiology of Malignant Salivary Gland Tumors

Salivary gland tumors are classified into 24 types as per WHO classification [3]. They are further subdivided into low-, intermediate-, and high-grade variety based on the histopathological criteria and behavior, such as intracystic component, lymphovascular invasion, and bone invasion. The long-term survival and metastatic

P.J. Shukla, MD (✉)
Department of Surgery, Weill Cornell Medical College
and New York Presbyterian Hospital, New York, NY 10021, USA

Department of Surgical Gastroenterology,
Tata Memorial Hospital, Parel, Mumbai, India
e-mail: pjshukla@doctors.org.uk

C. Merchant, MD
Section of Colon and Rectal Surgery, Department of Surgery,
Weill Cornell Medical College and New York Presbyterian Hospital,
New York, NY 10021, USA

I. Di Carlo (ed.), *Noncolorectal, Nonneuroendocrine Liver Metastases: Diagnosis and Current Therapies*, DOI 10.1007/978-3-319-09293-5_9

potential depend heavily on the tumor grade. Higher-grade tumors are associated with frequent metastases. The 5-year survival is 80–95 % for low-grade tumors and 30–50 % for high-grade tumors [2].

As mentioned the majority of salivary gland tumors are benign, and pleomorphic adenoma, a mixed tumor, is the most common type of benign tumor. The incidence of malignant tumors depends upon the type of salivary gland with a higher incidence of malignancy in minor salivary glands. In the parotid gland 20–25 % of tumors are malignant, with this incidence increasing to 40 % in the submandibular salivary gland and reaching to 90 % in the minor salivary glands [2].

Mucoepidermoid carcinoma is the most frequent malignant tumor of the salivary glands (29 %). MEC is also reported to be the most common malignant tumor of the minor salivary glands (49.8 %). Adenoid cystic tumor accounts for 26.3 % of malignant tumors arising from the minor salivary gland. In fact MEC and ACC combined account for the majority of the malignant tumors arising from the major and minor salivary glands [1].

MEC is composed of three cell types: mucoid, squamoid, and undifferentiated. Classically MEC will have a variable composition of various cell types, but often one cell type dominates. MEC where the squamoid cell type dominates is the high-grade version and has the worst outcome, with a 5-year survival of only 30 % [1].

ACC is a highly aggressive tumor with indolent behavior. It is characterized in different subtypes based on the growth pattern: tubular, cribriform, and solid. The solid type of growth pattern is the high-grade ACC and has the worst outcome. ACC undergoes perineural invasion very early during its growth. It spreads extensively to the local lymph nodes and to the distant organs [4].

9.3 Distant Metastasis from Malignant Salivary Gland Tumors

Malignant salivary gland tumors are known for both locoregional and distant metastases [4]. The incidence of distant metastasis ranges from 24 to 61 % [5]. They metastasize through perineural invasion, lymphatic spread, and hematogenous dissemination. The lung is the most common site for distant spread (75–90 %), followed by the bone, CNS, liver, and other organs [5]. Both MEC and ACC are known to metastasize to distant organs. MEC metastasizes in 10–15 % of cases and ACC in 24–31 % of patients. Metastasis from ACC is particularly of interest because the metastasis can occur early during the development of the tumor and may present years after the primary tumor has been treated. Cases have been reported where distant metastasis has been detected 10 years after the initial diagnosis of the primary tumor [6]. On most occasions, distant lesions are associated with locoregional recurrence.

Distant metastases highly depend upon the type of tumor, T-stage, and the grade of the tumor. Large tumors with higher grade tend to metastasize more frequently. Positive margins and perineural invasion on histopathological examination of the resected specimen are positive predictors of distant metastases [7].

9.4 Metastasis to Liver

The liver is an infrequent site for distant metastasis from salivary gland tumors. Published data on salivary gland liver metastases includes individual case reports and few studies which report that these account for <1 % cases with liver metastases. ACC is the most common tumor to metastasize to the liver [8]. The tumor metastasizes to the liver hematogenously, and the lesions in the liver and their locations are consistent with the hematogenous spread to the liver from more common secondaries to the liver from colorectal and neuroendocrine tumors. Generally one tends to find multiple lesions, and there is no dominance toward any specific site or lobe of the liver.

Liver lesions are generally detected during metastatic work-up of a patient with locoregional recurrence. Rarely they may be the initial presentation of a malignant salivary tumor. The symptoms are similar to secondaries to the liver from any other tumor, and these symptoms are dictated by the size and site of these lesions. The derangements in liver functions also depend upon the size and location of the secondaries. The most common derangement to expect is mild elevation in the hepatic transaminases.

ACC may metastasize early during the course of the tumor development and present months or even years later, as secondary lesions in the liver.

9.5 Management of Liver Metastases

Early metastasis, indolent growth, and delayed presentation make liver secondaries from salivary gland tumors a diagnostic challenge. In view of these features, any surgeon treating these tumors should have a high degree of suspicion for liver metastasis in any patient treated previously for salivary gland tumors, especially for ACC, irrespective of the time lapse between the initial disease and presentation of metastatic disease.

Ultrasound (USG) is most frequently the first step in the evaluation of liver lesions, guiding fine-needle aspirations or core biopsies. However a more detailed evaluation warrants using either CT scan or MRI. Though MRI is the preferred modality for evaluation of locoregional disease, CT scan is relatively more efficient in evaluating liver lesions. CT scan when used for ACC may have a drop in specificity due to the lack of sufficient contrast absorption. All patients with recurrence from salivary gland tumors should receive some form of imaging of their chest, the more frequent site of metastasis [9]. Though there are no clear guidelines on the usage of whole-body FDG18-labeled PET CT scan in literature, a sensitivity of 74.4 % and a specificity of 100 %, with positive predictive value of 100 % and a negative predictive value of 61 %, have been reported [1, 10].

FNAC is most commonly used for determining the histology of the liver lesion. However when feasible a biopsy should be performed to accurately determine not only the type but also the grade of the tumor [1].

The management of distant metastases with salivary gland tumor is dependent upon the type and grade of the tumor and the performance status of the patient. Surgery, which is the preferred method of treatment for primary tumors, is not the first line of treatment for metastatic disease. However in selected cases with either a solitary liver lesion or well-compartmentalized liver lesion, hepatic resection is justified [6]. A tumor which is of a rare type should be treated as a part of a clinical trial [11]. It is felt that such tumors are best benefited by clinical trials because of their rarity and paucity of published data; hence, the formulation of established guidelines is not feasible. Tumors which have rapid growth and are of higher grade are treated with chemotherapy [1]. The chemotherapeutic agents commonly used for tumors other than ACC are cisplatin, paclitaxel, or gemcitabine. The response rate with these agents is 20–25 % [1]. For ACC, mitoxantrone, vinorelbine, or anthracycline as single agents or in combination with cisplatin have been advised from small published data [12]. Indolent tumors such as ACC can also be carefully observed without initiating any specific treatment regime. Radiotherapy or combined radiochemotherapy is generally used for management of the locoregional disease.

Recently newer targeted therapies have been used for management of salivary gland tumors. This includes the use of biological agents such as inhibitors of C-KIT, HER2, and EGFR or a combination of inhibitors against both HER2 and EGFR. The preliminary results with these therapies have not been very promising, and results from future studies should help in clarifying their role [1, 12].

9.6 Follow-Up and Outcome

Long-term follow-up is essential in patients with salivary gland tumors. Every patient should undergo a chest radiograph and an abdominal ultrasound as part of the evaluation, apart from the detailed clinical examination. New molecular markers like C-KIT, p53, EGRF, and others are still under evaluation.

The prognosis in patients with salivary gland tumors depends on the histological type, stage and grade of the tumor, site of origin, completeness of primary resection, and the presence or absence of distant metastasis. For some low-grade tumors 5-year survival may be as high as 75–100 %, but for tumors undergoing distant metastasis like ACC, the 5-, 10-, 15-, and 20-year survival is 69.1, 45.7, 26.5, and 14.3 % [13].

9.7 Conclusion

Liver metastasis from salivary gland tumors is rare and may present years after the initial tumor has been treated. ACC is the most common tumor to metastasize. Once detected the management depends upon the type of tumor, stage of the disease, and physical condition of the patient. Surgery may be used for lesions detected early during the course of the disease, and chemotherapy is generally used as a palliative option for advanced conditions. Overall survival may vary from 60 to 15 % and is generally poor for high-grade tumors like ACC.

References

1. Ettl T, Schwarz-Furlan S, Gosau M, Reichert TE (2012) Salivary gland carcinomas. Oral Maxillofac Surg 16(3):267–283
2. To VS, Chan JY, Tsang RK, Wei WI (2012) Review of salivary gland neoplasms. ISRN Otolaryngol 2012:872982
3. Seifert G, Sobin LH (1992) The World Health Organization's histological classification of salivary gland tumors. Cancer 70(2):379–385
4. Spiro RH (1997) Distant metastasis in adenoid cystic carcinoma of salivary origin. Am J Surg 174(5):495–498
5. Schwentner I, Obrist P, Thumfart W, Sprinzl G (2006) Distant metastasis of parotid gland tumors. Acta Otolaryngol 126(4):340–345
6. Qureshi SS, Nadkarni MS, Shrikhande SV, Desai S, Deodhar K, Ramadwar M et al (2005) Hepatic resection for metastasis from adenoid cystic carcinoma of parotid gland. Indian J Gastroenterol 24(1):29–30
7. Shingaki S, Kanemaru S, Oda Y, Niimi K, Mikami T, Funayama A et al (2014) Distant metastasis and survival of adenoid cystic carcinoma after definitive treatment. J Oral Maxillofac Surg Med Pathol. 26(3):312–316
8. Akhavan A, Binesh F, Navabii H (2013) Adenoid cystic carcinoma of hard palate with coincidental metastases to lung and liver. BMJ Case Rep. Feb 2014
9. Lee YY, Wong KT, King AD, Ahuja AT (2008) Imaging of salivary gland tumours. Eur J Radiol 66(3):419–436
10. Sharma P, Jain TK, Singh H, Suman SK, Faizi NA, Kumar R et al (2013) Utility of (18)F-FDG PET-CT in staging and restaging of patients with malignant salivary gland tumours: a single-institutional experience. Nucl Med Commun 34(3):211–219
11. Network NCC (2013) NCCN Guidelines, nccn.org
12. Papaspyrou G, Hoch S, Rinaldo A, Rodrigo JP, Takes RP, van Herpen C et al (2011) Chemotherapy and targeted therapy in adenoid cystic carcinoma of the head and neck: a review. Head Neck 33(6):905–911
13. Gao M, Hao Y, Huang MX, Ma DQ, Luo HY, Gao Y et al (2013) Clinicopathological study of distant metastases of salivary adenoid cystic carcinoma. Int J Oral Maxillofac Surg 42(8): 923–928

Hepatic Metastases from Sarcomas

10

Adriana Toro and Isidoro Di Carlo

10.1 Introduction

Soft-tissue sarcomas (STSs) are rare malignant tumors with an incidence of approximately 1 % of all malignancies [1]. Their treatment is complex, requiring a multidisciplinary approach that includes surgeons, radiologists, pathologists, and medical oncologists. Curative surgical resection with negative histological margins is the best treatment. However, distant metastases develop in up to 50 % of cases in which the resected margin shows cancerous cells [2]. Although the liver is one of the target organs for STS metastases, the spread from the primary STS to the hepatic parenchyma is not currently well understood as compared with retroperitoneal and primary visceral abdominal sarcomas, which are known to metastasize to the liver through the abdominal lymphatic system, by dissemination through the portal vein or through direct invasion [3].

Gastrointestinal organ sarcomas such as gastrointestinal stromal tumors (GISTs) and leiomyosarcomas (LMS) commonly metastasize to the liver, with a reported incidence of 55–72 % in patients who underwent a curative resection of the primary tumor [4–6]. GISTs occur most commonly in the stomach, small intestine, and rectum. LMSs are rare in the digestive tract, except in the esophagus and the muscularis mucosae of the colon and rectum [7].

After complete resection of liver metastases, the median overall survival range is between 30 and 57 months, the 5-year survival range is between 27 and 49 %, and

A. Toro, MD, PhD,
Department of Surgery, Taormina Hospital, Messina, Italy

I. Di Carlo, MD, PhD, FACS (✉)
Department of Surgical Sciences, Organ Transplantation,
and Advanced Technologies, University of Catania,
Cannizzaro Hospital, via Messina 826, Catania 95126, Italy
e-mail: idicarlo@unict.it

I. Di Carlo (ed.), *Noncolorectal, Nonneuroendocrine Liver Metastases: Diagnosis and Current Therapies*, DOI 10.1007/978-3-319-09293-5_10

Table 10.1 Principal types of STS

Tissue of origin	Type of sarcoma
Adipose tissue	Liposarcoma
Smooth muscle tissue	Leiomyosarcoma
Striated muscle tissue	Rhabdomyosarcoma
Vascular endothelium	Kaposi's sarcoma and hemangiosarcoma
Bone	Osteosarcoma
Cartilage	Chondrosarcoma
Connective tissue	Fibrosarcoma
Nerve	Malignant tumor of the nerve sheaths and Ewing's sarcoma
Interstitial cells of Cajal	Gastrointestinal stromal tumor

the median disease-free survival range is between 14 and 32 months [3]. The prognosis for patients with advanced and unresectable disease is poor, with a median survival between 8 and 13 months [2].

10.2 Epidemiology

STSs originate mostly from the embryonic mesoderm and are a heterogeneous group of rare malignant tumors that affect patients of all ages. The principal types of STS are presented in Table 10.1. GISTs are the most common STS. In 1995, the annual incidence of GIST was 2.1 per million inhabitants; in 2003, the annual incidence was 12.7 per million inhabitants. This increased incidence reflects improved understanding and better diagnosis of GISTs [8]. GISTs occur predominantly in the middle-aged or older population, with a peak incidence in the fifth and sixth decades of life. No significant sex difference exists, although some articles report a male predominance [9]. A rare association with neurofibromatosis type 1 was reported [10].

GISTs are morphologically characterized by epithelioid or mixed spindle cells and, in approximately 95 % of cases, by the immunophenotypic expression of both growth factor receptor c-Kit (CD117) and platelet-derived growth factor receptor-alpha (PDGFRA). The biological behavior of the tumor depends on its size, growth rate (expressed by the mitotic index), and mutations [11]. With the same size and mitotic index, gastric GISTs have lower clinical aggressiveness than small intestine GISTs [12]. The clinical aggressiveness is expressed predominantly in the form of peritoneal dissemination and liver metastasis [13].

GISTs are characterized molecularly by the presence of activating mutations of the *KIT* gene (75–80 % of cases) and, in a minority of cases (5–10 %), of the *PDGFRA* gene. Mutations predominantly involve exon 11 of the *KIT* gene. Exons 9, 13, 14, and 17 of the *KIT* gene and exons 12 and 18 of the *PDGFRA* gene are mutated with lower frequency [12]. Mutational analysis of the *KIT* and *PDGFRA* genes is a prognostic parameter (GISTs with mutation of exon 9 and 11 tend to have a more aggressive biological behavior) and a prediction of response to drugs that inhibit receptor tyrosine kinase activities [14].

The pathological diagnosis of GISTs should include the mitotic index, size, and anatomic site; all three of these factors contribute to the prognosis of the patient [15].

LMS is the second most common retroperitoneal tumor in adults after liposarcoma [16]. LMS is a rare malignant neoplasm of smooth muscle that can originate in the retroperitoneum, particularly from the genitourinary tract, the gastrointestinal tract, the large vessels, and, rarely, the bones [17]. LMS occur predominantly in the middle-aged or older population. Retroperitoneal LMS are more common in women [17].

The etiology of LMS is not clear. Some authors report that Epstein–Barr virus and prior irradiation can be implicated [18]. Today it is assumed that the majority of alimentary tract LMS are GISTs with different immunohistochemistry [19]. Immunohistochemistry allows diagnosis of LMS when smooth muscle actin and desmin are expressed by tumor cells [20]. H-caldesmon and DGFRA protein are additional muscle cell markers that may be expressed by the tumor [21].

10.3 Diagnosis

10.3.1 GIST

Because GISTs often occur with nonspecific symptoms, the diagnosis is frequently delayed. The clinical manifestations of GIST depend on the anatomic location and the size of the tumor and include gastrointestinal bleeding, hematemesis, melena, hematochezia, a palpable mass, abdominal pain, vomiting, weight loss, signs and symptoms of anemia, abdominal distention, and intestinal obstruction [22]. Ileal GISTs may mimic gynecological disease [23].

GISTs occur most frequently in the stomach (70 %), followed by the small intestine (30–35 %) and anorectum (7 %). They are rare in the esophagus and colon [24]. Between 60 and 70 % of GISTs are benign [9]. GISTs of the stomach that have a high mitotic rate (>50 mitoses per high-power field), and that present with ulcers, mesenteric fat infiltration, direct organ invasion, and metastasis have a lower tendency for malignant behavior compared with GISTs in the small bowel [25]. The primary tumor may be >20 cm. The more common sites of metastases are the liver, lungs, and peritoneum. Unfortunately, 61 % of patients have metastases at the time of diagnosis [9].

Imaging

Hepatic metastases of sarcomas have similar appearances to other liver metastases on imaging, except for certain specific types of sarcoma metastases. Examples of such specific types are metastases of osteosarcomas and liposarcomas. Osteosarcoma metastases may show ossification or calcification, which is recognized by high attenuation values on computer tomography (CT) scans and uptake of bone tracers on bone scintigraphy [26]. Liposarcoma metastases may show fat content, recognized as low attenuation values on CT scans and hyperintense signal intensity on T1-weighted magnetic resonance imaging (MRI) scans that is suppressed on fat-saturated images [27]. These features, however, do not occur in all cases of osteosarcoma and liposarcoma metastases [26, 28, 29].

CT Scan

On unenhanced CT scan, liver metastases from other sarcomas appear hypodense. On the early phase of contrast-enhanced CT scans, they are either hypovascular or hypervascular. Hypovascular metastases remain hypodense on the late phase of contrast-enhanced CT scans, whereas hypervascular metastases tend to show peripheral washout [30]. CT scans with contrast of GIST liver metastases show typically well-defined heterogeneous masses with a peripheral enhancing border of variable thickness and central low attenuation, the result of necrosis, hemorrhage, or cystic change [25].

Ultrasonography

On ultrasonography, hepatic metastases may appear hypoechoic, hyperechoic, or target-like.

MRI

On MRI scans, metastases appear hypointense on T1-weighted images and moderately hyperintense on T2-weighted images. They show restricted diffusion on diffusion-weighted images. As with dynamic gadolinium-enhanced CT scans, metastases are either hypervascular or hypovascular on the early phase of dynamic gadolinium-enhanced MRI scans. Hypovascular metastases tend to remain hypointense on the delayed images whereas hypervascular metastases tend to show peripheral washout [30, 31]. Metastases appear hypointense on the hepatocyte-uptake phase after injection of the hepatocyte-specific contrast agent on MRI [32]. Metastases tend to show avid uptake of fluorodeoxyglucose (FDG) on positron emission tomography (PET)/CT scans [33].

10.4 Treatment

10.4.1 Surgery and Imatinib

Liver Metastases from Visceral Sarcomas

Approximately 25–40 % of all patients with abdominal and pelvic STS develop metastases to the liver. Because systemic chemotherapy does not prolong survival remarkably, hepatic metastasis is generally associated with a poor prognosis [34]. Liver resection is the curative treatment of choice for hepatic metastases from GIST or LMS. Patients who undergo complete resection for GIST or LMS can have actuarial survival rates of 80 and 50 % after 1 and 3 years, respectively; patients who do not undergo liver resection have a poor overall survival of 4 % [35].

In 1998, Hirota et al. discovered gain-of-function mutations in exon 11 of the *c-Kit* proto-oncogene [36]. The cell surface transmembrane receptor c-Kit has tyrosine kinase activity and production of the protein c-Kit proto-oncogene is present in the majority of GISTs. The activated c-Kit receptor tyrosine kinase (CD117) stimulates the proliferation and the survival of neoplastic GIST tumor cells [37]. In 2001, DeMatteo et al. analyzed a tyrosine kinase inhibitor (TKI), STI571 (imatinib mesylate), used as an anticancer drug. In GISTs, there is a somatic mutation in the *c-Kit* proto-oncogene that activates its product, the c-Kit receptor tyrosine kinase. STI571 is a TKI that blocks c-Kit [35] and has demonstrated efficacy, minimal toxicity, and a partial response rate of 69 % [38]. The therapeutic use of STI571 has been extended to include being used in conjunction with hepatectomy for liver metastases arising from GISTs. STI571 is used before hepatectomy to permit resection in patients with unresectable disease and after liver resection to prevent tumor recurrence [35].

Before imatinib mesylate, the median survival reported was 19 months in patients with metastatic GIST and only 12 months in patients who also had local recurrences [39]. In patients with CD117-positive tumors, a 5-year survival of 80 % was reported compared with 33 % in patients with CD117-negative tumors [3]. Although tumors recurred in most patients; overall 1-, 2-, and 3-year survivals have been reported with rates of 96.7 %, 76.8 %, and 67.4 %, respectively [40]. In long-term follow-up, tumor recurrence or progression can occur despite an initial response to imatinib mesylate therapy [41]. For this reason, surgical resection should remain the mainstay of treatment for GIST liver metastasis (Table 10.2).

Liver metachronous metastases that arise 24 months after a curative resection are associated with a better prognosis in multivariate analysis. The time of development of liver metastasis is an important prognostic factor in the surgical treatment and in the selection of patients for treatment of recurrence after hepatectomy [47]. However, even patients with liver metachronous metastases that arise before 24 months after a curative resection have a median survival of 31 months [12].

In the largest series reported in the literature, only 17 % of patients were able to undergo resection because liver metastases from visceral STS tend to be diffuse and bilobar, rendering the disease of many patients unresectable [35]. Without hepatic resection, the reported survival rate for these patients is 14 months [53].

Timing of Surgical Resection and TKI Therapy

It is currently well confirmed that surgical resection in association with postoperative TKI treatment improves survival for patients affected by hepatic metastases from GIST. However, two aspects are not well clarified: the timing of TKI therapy and primary resection, and the GIST resistance mechanism. Because these two aspects are not well understood, different therapeutic approaches are currently proposed. Haller et al. [54] treat recurrence of GIST with systemic TKIs and emphasize surgery for patients who demonstrate early signs of TKI resistance such as "stagnation of tumor shrinkage" on radiographic imaging. On the other hand, the group of Memorial Sloan Kettering Cancer Center (MSKCC) [55, 56] reserves surgery for recurrent disease within 6 months of initiating TKI therapy to minimize the risk of acquiring secondary mutations responsible for TKI resistance. The strategy of this second approach depends on the fact that the response to imatinib from GISTs is maximized after 6 months; therefore, tumor debulking will delay the development

Table 10.2 Patients with metastases of STS treated with hepatic resection

Author	Year	Number of patients	Sex male/female	Age (years)	Majority of primary tumor type	Time primary tumor syn/met (months)	MTS unilob/bilob	Disease-free interval (months)	Survival (months)	5-year survival
Jaques [42]	1995	14	ND	52	LMS	ND	ND	ND	12	0 %
Elias [43]	1998	13	ND	ND	ND	ND	ND	ND	ND	18 %
Chen [44]	1998	11	2/9	57	LMS	0/11	ND	ND	39	ND
Lang [45]	2000	23	16/7	54	LMS	8/15	9/14	ND	32	13 %
DeMatteo [35]	2001	56	25/31	50	GIST/LMS/OTH	11/45	ND	38	39	30 %
Shima [46]	2003	10	4/6	61	LMS	ND	ND	46	39	11 %
Nunobe [47]	2005	18	10/8	58	GIST	6/12	ND	13.5	38	34 %
Ercolani [48]	2005	10	ND	ND	ND	ND	ND	ND	44	36 %
Adam [49]	2006	125	ND	ND	ND	ND	ND	ND	32	31 %
Teo [50]	2006	7	1/6	47	GIST/LMS	3/4	ND	15	24	ND
Lendoire [51]	2007	23	ND	57	ND	ND	ND	ND	19	9 %
Rehders [1]	2009	27	11/16	47	GIST/LMS	11/16	4/27	23	44	49 %
Chua [3]	2011	15	6/9	57	GIST	3/12	3/12	14	ND	80 % (CD117+) 33 % (CD117–)
Zacherl [52]	2011	15	5/10	62	GIST/LMS/OTH	5/10	7/8	33	34	27 %
Turley [40]	2012	39	28/11	60	GIST	ND	ND	25	ND	ND

Syn synchronous, *met* metachronous, *MTS* metastases, *unilob* unilobar, *bilob* bilobar, *ND* no data, *LMS* leiomyosarcoma, *GIST* gastrointestinal stromal tumor, *OTH* others

of secondary Kit mutations that lead to TKI resistance [57]. This second approach is also validated by a second study in which patients who were treated with imatinib alone had a poorer survival than patients who received 6 months of preoperative TKI therapy before surgery [58].

Currently the evidence of long-term survival based only on TKI therapy in case of recurrent or metastatic GIST is critical. Therefore, measures to prevent acquired resistance are vitally important, and because tumor cell exposure to the TKI cannot be decreased, resection of the tumor whenever that is feasible is the best strategy to minimize the risk of developing secondary TKI resistance mutations.

Liver Metastases from Nonvisceral Sarcomas

In contrast to pulmonary metastases of nonvisceral STS, which are treated with aggressive surgery in many centers, the attitude toward hepatic metastases seems to discourage aggressive surgery. However, some groups have adopted an aggressive surgical approach that is in contrast with the current typical management. Of 45 patients reported in the literature as affected by hepatic metastases arising from nonvisceral sarcomas, 27 patients underwent hepatic resection. Some of the patients had a "liberal" indication; that is, in eight patients, extrahepatic abdominal recurrence and hepatic metastases were diagnosed and were resected simultaneously. The results were encouraging because the 5-year survival was 49 %, which is much better than found in other series, which report 5-year survivals of between 20 and 39 % [35, 45, 47]. These results encourage the use of hepatic resection in this category of metastases arising from nonvisceral sarcomas, when the procedure is technically and functionally feasible.

Chemotherapy

The first-line chemotherapy in STS metastases is doxorubicin and/or ifosfamide, with radiological response rates of approximately 20–30 %. The second-line chemotherapies include gemcitabine and gemcitabine plus docetaxel. Trabectedin is a tetrahydroisoquinoline alkaloid isolated from the Caribbean marine tunicate, Ecteinascidia turbinata. Trabectedin treatment was comparable with second-line treatments and showed favorable 6-month progression-free survival. In particular, some distinct histological subtypes seem to show major responses to trabectedin, e.g., LMS [3].

10.4.2 Transplantation

The major report in the literature regarding the use of transplantation concerns 13 patients who received transplants for metastatic disease from predominantly gastrointestinal LMS. Recurrence was 95 % (18 of 19 patients) after a median survival of 6 months (range, 2–90 months). Survival for the group as a whole was 47 % for 1 year, 15 % for 3 years, and 5 % for 5 years. Therefore, because better results can be achieved using surgery and TKI treatment, use of transplantation as a therapy is discouraged and has very limited indications [59].

10.4.3 TACE

Patients with hepatic recurrence after liver resection or patients with unresectable liver metastases may be treated with transcatheter arterial chemoembolization (TACE). TACE allows the delivery of high concentrations of chemotherapeutic agents through the artery that feeds directly into the tumor mass, with minimal systemic toxicity [60]. Embolic particles are used to reduce arterial inflow and drug washout and to maximize contact time with the drugs, thus causing significant necrosis in the tumor cells [7]. This technique is effective because these metastatic tumors tend to be hypervascular. The median survival time after first TACE application was reported to be 18 months [61]. Use of TACE was reported in 14 patients with hepatic metastases secondary to gastrointestinal LMS. Following an average of two chemoembolizations, ten of these patients achieved a greater than 50 % regression of the tumoral mass, which was stable for a median period of 2 years [61]. An additional four patients affected by liver metastases from GIST and not suitable for surgery were reported by Shima as being treated by TACE [46]. Three of the patients had survivals of 17, 23, and 28 months and the last patient was still alive at the time the data was published.

10.4.4 Radiofrequency Ablation (RFA)

Radiofrequency ablation (RFA) is used as an ablative therapeutic technique for patients who are not candidates for hepatic resection [62]. RFA may play a role especially in patients with stable disease elsewhere and with progressive disease limited to a single liver metastasis, presumably caused by a resistant clone. In patients with liver metastases from GIST sarcomas, the progression after RFA treatment is slower relative to metastases arising from non-GIST sarcomas (28 months versus 9 months). The overall survival is longer for patients with GIST liver metastases relative to patients with liver metastases from non-GIST sarcomas [63]. RFA may be used as an isolated technique or may be combined with hepatic resection so that more patients may become candidates for surgical treatment. The surgeon can resect larger tumors and use RFA for residual smaller lesions. RFA can be also used in unfavorable locations or for patients who were judged to be unable to tolerate a major parenchymal resection. In one study, patients treated with RFA alone or in combination with surgical resection had a significantly higher rate of recurrence (90.9 %) compared with patients who underwent resection alone (57.1 %) [64].

10.4.5 Selective Internal Radiation Therapy (SIRT)

Selective internal radiation therapy (SIRT) is based on providing radiation that is limited to the liver. Microscopic beads are injected into the liver, reaching a maximum concentration within the tumor [65]. This treatment makes use of the new microvascularization of the tumor, which is at a 3- to 200-times greater density within the tumor compared with the healthy liver parenchyma, and the difference in the source of blood supply between the liver, which receives flow prevalently from the portal vein, and malignant tumors, which get their blood primarily from the arterial supply. Thus, the tumor is a perfect target for this treatment because the technique concentrates the beads in the tumoral cells while sparing the healthy liver cells, making this technique useful in liver metastases from GIST. ^{90}Yttrium may be delivered through biocompatible resin microspheres (SIR-Spheres® made by SirTex Medical, Sidney Australia) or glass beads (Theraspheres made by MDS Nordion, Ottawa, Canada). Because these particles concentrate in the microvasculature of the tumors, they offer a dual benefit with high-dose interstitial radiotherapy. ^{90}Yttrium (^{90}Y) emits beta rays that have a half-life of approximately 64 h and an average energy below 1 MeV (one gigabecquerel (27 mCi) delivers a total absorbed radiation dose of 50 Gy/kg). Hence, the interstitial radiation penetrates to a mean distance of 2.5 mm (maximum 1.1 cm). ^{90}Y decays to stable zirconium-90; during this decay, 94 % of the radiation is delivered in the first 11 days [11, 66]. SIRT is a technique that allows high average doses of radiation (200–300 Gy) to be administered to liver tumors with minimal serious effect on the nontumorous liver [11]. This method can be used for liver metastases from GIST but, until now, few cases have been reported in the literature and, thus, they do not yet permit any conclusion.

10.4.6 Chemosaturation with Percutaneous Hepatic Perfusion (CS-PHP)

The new technique of chemosaturation with percutaneous hepatic perfusion (CS-PHP) is performed via a specialized double-balloon catheter that occludes the intrahepatic inferior vena cava adjacent to the hepatic venous outflow. This allows extracorporeal filtration of the chemotherapeutic agent in the effluent venous blood, with subsequent return to the systemic circulation via a veno–veno bypass into the internal jugular vein. CS-PHP may represent an additional treatment option for hepatic STS metastases because it avoids an extensive surgical procedure and can maximize treatment to the entire liver. This technique is repeatable and has a low toxicity profile [4]. However, for this technique also, the paucity of reported cases does not yet permit any conclusion.

Acknowledgment The Authors are very grateful to doctor Ahmed Mafhouz from Weill Cornell Medical College-Q, New York, USA for his contribution for the part of diagnosis in the present chapter.

References

1. Rehders A, Peiper M, Stoecklein NH, Alexander A, Boelke E, Knoefel WT, Rogiers X (2009) Hepatic metastasectomy for soft-tissue sarcomas: is it justified? World J Surg 33:111–117
2. Schmitt T, Keller E, Dietrich S, Wuchter P, Ho AD, Egerer G (2010) Trabectedin for metastatic soft tissue sarcoma: a retrospective single center analysis. Mar Drugs 8:2647–2658

3. Chua TC, Chu F, Morris DL (2011) Outcomes of single-centre experience of hepatic resection and cryoablation of sarcoma liver metastases. Am J Clin Oncol 34:317–320
4. Deneve JL, Choi J, Gonzalez RJ, Conley AP, Stewart S, Han D, Werner P, Chaudhry TA, Zager JS (2012) Chemosaturation with percutaneous hepatic perfusion for unresectable isolated hepatic metastases from sarcoma. Cardiovasc Intervent Radiol 35:1480–1487
5. DeMatteo RP, Lewis JJ, Leung D, Mudan SS, Woodruff JM, Brennan MF (2000) Two hundred gastrointestinal stromal tumors: recurrence patterns and prognostic factors for survival. Ann Surg 231:51–58
6. Mudan SS, Conlon KC, Woodruff JM, Lewis JJ, Brennan MF (2000) Salvage surgery for patients with recurrent gastrointestinal sarcoma: prognostic factors to guide patient selection. Cancer 88:66–74
7. Miettinen M, Kopczynski J, Makhlouf HR, Sarlomo-Rikala M, Gyorffy H, Burke A, Sobin LH, Lasota J (2003) Gastrointestinal stromal tumors, intramural leiomyomas, and leiomyosarcomas in the duodenum: a clinicopathologic, immunohistochemical, and molecular genetic study of 167 cases. Am J Surg Pathol 27:625–641
8. Goettsch WG, Bos SD, Breekveldt-Postma N, Casparie M, Herings RM, Hogendoorn PC (2005) Incidence of gastrointestinal stromal tumours is underestimated: results of a nationwide study. Eur J Cancer 41:2868–2872
9. Burkill GJ, Badran M, Al-Muderis O, Meirion Thomas J, Judson IR, Fisher C, Moskovic EC (2003) Malignant gastrointestinal stromal tumor: distribution, imaging features, and pattern of metastatic spread. Radiology 226:527–532
10. Giuly JA, Picand R, Giuly D, Monges B, Nguyen-Cat R (2003) Von Recklinghausen disease and gastrointestinal stromal tumors. Am J Surg 185:86–87
11. Miettinen M, Lasota J (2006) Gastrointestinal stromal tumors: review on morphology, molecular pathology, prognosis, and differential diagnosis. Arch Pathol Lab Med 130: 1466–1478
12. Miettinen M, Lasota J (2006) Gastrointestinal stromal tumors: pathology and prognosis at different sites. Semin Diagn Pathol 23:70–83
13. Fletcher CD, Berman JJ, Corless C, Gorstein F, Lasota J, Longley BJ, Miettinen M, O'Leary TJ, Remotti H, Rubin BP, Shmookler B, Sobin LH, Weiss SW (2002) Diagnosis of gastrointestinal stromal tumors: a consensus approach. Hum Pathol 33:459–465
14. Rossi S, Miceli R, Messerini L, Bearzi I, Mazzoleni G, Capella C, Arrigoni G, Sonzogni A, Sidoni A, Toffolatti L, Laurino L, Mariani L, Vinaccia V, Gnocchi C, Gronchi A, Casali PG, Dei Tos AP (2011) Natural history of imatinib-naive GISTs: a retrospective analysis of 929 cases with long-term follow-up and development of a survival nomogram based on mitotic index and size as continuous variables. Am J Surg Pathol 35:1646–1656
15. Joensuu H, Vehtari A, Riihimäki J, Nishida T, Steigen SE, Brabec P, Plank L, Nilsson B, Cirilli C, Braconi C, Bordoni A, Magnusson MK, Linke Z, Sufliarsky J, Federico M, Jonasson JG, Dei Tos AP, Rutkowski P (2012) Risk of recurrence of gastrointestinal stromal tumour after surgery: an analysis of pooled population-based cohorts. Lancet Oncol 13:265–274
16. Hartman DS, Hayes WS, Choyke PL, Tibbetts GP (1992) From the archives of the AFIP. Leiomyosarcoma of the retroperitoneum and inferior vena cava: radiologic-pathologic correlation. Radiographics 12:1203–1220
17. O'Sullivan PJ, Harris AC, Munk PL (2008) Radiological imaging features of non-uterine leiomyosarcoma. Br J Radiol 81:73–81
18. Rogatsch H, Bonatti H, Menet A, Larcher C, Feichtinger H, Dirnhofer S (2000) Epstein-Barr virus-associated multicentric leiomyosarcoma in an adult patient after heart transplantation: case report and review of the literature. Am J Surg Pathol 24:614–621
19. Barbetakis N, Paliouras D, Asteriou C, Samanidis G, Kleontas A, Anestakis D, Kaplanis K, Tsilikas C (2009) Cutaneous skull metastasis from uterine leiomyosarcoma: a case report. World J Surg Oncol 7:45
20. Miettinen M, Sobin LH, Lasota J (2009) True smooth muscle tumors of the small intestine: a clinicopathologic, immunhistochemical, and molecular genetic study of 25 cases. Am J Surg Pathol 33:430–436

21. Ceballos KM, Nielsen GP, Selig MK, O'Connell JX (2000) Is anti-h-caldesmon useful for distinguishing smooth muscle and myofibroblastic tumors? An immunohistochemical study. Am J Clin Pathol 114:746–753
22. Levy AD, Remotti HE, Thompson WM, Sobin LH, Miettinen M (2003) Gastrointestinal stromal tumors: radiologic features with pathologic correlation. Radiographics 23:283–304
23. Miettinen M, Sarlomo-Rikala M, Lasota J (1998) Gastrointestinal stromal tumours. Ann Chir Gynaecol 87(4):278–281
24. O'Sullivan PJ, Harris AC, Ho SG, Munk PL (2006) The imaging features of gastrointestinal stromal tumours. Eur J Radiol 60:431–438
25. Levy AD, Remotti HE, Thompson WM, Sobin LH, Miettinen M (2003) Anorectal gastrointestinal stromal tumors: CT and MR imaging features with clinical and pathologic correlation. AJR Am J Roentgenol 180:1607–1612
26. Kim SJ, Choi JA, Lee SH, Choi JY, Hong SH, Chung HW, Kang HS (2004) Imaging findings of extrapulmonary metastases of osteosarcoma. Clin Imaging 28:291–300
27. Prasad SR, Wang H, Rosas H, Menias CO, Narra VR, Middleton WD, Heiken JP (2005) Fat-containing lesions of the liver: radiologic-pathologic correlation. Radiographics 25:321–331
28. Chan HH, Chan JK, Ng WM, Shek TW, Chan FL (2001) Lace-like enhancement pattern of osteosarcoma of rib and liver metastasis in CT scans. Australas Radiol 45:305–308
29. Sheah K, Ouellette HA, Torriani M, Nielsen GP, Kattapuram S, Bredella MA (2008) Metastatic myxoid liposarcomas: imaging and histopathologic findings. Skelet Radiol 37:251–258
30. Mahfouz AE, Hamm B, Mathieu D (1996) Imaging of metastases to the liver. Eur Radiol 6:607–614
31. Mahfouz AE, Hamm B, Wolf KJ (1994) Peripheral washout: a sign of malignancy on dynamic gadolinium-enhanced MR images of focal liver lesions. Radiology 190:49–52
32. Lafaro KJ, Roumanis P, Demirjian AN, Lall C, Imagawa DK (2013) Gd-EOB-DTPA-Enhanced MRI for detection of liver metastases from colorectal cancer: a surgeon's perspective! Int J Hepatol 2013:572307
33. Chua SC, Groves AM, Kayani I, Menezes L, Gacinovic S, Du Y, Bomanji JB, Ell PJ (2007) The impact of 18F-FDG PET/CT in patients with liver metastases. Eur J Nucl Med Mol Imaging 34:1906–1914
34. Le Cesne A, Judson I, Crowther D, Rodenhuis S, Keizer HJ, Van Hoesel Q, Blay JY, Frisch J, Van Glabbeke M, Hermans C, Van Oosterom A, Tursz T, Verweij J (2000) Randomized phase III study comparing conventional-dose doxorubicin plus ifosfamide versus high-dose doxorubicin plus ifosfamide plus recombinant human granulocyte-macrophage colony-stimulating factor in advanced soft tissue sarcomas: a trial of the european organization for research and treatment of cancer/soft tissue and bone sarcoma group. J Clin Oncol 18:2676–2684
35. DeMatteo RP, Shah A, Fong Y, Jarnagin WR, Blumgart LH, Brennan MF (2001) Results of hepatic resection for sarcoma metastatic to liver. Ann Surg 234:540–547
36. Hirota S, Isozaki K, Moriyama Y, Hashimoto K, Nishida T, Ishiguro S, Kawano K, Hanada M, Kurata A, Takeda M, Muhammad Tunio G, Matsuzawa Y, Kanakura Y, Shinomura Y, Kitamura Y (1998) Gain-of-function mutations of c-kit in human gastrointestinal stromal tumors. Science 279:577–580
37. Demetri GD, von Mehren M, Blanke CD, Van den Abbeele AD, Eisenberg B, Roberts PJ, Heinrich MC, Tuveson DA, Singer S, Janicek M, Fletcher JA, Silverman SG, Silberman SL, Capdeville R, Kiese B, Peng B, Dimitrijevic S, Druker BJ, Corless C, Fletcher CD, Joensuu H (2002) Efficacy and safety of imatinib mesylate in advanced gastrointestinal stromal tumors. N Engl J Med 347:472–480
38. van Oosterom AT, Judson I, Verweij J, Stroobants S, di Donato PE, Dimitrijevic S, Martens M, Webb A, Sciot R, Van Glabbeke M, Silberman S, Nielsen OS, European Organisation for Research and Treatment of Cancer Soft Tissue and Bone Sarcoma Group (2001) Safety and efficacy of imatinib (STI571) in metastatic gastrointestinal stromal tumours: a phase I study. Lancet 358:1421–1423
39. Rubin BP, Fletcher JA, Fletcher CD (2000) Molecular insights into the histogenesis and pathogenesis of gastrointestinal stromal tumors. Int J Surg Pathol 8:5–10

40. Turley RS, Peng PD, Reddy SK, Barbas AS, Geller DA, Marsh JW, Tsung A, Pawlik TM, Clary BM (2012) Hepatic resection for metastatic gastrointestinal stromal tumors in the tyrosine kinase inhibitor era. Cancer 118:3571–3578
41. Wu PC, Langerman A, Ryan CW, Hart J, Swiger S, Posner MC (2003) Surgical treatment of gastrointestinal stromal tumors in the imatinib (STI-571) era. Surgery 134:656–665
42. Jaques DP, Coit DG, Casper ES, Brennan MF (1995) Hepatic metastases from soft-tissue sarcoma. Ann Surg 221:392–397
43. Elias D, de Cavalcanti AA, Eggenspieler P, Plaud B, Ducreux M, Spielmann M, Theodore C, Bonvalot S, Lasser P (1998) Resection of liver metastases from a noncolorectal primary: indications and results based on 147 monocentric patients. J Am Coll Surg 187:487–493
44. Chen H, Pruitt A, Nicol TL, Gorgulu S, Choti MA (1998) Complete hepatic resection of metastases from leiomyosarcoma prolongs survival. J Gastrointest Surg 2:151–155
45. Lang H, Nussbaum KT, Kaudel P, Frühauf N, Flemming P, Raab R (2000) Hepatic metastases from leiomyosarcoma: a single-center experience with 34 liver resections during a 15-year period. Ann Surg 231:500–505
46. Shima Y, Horimi T, Ishikawa T, Ichikawa J, Okabayashi T, Nishioka Y, Hamada M, Shibuya Y, Ishii T, Ito M (2003) Aggressive surgery for liver metastases from gastrointestinal stromal tumors. J Hepato Pancreat Surg 10:77–80
47. Nunobe S, Sano T, Shimada K, Sakamoto Y, Kosuge T (2005) Surgery including liver resection for metastatic gastrointestinal stromal tumors or gastrointestinal leiomyosarcomas. Jpn J Clin Oncol 35:338–341
48. Ercolani G, Grazi GL, Ravaioli M, Ramacciato G, Cescon M, Varotti G, Del Gaudio M, Vetrone G, Pinna AD (2005) The role of liver resections for noncolorectal, nonneuroendocrine metastases: experience with 142 observed cases. Ann Surg Oncol 12:459–466
49. Adam R, Chiche L, Aloia T, Elias D, Salmon R, Rivoire M, Jaeck D, Saric J, Le Treut YP, Belghiti J, Mantion G, Mentha G, Association Française de Chirurgie (2006) Hepatic resection for noncolorectal nonendocrine liver metastases: analysis of 1,452 patients and development of a prognostic model. Ann Surg 244:524–535
50. Teo MC, Tan YM, Chung AY, Chow PK, Cheow PC, Soo KC, Hee SW, Ooi LL (2006) Metastectomy for non-colorectal, non-neuroendocrine liver secondaries. ANZ J Surg 76: 575–578
51. Lendoire J, Moro M, Andriani O, Grondona J, Gil O, Raffin G, Silva J, Bracco R, Podestá G, Valenzuela C, Imventarza O, Pekolj J, De Santibañes E (2007) Liver resection for non-colorectal, non-neuroendocrine metastases: analysis of a multicenter study from Argentina. HPB (Oxford) 9:435–439
52. Zacherl M, Bernhardt GA, Zacherl J, Gruber G, Kornprat P, Bacher H, Mischinger HJ, Windhager R, Jakesz R, Grünberger T (2011) Surgery for liver metastases originating from sarcoma-case series. Langenbecks Arch Surg 396:1083–1091
53. Ng EH, Pollock RE, Romsdahl MM (1992) Prognostic implications of patterns of failure for gastrointestinal leiomyosarcomas. Cancer 69:1334–1341
54. Haller F, Detken S, Schulten HJ, Happel N, Gunawan B, Kuhlgatz J, Füzesi L (2007) Surgical management after neoadjuvant imatinib therapy in gastrointestinal stromal tumours (GISTs) with respect to imatinib resistance caused by secondary KIT mutations. Ann Surg Oncol 14:526–532
55. Joensuu H (2006) Gastrointestinal stromal tumor (GIST). Ann Oncol 17(Suppl 10):x280–x286
56. Steeghs N, Nortier JW, Gelderblom H (2007) Small molecule tyrosine kinase inhibitors in the treatment of solid tumors: an update of recent developments. Ann Surg Oncol 14:942–953
57. Verweij J, Casali PG, Zalcberg J, LeCesne A, Reichardt P, Blay JY, Issels R, van Oosterom A, Hogendoorn PC, Van Glabbeke M, Bertulli R, Judson I (2004) Progression-free survival in gastrointestinal stromal tumours with high-dose imatinib: randomised trial. Lancet 364: 1127–1134
58. Xia L, Zhang MM, Ji L, Li X, Wu XT (2010) Resection combined with imatinib therapy for liver metastases of gastrointestinal stromal tumors. Surg Today 40:936–942
59. Husted TL, Neff G, Thomas MJ, Gross TG, Woodle ES, Buell JF (2006) Liver transplantation for primary or metastatic sarcoma to the liver. Am J Transplant 6:392–397

60. Trevisani F, De Notariis S, Rossi C, Bernardi M (2001) Randomized control trials on chemoembolization for hepatocellular carcinoma: is there room for new studies? J Clin Gastroenterol 32:383–389
61. Mavligit GM, Zukwiski AA, Ellis LM, Chuang VP, Wallace S (1995) Gastrointestinal leiomyosarcoma metastatic to the liver. Durable tumor regression by hepatic chemoembolization infusion with cisplatin and vinblastine. Cancer 75:2083–2088
62. Bleicher RJ, Allegra DP, Nora DT, Wood TF, Foshag LJ, Bilchik AJ (2003) Radiofrequency ablation in 447 complex unresectable liver tumors: lessons learned. Ann Surg Oncol 10:52–58
63. Jones RL, McCall J, Adam A, O'Donnell D, Ashley S, Al-Muderis O, Thway K, Fisher C, Judson IR (2010) Radiofrequency ablation is a feasible therapeutic option in the multi modality management of sarcoma. Eur J Surg Oncol 36:477–482
64. Pawlik TM, Vauthey JN, Abdalla EK, Pollock RE, Ellis LM, Curley SA (2006) Results of a single-center experience with resection and ablation for sarcoma metastatic to the liver. Arch Surg 141:537–543
65. Uthappa MC, Ravikumar R, Gupta A (2011) Selective internal radiation therapy: 90Y (yttrium) labeled microspheres for liver malignancies (primary and metastatic). Indian J Cancer 48:18–23
66. Hong X, Choi H, Loyer EM, Benjamin RS, Trent JC, Charnsangavej C (2006) Gastrointestinal stromal tumor: role of CT in diagnosis and in response evaluation and surveillance after treatment with imatinib. Radiographics 26:481–495

Liver Metastases from Stomach Cancer 11

Akio Saiura

11.1 Incidence

Gastric carcinoma is a malignant epithelial tumor of the stomach mucosa. Adenocarcinoma of the esophagogastric junction is another clinical entity and is difficult to distinguish from gastric carcinoma. Gastric cancer is estimated to be the fifth most common type of cancer with 952,000 cases worldwide (6.8 % of the total) and is the third leading cause of cancer death (723,000 deaths, 8.8 % of the total) worldwide, according to a report in GLOBOCAN 2012 by the World Health Organization [1]. The incidence of gastric cancer varies with geographic regions, with half of the cases worldwide occurring in Eastern Asia. The highest estimated mortality rates are in Eastern Asia (24 per 100,000 in men, 9.8 per 100,000 in women) and the lowest in Northern America (2.8 and 1.5 per 100,000, respectively) (Fig. 11.1). High mortality rates are also present in both sexes in Central and Eastern Europe and in Central and South America. Age-standardized incidence rates are about twice as high in men as in women, ranging from 3.3 per 100,000 in Western Africa to 35.4 per 100,000 in Eastern Asia for men and from 2.6 per 100,000 in Western Africa to 13.8 per 100,000 in Eastern Asia for women. However, there has been a rapid decline in the incidence of gastric cancer and a steady decline in gastric cancer mortality worldwide. In some Western countries, rates have decreased by more than one third within just one generation. There is about a 20-fold difference in the incidence rates when comparing the rates in Japan with those of some white populations from the USA and of some African countries. The intestinal type of adenocarcinoma is more common in high-risk areas, while the diffuse type is more common in low-risk areas [2].

A. Saiura, MD, PhD
Department of Gastroenterological Surgery, Cancer Institute Hospital,
Japanese Foundation for Cancer Research, Ariake Hospital,
3-8-31 Ariake, Koto-ku, Tokyo 135-8550, Japan
e-mail: saiura-tky@umin.ac.jp

I. Di Carlo (ed.), *Noncolorectal, Nonneuroendocrine Liver Metastases: Diagnosis and Current Therapies*, DOI 10.1007/978-3-319-09293-5_11

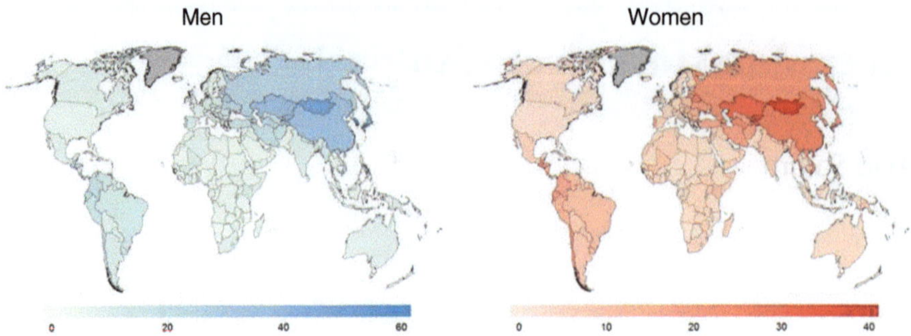

Fig. 11.1 Estimated stomach cancer incidence worldwide in 2012

Table 11.1 Clinical differences between GLM and CLM

	GLM	CLM
Efficacy of liver resection	Unknown (%)	Established (%)
Incidence of liver metastases	4.50	23–29
Rate of liver resection	<20	20–40
5-year survival after liver resection	20–30	30–50

CLM colorectal liver metastases, *GLM* gastric liver metastases

The etiology of gastric cancer is multifactorial. Previous studies show that adequate intake of fresh fruits and vegetables decreases the risk of gastric cancer, and excess intake of salt increases the risk [3]. Also, *helicobacter pylori* infection is strongly associated with the development of gastric cancer [4].

The liver is the most frequent site of distant metastases from colorectal cancer with a rate of 17–29 % [5, 6]. In these cases, liver resection is widely accepted as a treatment and potential cure. There are some differences between colorectal liver metastases and gastric liver metastases with regard to liver resection (Table 11.1). In patients with gastric cancer, the rate of synchronous and metachronous liver metastases was reported to be 3.5–11.1 %. Most patients with liver metastases from gastric cancer are multiple bilobar diseases accompanied with simultaneous peritoneal dissemination, widespread lymph node metastases, and direct invasion to adjacent structures [7–9]. In a previous RCT for advanced gastric cancer, 44 % of patients with liver metastases were included in the study [10].

11.2 Natural History

Liver metastasis is defined as a non-curative factor in patients with gastric cancer in classifications by both the Japanese Gastric Cancer Association and the American Joint Committee on Cancer Staging [11, 12] (Tables 11.2 and 11.3). The prognosis for gastric cancer patients with liver metastases is poor, with a 6-month survival rate of 20–50 % [7, 8, 13]. A previous RCT demonstrated the natural history of patients

Table 11.2 TNM classification of gastric tumors

TX	Primary tumor cannot be assessed
T0	No evidence of primary tumor
Tis	Carcinoma in situ: intraepithelial tumor without invasion of the lamina propria
T1	Tumor invades lamina propria, muscularis mucosae, or submucosa
T1a	Tumor invades lamina propria or muscularis mucosae
T1b	Tumor invades submucosa
T2	Tumor invades muscularis propria
T3	Tumor penetrates subserosal connective tissue without invasion of visceral peritoneum or adjacent structures.c,d
T4	Tumor invades serosa (visceral peritoneum) or adjacent structures.c,d
T4a	Tumor invades serosa (visceral peritoneum)
T4b	Tumor invades adjacent structures
NX	Regional lymph node(s) cannot be assessed
N0	No regional lymph node metastasis.b
N1	Metastases in 1–2 regional lymph nodes
N2	Metastases in 3–6 regional lymph nodes
N3	Metastases in ≥7 regional lymph nodes
N3a	Metastases in 7–15 regional lymph nodes
N3b	Metastases in ≥16 regional lymph nodes
M0	No distant metastasis
M1	Distant metastasis

Reprinted with permission from AJCC: Stomach [60]

with advanced gastric cancer including liver metastases, with a median survival time of 2–4 months (Table 11.4) [14–16]. However, systemic chemotherapy can prolong overall survival.

11.3 Diagnosis

Early diagnosis is crucial because of the possibility of early metastasis to the lymph nodes, liver, and peritoneal dissemination. Most patients in Western countries are diagnosed with inoperable advanced disease requiring palliative treatment. A screening system has been developed in Japan and has shown that early diagnosis is possible [17]. Currently, synchronous liver metastases can be detected at a rate of 2.2–4.8 % [18–20]. Upper endoscopy is the most sensitive and specific method for diagnosing gastric cancer compared to other diagnostic strategies such as barium studies. During endoscopy, any suspicious lesion can be biopsied easily and a final diagnosis can be done. Contrast-enhanced computed tomography (CE-CT) should be routinely performed for staging, especially for liver metastases and lymph node metastases (Fig. 11.2). Gross appearance of GLM as well as radiological finding is similar with other primary or metastatic adenocarcinoma (Fig. 11.3).

Table 11.3 Stage grouping

Stage	T	N	M
0	Tis	N0	M0
IA	T1	N0	M0
IB	T2	N0	M0
	T1	N1	M0
IIA	T3	N0	M0
	T2	N1	M0
	T1	N2	M0
IIB	T4a	N0	M0
	T3	N1	M0
	T2	N2	M0
	T1	N3	M0
IIIA	T4a	N1	M0
	T3	N2	M0
	T2	N3	M0
IIIB	T4b	N0	M0
	T4b	N1	M0
	T4a	N2	M0
	T3	N3	M0
IIIC	T4b	N2	M0
	T4b	N3	M0
	T4a	N3	M0
IV	Any T	Any N	M1

Reprinted with permission from AJCC: Stomach [60]

Table 11.4 Randomized controlled trials (RCTs) comparing best supportive care (BSC) in management of advanced gastric cancer

	Patients	RR	MST(months)	*P*-value	Author
FAMTX	30	50	9	$P<0.01$	Murad (1993)
BSC	10	–	2		
ELF	10	30	10	$P<0.02$	Glimelius (1994)
BSC	8	–	4		
FEMTX	21	29	12.3	$P<0.01$	Pyrhonen (1995)
BSC	20	–	3.1		

RR response rate (%), *FAMTX* 5-FU, ADM, methotrexate (MTX), *ELF* etoposide, 5-FU, leucovorin, *FEMTX* 5-FU, epirubicin, MTX

Lymph node metastases can be detected by CT and larger lymph nodes are highly related to metastases. Peritoneal metastases and liver metastases smaller than 5 mm are frequently missed by CT even with multidirector row CT [21]. The depth of tumor invasion is not accurately assessed with CT. Staging laparoscopy can detect radiographically occult peritoneal metastases and reduce the substantial morbidity and mortality associated with laparotomy [22]. The use of 18-fluorodexyglucose positron emission tomography (FDG-PET) CT can help detect occult extrahepatic

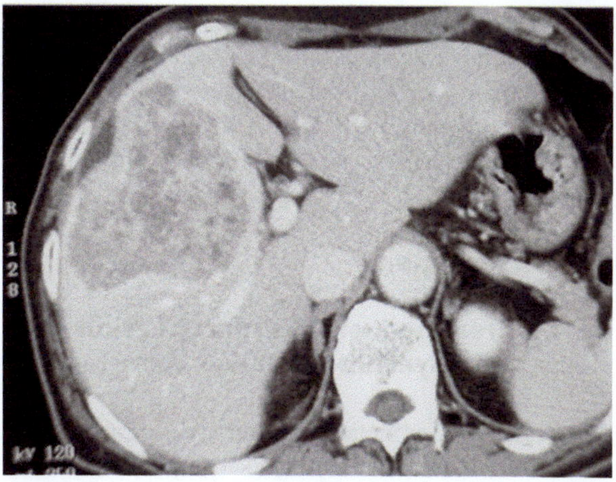

Fig. 11.2 Contrast-enhanced axial CT reveals a hypovascular tumor in segment 5 and 8 of the liver

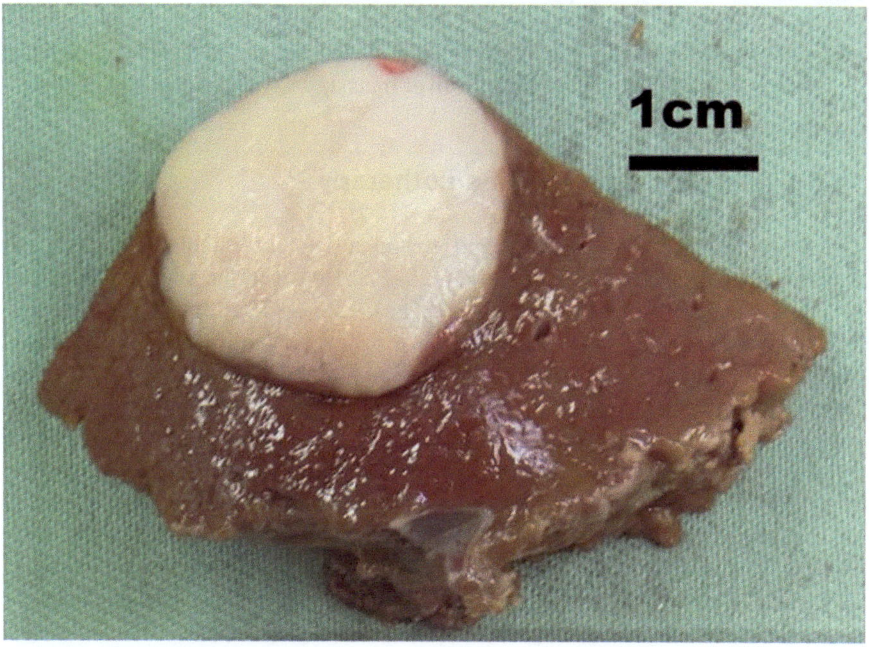

Fig. 11.3 Gross appearance of GLM

metastases; however, the detection rate of diffuse gastric cancers is very low [23]. Smyth et al. reported that FDG-PET/CT identified metastatic lesions in approximately 10 % of patients with locally advanced gastric cancer [24]. The current gold standard in preoperative diagnosis focusing on liver metastases from gastric cancer (GLM) is CE-CT and magnetic resonance imaging (MRI) using a gadolinium-based contrast agent. A novel imaging technique, gadolinium ethoxybenzyl diethylenetriamine pentaacetic acid-enhanced MRI (EOB-MRI), has been developed for identifying liver neoplasms. This technique enables not only a dynamic study evaluating tumor vascularity but also liver-specific imaging with the contrast agent taken up by the liver cells. EOB-MRI is therefore considered a more highly sensitive imaging modality over MRI and CE-CT for demonstrating and characterizing liver tumors.

11.4 Treatment

11.4.1 Treatment of the Primary Lesion with Synchronous Liver Metastases

Most cases of liver metastases from gastric cancer are considered to be an incurable advanced disease and are treated with palliative chemotherapy. The indication for gastrectomy in patients with incurable distant metastases should be determined after consideration of individual performance status and the surgical risk involved. In a particular patient with symptomatic gastric cancer such as bleeding or obstruction, gastrectomy can be indicated with the aim of palliation. In general, palliative systemic chemotherapy is indicated for liver metastases from gastric cancer.

11.5 Palliative Systemic Chemotherapy

There are different backgrounds and treatments for resectable gastric cancer between Eastern and Western countries [25–27]. However, the standard treatment for metastatic gastric cancer including most gastric liver metastases is systemic chemotherapy. Most liver metastases from gastric cancer are multiple and disseminated diseases with other non-curable factors such as peritoneal dissemination or extensive lymph node metastases [28]. The benefit of palliative chemotherapy over best supportive care for advanced gastric cancer has been demonstrated in RCTs [16, 29]. Systematic review and meta-analysis showed that systemic chemotherapy had a survival benefit compared with best supportive care in patients with advanced gastric cancer [30]. To date, a large number of chemotherapy regimens have been tested in randomized studies, including patients with liver metastases from gastric cancer. Due to the differences of tolerability to chemotherapy, standard chemotherapeutic treatments for advanced gastric cancer including liver metastases is heterogeneous throughout the world. There is no international consensus regarding which chemotherapy regimen should be used first.

In Western countries, many chemotherapy regimens are effective in the treatment of advanced gastric cancer [31–34], and to date, combination therapy is superior to single-agent chemotherapy. The current standard regimen in the treatment of advanced gastric cancer is combination therapy with ECF (epirubicin, cisplatin, and infused 5-FU) [35] (Table 11.5). In Japan, the current first-line chemotherapy regimen for metastatic gastric cancer (mGC) is a combination therapy of

Table 11.5 RCTs for advanced gastric cancer in Western countries

RCT	Regimen	Number of patients	RR (%)	MST(months)	*P* value
EORTC (1991)	FAM	103	9	7.2	0.04
	FAMTX	105	41	10.5	
Webb et al. [32]	FAMTX	130	21	5.7	0.0009
	ECF	126	45	8.9	
EORTC (2000)	FAMTX	133	12	6.7	NS
	ELF	132	9	7.2	
	FP	134	20	7.2	
V325 (2006)	DCF	221	38.7	9.2	0.02
	FP	224	23.2	8.6	

RR response rate (%), *FAMTX* 5-FU, ADM, methotrexate (MTX), *ELF* etoposide, 5-FU, leucovorin, *FEMTX* 5-FU, epirubicin, MTX

Table 11.6 RCTs for advanced gastric cancer in Japan

RCT	Regimen	Number of patients	RR	PFS	OS	*P* value
SPIRITS	S1	150	31	4	11	
	S1 + CDDP	148	54	6	13	0.0366
JCOG9912	5FU	234	9	2.9	10.8	
	Irinotecan + CDDP	236	38	4.8	12.3	0.055
	S-1	234	28	4.2	11.4	0.034
GC0301/TOP-002	S-1	160	27	3.6	10.5	
	S-1+ irinotecan	155	42	4.5	12.8	NS

fluoropyrimidine plus a platinum compound [36, 37] (Table 11.6). More recent phase III studies have focused on the benefit of adding a targeted therapy to XP therapy (capecitabine plus cisplatin) [38, 39]. A recent study identified human epidermal growth factor receptor 2 (HER2) as an important biomarker for gastric cancer prognosis. In a recent worldwide RCT (ToGA study), the addition of trastuzumab to XP improved survival in patients with advanced gastric cancer or gastroesophageal junction cancer compared with XP alone [38]. Trastuzumab in combination with chemotherapy is considered a new standard option for patients with HER2-positive mGC, although the HER2 status should be tested in liver metastases as well as in the primary lesion due to the heterogeneity of HER2 [40].

11.6 Surgical Treatment of Liver Metastases of Gastric Cancer

Reports on liver resection for non-colorectal non-neuroendocrine metastases (NCNN) from Western institutions include only very small numbers of patients with GLM (2–4 %) (Table 11.7). In contrast, liver resection of GLM comprises

Table 11.7 Rate of GLM undergoing liver resection for metastatic non-colorectal non-neuroendocrine tumors

Reference	Number of patients		%
	Total	GLM	
Weitz (2005)	141	3	2
Adam (2006)	1,452	64	4
Takemura (2013)	145	73	50

most cases of liver resection for NCNN in Japan. There is no prospective study to evaluate the efficacy of surgical treatment of GLM due to the small number of cases. Ochiai et al. reported the first case series to identify the predictive factors for GLM after liver resection [41]; however, to date only a limited number of retrospective analyses exist. Takemura et al. reported a retrospective analysis of the largest number of cases of GLM with liver resection ($n=64$) from a single center in Japan, with an overall survival rate after liver resection of 37 %. Adam et al. also reported on a series of 64 cases of surgically treated GLM, which was a subset of 1,452 patients with non-colorectal liver metastases from 41 institutions [42]. Elias et al. reported disappointing results with a 3-year survival rate of lower than 20 % [43]. However, conclusions cannot be drawn from the retrospective analysis of less than 100 cases. Therefore, the significance of liver resection for liver metastases from gastric cancer remains controversial due to the lack of evidence. Some consider that liver metastases from gastric cancer represent a systemic disease and surgery has no role in its treatment because the results of liver resections are still discouraging. In contrast to colorectal liver metastases, liver-limited metastases are a rare condition in patients with GLM, most of which have an accompanying extrahepatic disease such as peritoneal dissemination or extensive lymph node metastases. However, a retrospective study of a small number of highly selected cases reported that long-term survivors encouraged the surgical resection for gastric liver metastases.

It is important to identify the selection criteria for liver resection of gastric cancer. Romano et al. conducted a systematic review of surgical treatment of GLM and examined various factors affecting postoperative outcome after liver resection [44] and suggested that liver resection can improve the prognosis for patients suffering from GLM compared to supportive treatment alone, with a median survival time of 3–5 months. Although most studies were reported from Japan, Romano et al. described that the review can also apply to clinical practice in Western countries in centers with skills and experience in liver surgery.

In general, resection of liver metastases are indicated when all tumors can be resected safely with a clear margin and there is no extrahepatic disease. Specifically, a general rule suggests that liver resections are attempted in patients: (1) with primary tumors curatively treated or treatable, (2) with no extrahepatic disease, and (3) with a small number of liver metastases which can be resected safely with a clear margin [45]. However, liver resections were rarely indicated, even in specialized hospitals. In a retrospective study of the large database of resection for gastric cancer, the rate of liver metastases ranges from 15 to 17 % [18, 41, 45, 46]; however, liver resections were performed in only 0.3–2.3 % of all gastric resections.

Table 11.8 Previous reports of liver resection of liver metastases from gastric cancer

Author	Year	Number of patients	5-years survival (%)	Poor prognostic factor	
				Primary factor	Liver factor
Ochiai	1994	21	19	Serosal invasion, ly(+), v(+)	
Miyazaki	1997	21	20		Multiple, surgical margin <10 mm
Ambiru	2001	40	18		Synchronous metastases
Okano	2002	21	34	Poorly differentiated	Multiple, synchronous, serosal invasion
Saiura	2002	10	20	Lymph node metastases	
Zacherl	2002	15		Proximal lesion	Bilobar
Sakamoto	2003	22	38		Multiple, size >5 cm
Shirabe	2003	36	26	ly(+), v(+)	Number >2
Koga	2007	42	42	Serosal invasion	Multiple
Sakamoto	2007	37	11		Bilobar, size >4 cm
Makino	2010	16	10		Bilobar
Tsujimoto	2010	17	31	>6 cm, D2 LND (−)	
Takemura	2012	64	37	Serosal invasion	Size >5 cm

11.7 Prognostic Factors

Previous retrospective studies have identified numerous factors affecting prognosis after liver resection for GLM. These prognostic factors can be divided into two groups that are associated with (1) primary lesion and (2) live lesion.

11.7.1 Prognostic Factors Associated with the Primary Lesion

Various clinicopathological or surgical factors associated with the primary lesion were reported to affect the outcome after liver resection for GLM (Table 11.8). Ochiai et al. identified that serosal invasion, lymphatic invasion (ly+), and venous invasion (v+) in the primary lesion were associated with poor outcomes in liver resection for GLM using multivariate analysis [41]. Koga et al. and Takemura et al. also reported that serosal invasion (T4) of the primary lesion was an independent prognostic factor for poor survival after liver resection for GLM [18, 47], and Shirabe et al. reported that ly+ or v+ was associated with poorer survival after liver resection [28]. In other studies, the presence of venous, lymphatic, or serosal invasion in the primary lesion had no impact on survival [45, 48].

The presence and extent of lymph node metastases is also reported to be associated with the outcome for GLM after liver metastases. Saiura et al. reported that patients with lymph node metastases in the primary lesion had a significantly poorer survival rate compared with those without lymph node metastases in a univariate analysis [45]. Similar findings were reported by Miyazaki et al., in which the 5-year

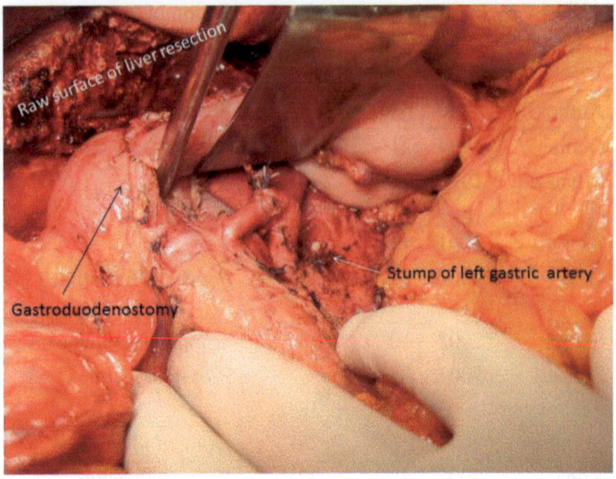

Fig. 11.4 Photo showing complete resection of synchronous GLM. Distal gastrectomy with D2 lymph nodes dissection and Billroth 1 gastroduodenostomy and left lateral sectionectomy of the liver

survival rate in patients with lymph node metastases was significantly worse than in patients without lymph node metastases [48]. Furthermore, Imamura et al. reported that the grade of histologic differentiation of the primary lesion has an impact on the outcome [49]. We can therefore characterize patients with metachronous GLM using these prognostic factors associated with the primary lesion. The limitation is the difficulty of how to apply these findings into clinical practice in patients with synchronous GLM.

Staging laparoscopy can help ensure precise diagnosis of serosal invasion of the primary lesion. The significance of lavage positive cytology of the primary lesion was poorly described in patients with surgically resected GLM. Those with positive peritoneal cytology of the primary lesion were thought to be excluded from the indication of liver resection for GLM because positive cytology is one of the non-curative factors in classifications by the Japanese Gastric Cancer Association and the American Joint Committee on Cancer Staging [11, 12]. Liver resection in patients with a non-curative factor of the primary lesion has no survival benefit in comparison to those treated with palliative chemotherapy [47]. In terms of surgical factors, D2 lymph node dissection has been accepted for the standard treatment for radical resection of advanced gastric cancer [50]. In patients with potentially curable GLM, radical resection of the primary lesion with D2 lymph node dissection should be done (Fig. 11.4).

11.7.2 Prognostic Factors Associated with a Hepatic Lesion

The size and number of the liver metastases is the most important prognostic factor; however, the cutoff value is not consistent among studies. Solitary metastasis is the best candidate for liver resection and most long-term survivors after liver resection for GLM had single liver metastasis [18, 28, 45, 48]. Okano et al. reported a 3-year overall survival after resection for solitary and multiple GLM was 56 and 0 %, respectively, strongly suggesting that the number of liver metastases is an important prognostic factor [45]. Shirabe et al. reported that three or more liver metastases were an independent negative prognostic factor for overall survival after liver resection for GLM [28]. However, there are reports of long-term survival after liver resection of multiple GLMs [47]. The upper limit is still unclear and will change with the development of a systemic chemotherapy as in colorectal cancer. In addition, a maximum size larger than 5 cm was reported as a negative prognostic factor in univariate and multivariate analysis.

The timing of liver resection in patients presenting with liver metastases during workup for the primary tumor is controversial. Some suggest that synchronous diagnosis of metastases presents a worse prognosis [28, 51, 52]. Ambiru et al. advocated that liver resection for GLM is indicated only in patients with a solitary metastases presenting metachronously [53, 54]; however, others have reported that liver resection has no difference in overall survival between synchronous and metachronous GLM [41, 47].

Delaying liver resection may increase survival in the surgically resected group by selecting out the patients with aggressive tumor biology who are likely to have a systemic disease. The timing of liver resection is still controversial in patients with colorectal liver metastases. To date, evidence related to the timing of liver resection for GLM is lacking. Adam et al. reported that a disease-free interval of longer than 1 year was a good prognostic factor after liver resection for NCNN hepatectomy [42]. Fujii et al. also suggested that hepatectomy should be attempted in patients where the disease-free interval was greater than or equal to 1 year [55].

The width of the surgical margin at the site of liver resection remains unknown; however, complete resection with a clear margin is strongly recommended for better survival. Miyazaki et al. reported that a significant difference in the tumor-free margin of the resection (<10 mm or >10 mm) was found between survivors and those who died with surgically resected GLM patients [48].

On the basis of prognostic factors, selection criteria are advocated. Takemura et al. identified that a maximum tumor size of larger than 5 cm and positive serosal invasion of the primary lesion were the two independent negative prognostic factors in a retrospective single center analysis in patients predominantly having three or less liver metastases. The study recommended that GLM patients with a maximum diameter of hepatic tumors of <5 cm and without serosal invasion of the primary gastric cancer were the best candidates for hepatectomy [47]. In a review of the literature in which numerous factors were examined, Romano et al. concluded that none of the reported predictive factors, alone or in combination, could deprive a patient of the possibility of long-term survival after liver resection, if we exclude cases presenting a bilobar spread of metastases [44].

11.7.3 Repeat Resection for Recurring Metastases

The liver is the most common site for recurrence of metastases after resection for gastric cancer, with the recurrence rate of 57–87 % [20, 28, 47, 48, 53, 56, 57]

Table 11.9 Previous reports of repeat liver resection of liver metastases from gastric cancer

Author	Year	No of patients	No of liver recurrence	Rate of liver recurrence (%)	Repeat resection	Number of survivor	
						3 years	5 years
Miyazaki	2001	16	14	88	NA	–	–
Ambiru	2001	31	21	68	0	–	–
Shirabe	2003	30	22	73	3	1	1
Sakamoto	2007	37	23	62	0	–	–
Cheon	2008	22	14	64	NA	–	–
Qui	2013	25	NA	NA	2	1	1
Takemura	2013	64	37	58	14	6	2

(Table 11.9). It is rare that it is the sole site of recurrence and most patients receive non-curable palliative treatment. As in patients with colorectal liver metastases, a repeat hepatectomy may be considered in the absence of extrahepatic disease and if the patient has a good performance status and adequate hepatic reserve; however, repeat resection for GLM has rarely been reported. Recently, Takemura et al. reported the result of an aggressive surgical approach for GLM including 14 repeat liver resections after 64 primary liver resections. In the report, the 5-year survival rate after repeat liver resections was 47 % which was comparable with those after the primary hepatectomy [58]. The mortality and morbidity rate were 0 and 29 %, respectively; however, the presence of severe adhesion around the liver hilum and the liver due to the previous primary lesion and liver resection concomitant with lymph node dissection makes repeat liver resection more challenging. The study demonstrated that a disease-free interval of >12 months after the initial hepatectomy predicts good patient survival after repeat hepatectomy.

11.8 Multidisciplinary Approach

Some studies report the use of radiofrequency ablation (RFA) in combination with or as an alternative to surgical resection for the treatment of liver metastases from gastric cancer. Chen et al. reported 21 cases of gastric liver metastases treated by RFA with a median survival time after RFA of 14 months. Patients with solitary metastases were considered appropriate candidates for RFA [59].

References

1. Ferlay J, Soerjomataram I, Ervik M, Dikshit R, Eser S, Mathers C, Rebelo M, Parkin DM, Forman D, Bray F (2013) GLOBOCAN 2012 v1.0, cancer incidence and mortality worldwide: IARC CancerBase No. 11 [internet]. International Agency for Research on Cancer, Lyon, Available from: http://globocan.iarc.fr, accessed on 10 April 2014
2. Munoz N, Correa P, Cuello C, Duque E (1968) Histologic types of gastric carcinoma in high- and low-risk areas. Int J Cancer 3(6):809–818

3. Gaddy JA, Radin JN, Loh JT, Zhang F, Washington MK, Peek RM Jr, Algood HM, Cover TL (2013) High dietary salt intake exacerbates Helicobacter pylori-induced gastric carcinogenesis. Infect Immun 81(6):2258–2267
4. Peek RM Jr, Blaser MJ (2002) Helicobacter pylori and gastrointestinal tract adenocarcinomas. Nat Rev Cancer 2(1):28–37
5. Leporrier J, Maurel J, Chiche L, Bara S, Segol P, Launoy G (2006) A population-based study of the incidence, management and prognosis of hepatic metastases from colorectal cancer. Br J Surg 93(4):465–474
6. Kobayashi H, Mochizuki H, Sugihara K, Morita T, Kotake K, Teramoto T, Kameoka S, Saito Y, Takahashi K, Hase K, Oya M, Maeda K, Hirai T, Kameyama M, Shirouzu K, Muto T (2007) Characteristics of recurrence and surveillance tools after curative resection for colorectal cancer: a multicenter study. Surgery 141(1):67–75
7. Koga S, Kawaguchi H, Kishimoto H, Tanaka K, Miyano Y, Kimura O, Takeda R, Nishidoi H (1980) Therapeutic significance of noncurative gastrectomy for gastric cancer with liver metastasis. Am J Surg 140(3):356–359
8. Okuyama K, Isono K, Juan IK, Onoda S, Ochiai T, Yamamoto Y, Koide Y, Satoh H (1985) Evaluation of treatment for gastric cancer with liver metastasis. Cancer 55(10):2498–2505
9. Ueda K, Iwahashi M, Nakamori M, Nakamura M, Naka T, Ishida K, Ojima T, Yamaue H (2009) Analysis of the prognostic factors and evaluation of surgical treatment for synchronous liver metastases from gastric cancer. Langenbeck's Arch Surg Deutsche Gesellschaft fur Chirurgie 394(4):647–653
10. Shitara K, Ikeda J, Kondo C, Takahari D, Ura T, Muro K, Matsuo K (2012) Reporting patient characteristics and stratification factors in randomized trials of systemic chemotherapy for advanced gastric cancer. Gastric Cancer 15(2):137–143
11. Japanese classification of gastric carcinoma: 3rd English edition (2011) Gastric Cancer 14(2): 101–112
12. Washington K (2010) 7th edition of the AJCC cancer staging manual: stomach. Ann Surg Oncol 17(12):3077–3079
13. Nakajima T, Nishi M, Kajitani T (1991) Improvement in treatment results of gastric cancer with surgery and chemotherapy: experience of 9,700 cases in the Cancer Institute Hospital, Tokyo. Semin Surg Oncol 7(6):365–372
14. Murad AM, Santiago FF, Petroianu A, Rocha PR, Rodrigues MA, Rausch M (1993) Modified therapy with 5-fluorouracil, doxorubicin, and methotrexate in advanced gastric cancer. Cancer 72(1):37–41
15. Glimelius B, Hoffman K, Haglund U, Nyren O, Sjoden PO (1994) Initial or delayed chemotherapy with best supportive care in advanced gastric cancer. Ann Oncol 5(2): 189–190
16. Pyrhonen S, Kuitunen T, Nyandoto P, Kouri M (1995) Randomised comparison of fluorouracil, epidoxorubicin and methotrexate (FEMTX) plus supportive care with supportive care alone in patients with non-resectable gastric cancer. Br J Cancer 71(3):587–591
17. Prolla JC, Kobayashi S, Kirsner JB (1969) Gastric cancer. Some recent improvements in diagnosis based upon the Japanese experience. Arch Intern Med 124(2):238–246
18. Koga R, Yamamoto J, Ohyama S, Saiura A, Seki M, Seto Y, Yamaguchi T (2007) Liver resection for metastatic gastric cancer: experience with 42 patients including eight long-term survivors. Jpn J Clin Oncol 37(11):836–842
19. Garancini M, Uggeri F, Degrate L, Nespoli L, Gianotti L, Nespoli A, Uggeri F, Romano F (2012) Surgical treatment of liver metastases of gastric cancer: is local treatment in a systemic disease worthwhile? HPB (Oxford) 14(3):209–215
20. Qiu JL, Deng MG, Li W, Zou RH, Li BK, Zheng Y, Lao XM, Zhou K, Yuan YF (2013) Hepatic resection for synchronous hepatic metastasis from gastric cancer. Eur J Surg Oncol 39(7):694–700
21. Kim SJ, Kim HH, Kim YH, Hwang SH, Lee HS, do Park J, Kim SY, Lee KH (2009) Peritoneal metastasis: detection with 16- or 64-detector row CT in patients undergoing surgery for gastric cancer. Radiology 253(2):407–415

22. Karanicolas PJ, Elkin EB, Jacks LM, Atoria CL, Strong VE, Brennan MF, Coit DG (2011) Staging laparoscopy in the management of gastric cancer: a population-based analysis. J Am Coll Surg 213(5):644–651, 651 e641
23. Mukai K, Ishida Y, Okajima K, Isozaki H, Morimoto T, Nishiyama S (2006) Usefulness of preoperative FDG-PET for detection of gastric cancer. Gastric Cancer 9(3):192–196
24. Smyth E, Schoder H, Strong VE, Capanu M, Kelsen DP, Coit DG, Shah MA (2012) A prospective evaluation of the utility of 2-deoxy-2-[(18) F]fluoro-D-glucose positron emission tomography and computed tomography in staging locally advanced gastric cancer. Cancer 118(22):5481–5488
25. Macdonald JS, Smalley SR, Benedetti J, Hundahl SA, Estes NC, Stemmermann GN, Haller DG, Ajani JA, Gunderson LL, Jessup JM, Martenson JA (2001) Chemoradiotherapy after surgery compared with surgery alone for adenocarcinoma of the stomach or gastroesophageal junction. N Engl J Med 345(10):725–730
26. Cunningham D, Allum WH, Stenning SP, Thompson JN, Van de Velde CJ, Nicolson M, Scarffe JH, Lofts FJ, Falk SJ, Iveson TJ, Smith DB, Langley RE, Verma M, Weeden S, Chua YJ, MAGIC Trial Participants (2006) Perioperative chemotherapy versus surgery alone for resectable gastroesophageal cancer. N Engl J Med 355(1):11–20
27. Sakuramoto S, Sasako M, Yamaguchi T, Kinoshita T, Fujii M, Nashimoto A, Furukawa H, Nakajima T, Ohashi Y, Imamura H, Higashino M, Yamamura Y, Kurita A, Arai K (2007) Adjuvant chemotherapy for gastric cancer with S-1, an oral fluoropyrimidine. N Engl J Med 357(18):1810–1820
28. Shirabe K, Shimada M, Matsumata T, Higashi H, Yakeishi Y, Wakiyama S, Ikeda Y, Ezaki T, Fukuzawa S, Takenaka K, Kishikawa K, Ikeda T, Taguchi K, Maehara Y, Sugimachi K (2003) Analysis of the prognostic factors for liver metastasis of gastric cancer after hepatic resection: a multi-institutional study of the indications for resection. Hepatogastroenterology 50(53):1560–1563
29. Glimelius B, Ekstrom K, Hoffman K, Graf W, Sjoden PO, Haglund U, Svensson C, Enander LK, Linne T, Sellstrom H, Heuman R (1997) Randomized comparison between chemotherapy plus best supportive care with best supportive care in advanced gastric cancer. Ann Oncol 8(2):163–168
30. Wagner AD, Grothe W, Haerting J, Kleber G, Grothey A, Fleig WE (2006) Chemotherapy in advanced gastric cancer: a systematic review and meta-analysis based on aggregate data. J Clin Oncol 24(18):2903–2909
31. Wils JA, Klein HO, Wagener DJ, Bleiberg H, Reis H, Korsten F, Conroy T, Fickers M, Leyvraz S, Buyse M et al (1991) Sequential high-dose methotrexate and fluorouracil combined with doxorubicin–a step ahead in the treatment of advanced gastric cancer: a trial of the European Organization for Research and Treatment of Cancer Gastrointestinal Tract Cooperative Group. J Clin Oncol 9(5):827–831
32. Webb A, Cunningham D, Scarffe JH, Harper P, Norman A, Joffe JK, Hughes M, Mansi J, Findlay M, Hill A, Oates J, Nicolson M, Hickish T, O'Brien M, Iveson T, Watson M, Underhill C, Wardley A, Meehan M (1997) Randomized trial comparing epirubicin, cisplatin, and fluorouracil versus fluorouracil, doxorubicin, and methotrexate in advanced esophagogastric cancer. J Clin Oncol 15(1):261–267
33. Vanhoefer U, Rougier P, Wilke H, Ducreux MP, Lacave AJ, Van Cutsem E, Planker M, Santos JG, Piedbois P, Paillot B, Bodenstein H, Schmoll HJ, Bleiberg H, Nordlinger B, Couvreur ML, Baron B, Wils JA (2000) Final results of a randomized phase III trial of sequential high-dose methotrexate, fluorouracil, and doxorubicin versus etoposide, leucovorin, and fluorouracil versus infusional fluorouracil and cisplatin in advanced gastric cancer: a trial of the European Organization for Research and Treatment of Cancer Gastrointestinal Tract Cancer Cooperative Group. J Clin Oncol 18(14):2648–2657
34. Van Cutsem E, Moiseyenko VM, Tjulandin S, Majlis A, Constenla M, Boni C, Rodrigues A, Fodor M, Chao Y, Voznyi E, Risse ML, Ajani JA (2006) Phase III study of docetaxel and cisplatin plus fluorouracil compared with cisplatin and fluorouracil as first-line therapy for advanced gastric cancer: a report of the V325 Study Group. J Clin Oncol 24(31):4991–4997

35. Allum WH, Blazeby JM, Griffin SM, Cunningham D, Jankowski JA, Wong R (2011) Guidelines for the management of oesophageal and gastric cancer. Gut 60(11):1449–1472
36. Koizumi W, Narahara H, Hara T, Takagane A, Akiya T, Takagi M, Miyashita K, Nishizaki T, Kobayashi O, Takiyama W, Toh Y, Nagaie T, Takagi S, Yamamura Y, Yanaoka K, Orita H, Takeuchi M (2008) S-1 plus cisplatin versus S-1 alone for first-line treatment of advanced gastric cancer (SPIRITS trial): a phase III trial. Lancet Oncol 9(3):215–221
37. Okines AF, Norman AR, McCloud P, Kang YK, Cunningham D (2009) Meta-analysis of the REAL-2 and ML17032 trials: evaluating capecitabine-based combination chemotherapy and infused 5-fluorouracil-based combination chemotherapy for the treatment of advanced oesophago-gastric cancer. Ann Oncol 20(9):1529–1534
38. Bang YJ, Van Cutsem E, Feyereislova A, Chung HC, Shen L, Sawaki A, Lordick F, Ohtsu A, Omuro Y, Satoh T, Aprile G, Kulikov E, Hill J, Lehle M, Ruschoff J, Kang YK (2010) Trastuzumab in combination with chemotherapy versus chemotherapy alone for treatment of HER2-positive advanced gastric or gastro-oesophageal junction cancer (ToGA): a phase 3, open-label, randomised controlled trial. Lancet 376(9742):687–697
39. Ohtsu A, Shah MA, Van Cutsem E, Rha SY, Sawaki A, Park SR, Lim HY, Yamada Y, Wu J, Langer B, Starnawski M, Kang YK (2011) Bevacizumab in combination with chemotherapy as first-line therapy in advanced gastric cancer: a randomized, double-blind, placebo-controlled phase III study. J Clin Oncol 29(30):3968–3976
40. Onsum MD, Geretti E, Paragas V, Kudla AJ, Moulis SP, Luus L, Wickham TJ, McDonagh CF, Macbeath G, Hendriks BS (2013) Single-cell quantitative HER2 measurement identifies heterogeneity and distinct subgroups within traditionally defined HER2-positive patients. Am J Pathol 183(5):1446–1460
41. Ochiai T, Sasako M, Mizuno S, Kinoshita T, Takayama T, Kosuge T, Yamazaki S, Maruyama K (1994) Hepatic resection for metastatic tumours from gastric cancer: analysis of prognostic factors. Br J Surg 81(8):1175–1178
42. Adam R, Chiche L, Aloia T, Elias D, Salmon R, Rivoire M, Jaeck D, Saric J, Le Treut YP, Belghiti J, Mantion G, Mentha G (2006) Hepatic resection for noncolorectal nonendocrine liver metastases: analysis of 1,452 patients and development of a prognostic model. Ann Surg 244(4):524–535
43. Elias D, Cavalcanti de Albuquerque A, Eggenspieler P, Plaud B, Ducreux M, Spielmann M, Theodore C, Bonvalot S, Lasser P (1998) Resection of liver metastases from a noncolorectal primary: indications and results based on 147 monocentric patients. J Am Coll Surg 187(5):487–493
44. Romano F, Garancini M, Uggeri F, Degrate L, Nespoli L, Gianotti L, Nespoli A, Uggeri F (2012) Surgical treatment of liver metastases of gastric cancer: state of the art. World J Surg Oncol 10:157
45. Okano K, Maeba T, Ishimura K, Karasawa Y, Goda F, Wakabayashi H, Usuki H, Maeta H (2002) Hepatic resection for metastatic tumors from gastric cancer. Ann Surg 235(1): 86–91
46. Saiura A, Umekita N, Inoue S, Maeshiro T, Miyamoto S, Matsui Y, Asakage M, Kitamura M (2002) Clinicopathological features and outcome of hepatic resection for liver metastasis from gastric cancer. Hepatogastroenterology 49(46):1062–1065
47. Takemura N, Saiura A, Koga R, Arita J, Yoshioka R, Ono Y, Hiki N, Sano T, Yamamoto J, Kokudo N, Yamaguchi T (2012) Long-term outcomes after surgical resection for gastric cancer liver metastasis: an analysis of 64 macroscopically complete resections. Langenbeck's Arch Surg Deutsche Gesellschaft fur Chirurgie 397(6):951–957
48. Miyazaki M, Itoh H, Nakagawa K, Ambiru S, Shimizu H, Togawa A, Shiobara M, Ohtsuka M, Sasada K, Shimizu Y, Yoshioka S, Nakajima N, Suwa T, Kimura F (1997) Hepatic resection of liver metastases from gastric carcinoma. Am J Gastroenterol 92(3):490–493
49. Imamura H, Matsuyama Y, Shimada R, Kubota M, Nakayama A, Kobayashi A, Kitamura H, Ikegami T, Miyagawa SI, Kawasaki S (2001) A study of factors influencing prognosis after resection of hepatic metastases from colorectal and gastric carcinoma. Am J Gastroenterol 96(11):3178–3184

50. Songun I, Putter H, Kranenbarg EM, Sasako M, van de Velde CJ (2010) Surgical treatment of gastric cancer: 15-year follow-up results of the randomised nationwide Dutch D1D2 trial. Lancet Oncol 11(5):439–449
51. Yamakado K, Nakatsuka A, Takaki H, Mori Y, Tonouchi H, Kusunoki M, Kida H, Takeda K (2005) Prospective study of arterial infusion chemotherapy followed by radiofrequency ablation for the treatment of liver metastasis of gastric cancer. J Vasc Interv Radiol 16(12): 1747–1751
52. Bines SD, England G, Deziel DJ, Witt TR, Doolas A, Roseman DL (1993) Synchronous, metachronous, and multiple hepatic resections of liver tumors originating from primary gastric tumors. Surgery 114(4):799–805; discussion 804–795
53. Ambiru S, Miyazaki M, Ito H, Nakagawa K, Shimizu H, Yoshidome H, Shimizu Y, Nakajima N (2001) Benefits and limits of hepatic resection for gastric metastases. Am J Surg 181(3): 279–283
54. Roh HR, Suh KS, Lee HJ, Yang HK, Choe KJ, Lee KU (2005) Outcome of hepatic resection for metastatic gastric cancer. Am Surg 71(2):95–99
55. Fujii K, Fujioka S, Kato K, Machiki Y, Kutsuna Y, Ishikawa A, Takamizawa J, Ko K, Yoshida K, Nimura Y (2001) Resection of liver metastasis from gastric adenocarcinoma. Hepatogastroenterology 48(38):368–371
56. Sakamoto Y, Ohyama S, Yamamoto J, Yamada K, Seki M, Ohta K, Kokudo N, Yamaguchi T, Muto T, Makuuchi M (2003) Surgical resection of liver metastases of gastric cancer: an analysis of a 17-year experience with 22 patients. Surgery 133(5):507–511
57. Cheon SH, Rha SY, Jeung HC, Im CK, Kim SH, Kim HR, Ahn JB, Roh JK, Noh SH, Chung HC (2008) Survival benefit of combined curative resection of the stomach (D2 resection) and liver in gastric cancer patients with liver metastases. Ann Oncol 19(6):1146–1153
58. Takemura N, Saiura A, Koga R, Yoshioka R, Yamamoto J, Kokudo N (2013) Repeat hepatectomy for recurrent liver metastasis from gastric carcinoma. World J Surg 37(11):2664–2670
59. Chen J, Tang Z, Dong X, Gao S, Fang H, Wu D, Xiang D, Zhang S (2013) Radiofrequency ablation for liver metastasis from gastric cancer. Eur J Surg Oncol 39(7):701–706
60. Edge SB, Byrd DR, Compton CC Fritz AG, Greene FL, Trotti A AJCC: Stomach (2010) In: Edge SB, Byrd DR, Compton CC, et al (eds) AJCC cancer staging manual. 7th edn. Springer, New York, pp 117-126

Management of Liver Metastases from Testicular Cancer

12

Hishaam Ismael and Thomas A. Aloia

12.1 Introduction

For most hepatobiliary surgeons, gastrointestinal malignancies and their metastases dominate practice. A small proportion of cases will focus on non-gastrointestinal, non-neuroendocrine metastatic tumors. Among these rarer presentations are liver metastases from testicular cancer.

Testicular cancer is a relatively rare but diverse set of tumor types that effect males, typically within the first several decades of life [1, 2]. They are generally divided by pure seminomatous and non-seminomatous germ cell histological types. They are further subdivided by the production of hormonal tumor markers. They typically spread to axial (i.e., iliac, para-aortic) nodal chains and systemically to distant organ sites with the lungs predominating. Metastatic disease patients are typically treated with systemic chemotherapy, with surgery at local-regional and metastatic sites reserved for staging and consolidation of therapy. Even in advanced stages, 95 % cure rates have been achieved with modern systemic therapies [1, 2]. Given the rarity of these tumors, their mode and distribution of spread, and the efficacy of systemic therapies, there is a very narrow indication for liver-directed therapies.

This epidemiology explains the relative paucity of reports on outcomes of aggregated patients with resected liver metastases from testicular primary tumors.

H. Ismael
Hepatobiliary Surgery Section, Department of Surgical Oncology,
MD Anderson Cancer Center, 1400 Pressler Drive, Unit 1484,
Houston, TX 77030, USA

T.A. Aloia (✉)
Department of Surgical Oncology, The University of Texas
MD Anderson Cancer Center, Houston, TX 77030, USA
e-mail: taaloia@mdanderson.org

I. Di Carlo (ed.), *Noncolorectal, Nonneuroendocrine Liver Metastases: Diagnosis and Current Therapies*, DOI 10.1007/978-3-319-09293-5_12

This chapter will review the international literature on the topic, including multimodality therapies, indications for liver surgery, and outcomes following liver-directed therapy in patients with metastases from testicular cancer.

12.2 Diagnosis

Patients with testicular cancer can present in early stages with a testicular mass, and at later stages with symptoms of metastatic disease, including cachexia and abdominal pain. Even in patients with liver metastases, liver failure is rarely the presenting symptom. Staging evaluation includes testicular exam with ultrasound, chest x-ray, and CT scanning of the chest, abdomen, and pelvis. Serologic evaluation must include measurement of alpha-fetoprotein (AFP), beta-human chorionic gonadotropin (β-HCG) hormone, and lactate dehydrogenase [3]. Primary diagnosis is usually confirmed with inguinal orchiectomy and concomitant lymphadenectomy. Elevated tumor markers are an ominous sign for at least micrometastatic spread of tumor to distant sites [2].

Even patients who present with technically resectable liver metastases require medical oncology evaluation and initiation of systemic therapy prior to liver-directed therapies [1]. Hepatobiliary surgeons are usually consulted after these therapies have been given and the oncologic and serologic response has been evaluated.

12.2.1 Global Prognostic Factors

There are a number of global prognostic factors for patients with testicular cancer that the hepatobiliary surgeon should be familiar with. Of course, the fact that a liver surgeon would be involved indicates the presence of distant visceral metastases, which places the patient in a poor prognosis category. However, within this subgroup better prognostic features include lower tumor marker levels, significant decline in tumor marker levels following orchiectomy, and the absence of pulmonary metastases [2–4].

12.3 Multidisciplinary Management

In addition to prognostic factors, it is also critical for surgeons to understand the type and side effects associated with the common systemic therapies given for testicular cancer that may impact subsequent surgery, anesthesia, and recovery. The most common systemic regimens include EP (etoposide/cisplatin), BEP (bleomycin/etoposide/cisplatin), and VIP (ifosfamide/mesna/etoposide/cisplatin) [1, 3]. As very few of these drugs are used to treat the malignancies that hepatobiliary surgeons typically encounter in routine practice, awareness of their unique risk profiles is important. All of the platinum-based regimens can have significant bone marrow suppression effects, and adequate hematologic recovery is required prior to surgery. Likewise, bleomycin can lead to pulmonary fibrosis, and pulmonary function tests to determine lung capacity prior to anesthesia are warranted when this drug has been included [5].

12.4 Selection of Patients for Surgery

Selection of patients for hepatectomy requires a three-part stepwise evaluation including assessment for medical, oncological, and technical resectability. Obviously, patients must be medically fit for prolonged anesthesia and recovery. As testicular cancer patients tend to be otherwise healthy young males with normal liver parenchyma, medical resectability is rarely an issue, although neoadjuvant chemotherapy toxicities may create nutritional and healing deficits. As such, performance status should be optimized by appropriate withdrawal of chemotherapy prior to surgery.

Oncological resectability is the next factor to consider. Patients need to be assessed for their response to systemic therapy and their burden of extrahepatic disease. Unlike liver metastases from gastrointestinal primary tumors, testicular tumors are far more likely to involve axial lymph nodes and systemic sites of disease, such as the lungs. Only a select group of patients with exceptional responses to systemic therapy and local-regional surgery would have an oncological rationale for liver-directed therapies. As testicular cancer is not typically treated by hepatobiliary surgeons, it is wise to consult with urologists and medical oncology specialists to best understand global prognosis, chemotoxicities, and novel therapeutics that may impact the decision, timing, and conduct of liver surgery.

Finally, for patients with a multidisciplinary review that has determined medical fitness and oncological rationale, technical resectability should be assessed. Given the typical multifocality of liver metastases from testicular cancer, a detailed review of high-quality cross-sectional imaging from pretreatment to present is requisite. This can be accomplished with multiphasic liver protocol CT scans and/or liver MR, preferably aided by newer hepatocyte-specific MR contrast agents.

The fundamental rules of hepatobiliary surgery regarding liver resection and the future liver remnant should be followed, including the ability to resect all sites of disease while retaining at least two contiguous liver segments of adequate functional volume with adequate inflow, outflow, and biliary drainage [6]. As testicular liver metastases tend to be bilateral and multifocal, accurate measurement of liver volumes [7] is critical, and liberal usage of two-stage surgery and portal vein embolization should be considered as needed [8].

Only after patients meet all three criteria for resectability should they be considered candidates for liver surgery. In addition, NCCN Guidelines recommend "referral to high-volume centers for surgical resection of masses post-chemotherapy" [3].

12.5 Other Liver-Directed Therapies

Theoretically, other common modalities for the treatment of liver tumors could apply to the nonsurgical treatment of testicular tumors. However, the multiplicity of these lesions makes ablative strategies obsolete in many cases. Likewise, only select subsets are radiosensitive, limiting the role for external beam, proton beam, and radioembolization. Combined these factors explain a near-complete absence of reports for nonsurgical liver-directed therapy in this disease [9, 10].

12.6 Long-Term Outcomes After Surgical Resection

A review of the world literature on the topic of outcomes following liver resection for testicular cancer metastases finds very few publications. In many cases, outcomes for testicular cancer patients are bundled with those with other, more common, genitourinary primary malignancies [11–13]. With the available data in the literature, several general comments and a few specific comments can be made.

In general, there are very few case reports in the literature. Table 12.1 outlines the 14 available studies reporting on a total of 317 patients specifically with testicular cancer liver metastases. Common demographic and tumor-specific features contained in these reports indicate a tendency toward unilateral metastatic disease.

Taking into account what must be significant selection bias toward patients with demonstrated favorable tumor biology and anatomy, long-term outcomes are generally positive with some reporting 70+ % survivals at 3 years and a range of 30–60 % 5-year postoperative survivals. For example, the largest reported experience compiled from the French multicenter cohort comprised 78 patients and indicated a 51 % 5-year survival post liver resection [14]. These survival figures placed testicular cancer liver metastases in a "good" prognosis category relative to the larger cohort of 1,452 non-colorectal, non-endocrine metastases surgically treated patients who shared a 36 % overall 5-year survival.

Also of note is the study by Hartmann et.al. that focused on only males with non-seminomatous germ cell tumor metastases and reported long-term outcomes following liver resection in 43 patients who received preoperative systemic therapy. With such a focused cohort, they reported a 63 % pathologic complete response rate with a 79 % 3-year survival, including 27 of 34 patients remaining free of disease at a median follow-up interval of 37 months (Fig. 12.1). There were no factors identified that could predict complete response to chemotherapy, so resection was advocated for all resectable patients. Long-term survivals were closely correlated with refractoriness to preoperative systemic chemotherapy.

Although it is difficult to develop a cohesive set of prognostic factors for liver surgery candidates from the available literature, several studies suggested that prolonged disease-free interval, smaller tumors, response to systemic therapy, and R0 resection were favorable attributes.

Table 12.1 Literature review including long-term outcomes reported following liver resection for testicular cancer metastases

Title	Author	Journal	Year	Time period	Testicular CA	Mortality	Prognostic factors	Survivals	Additional points
Hepatic resection for disseminated germ cell carcinoma	Goulet et al. [15]	*Annals of Surgery*	1990	1976–1989	28	0 %		54 % in the last 5 years	
Hepatic resection for noncolorectal nonneuroendocrine metastases: a 15-year experience with 96 patients	Harrison et al. [16]	*Surgery*	1997	1980–1995	34 GU 9 testicular	0 %	Disease-free interval, R0, primary tumor site	GU tumors have a 60 % 5-year survival	
Comparison of histological results from the resection of residual masses at different sites after chemotherapy for metastatic non-seminomatous germ cell tumors	Hartmann et al. [17]	*European Journal of Cancer*	1997	1980–1995	4	0 %	R0 resection, necrosis/mature teratoma on histology associated with improved disease-free and overall survival	73 % alive after 33 months	30 % had dissimilar histologic findings. 27 patients were eligible (2 sites of resection)

(continued)

Table 12.1 (continued)

Title	Author	Journal	Year	Time period	Testicular CA	Mortality	Prognostic factors	Survivals	Additional points
Resection of liver metastases from a noncolorectal primary: indications and results based on 147 monocentric patients	Elias et al. [18]	*Journal of the American College of Surgeons*	1998	1984–1996	20	2 %		36 %	50 % 3-year survival for testicular CA. 46 % 5-year survival. No difference between curative and palliative resection. Neuroendocrine tumors included in study
Hepatic resection of metastatic testicular carcinoma: a further update	Hahn et al. [19]	*Annals of Surgical Oncology*	1999	1974–1996	57	0 %	Group 1 and 2	Group 1: 8/9 alive, Group 2 23/29, Group 3a 6/14, Group 3b 2/5	Group 1 had necrosis on pathology; group 2 showed a mature teratoma; 3a had active disease with normal preop tumor markers; 3b had elevated preop markers

Hepatic resection for noncolorectal nonendocrine liver metastasis	Hemming et al. [20]	*Liver Transplantation*	2000	1978–1998	1	0 %	Primary tumor (GI vs non-GI) and R0 resection	45 %	Most were in the right hemiliver
Resection of noncolorectal and nonendocrine liver metastases: late metastases are the only chance of cure	Laurent et al. [21]	*World Journal of Surgery*	2001	1980–1997	2	0 %	Disease-free interval >24 months, GU primary	35 %	Encouraged re-hepatectomy
Multimodality treatment of patients with liver metastases from germ cell tumors. The role of surgery	Rivoire et al. [22]	*Cancer*	2001	1984–1997	37	3 %	Tumor less than 10 mm. Poor outcome associated with lesions greater than 30 mm, presence of viable disease or embryonal CA	62 %	18 had necrosis, 7 had mature teratoma, and 12 had active disease
Partial hepatectomy for metastases from noncolorectal nonneuroendocrine carcinoma	Weitz et al. [23]	*Annals of Surgery*	2005	1981–2002	20	0 %	Disease-free interval >24 months, reproductive tract primary, R0 resection	72 % 3-year survival	

(continued)

Table 12.1 (continued)

Title	Author	Journal	Year	Time period	Testicular CA	Mortality	Prognostic factors	Survivals	Additional points
Role of postchemotherapy surgery in the management of patients with liver metastases from germ cell tumors	Hartmann et al. [24]	*Annals of Surgery*	2005	1990–1998	43	0 %	Refractoriness to chemo was associated with a shorter survival, and a trend was established with elevated AFP	70.9 %	Necrosis in 67 %, teratoma in 12 %, and cancer in 21 %. Histologic discrepancy in 39 %
Hepatic resection for noncolorectal nonendocrine liver metastases	Adam et al. [14]	*Annals of Surgery*	2006	1983–2004	78	2.3 %	Limited resection, R0, disease-free interval, younger age, response to chemotherapy	36 %	Mortality was over 60 days. Repeat hepatectomy has benefit 69 % vs 33 %
Long-term results of liver resection for non-colorectal, nonneuroendocrine metastases	O'Rouke et al. [25]	*Annals of Surgical Oncology*	2007	1986–2006	1	0.8 %	Tumor size less than 5 cm in diameter, absence of extrahepatic disease/nodal disease and R0 resection had better outcomes – univariate analysis	38.5 %	Review of 2 prospective databases. Diameter greater than 5 cm and extrahepatic nodal disease were the only two positive variables on multivariate analysis

Resection of noncolorectal nonneuroendocrine metastases: a comparative analysis	Reddy et al. [26]	*Journal of the American College of Surgeons*	2007	1995–2005	GU 18–2 testicular Ca	4 %	Chemoradiation and delayed liver resection >6 months associated with improved survival	37 %	
Hepatic metastasectomy for germ cell tumors: is it worth it?	You et al. [27]	*Journal of Gastrointestinal Surgery*	2009	1975–2002	36–15 underwent surgery	0 %		65 %	33 % 5-year survival for patients with active disease on pathology (poor response to chemotherapy – more aggressive). Review of literature: mortality 0–3 % and morbidity 28–30 %

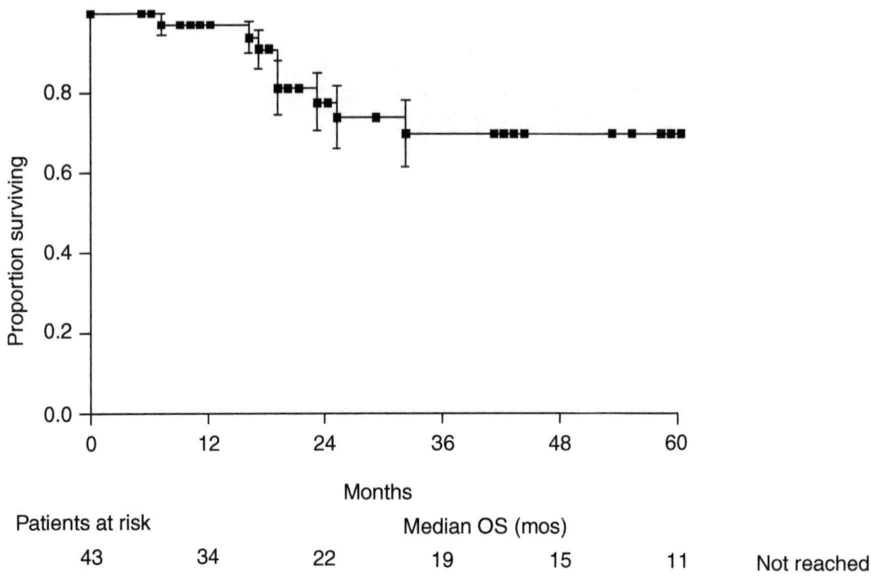

Fig. 12.1 Overall survival of 43 patients with metastatic GCT who underwent postchemotherapy hepatic surgery (Reprinted with permission from Hartmann et al. [24])

Conclusions

Testicular cancer is a rare malignancy with a unique metastatic phenotype. Patients with visceral metastases are universally managed with induction systemic chemotherapy. A small subset of these patients, particularly those with low volume or absent pulmonary disease, may become candidates for liver-directed therapy. For patients with testicular cancer liver metastases who are considered for metastasectomy, the general principles of liver surgery resectability apply to these patients. However, hepatobiliary surgeons must understand the toxicities of the systemic therapies commonly used to treat testicular cancer patients, as these drugs are usually foreign to liver surgeons and may impact surgery, anesthesia, and recovery. Reported outcomes after liver resection indicate that in highly selected patients, 30–60 % long-term survivals can be achieved. Clearly, integration of the hepatobiliary surgery consultant into a multidisciplinary urologic oncology group maximizes the opportunity to aid the patient and minimizes the risk of injury.

References

1. Shelley MD, Burgon K, Mason MD (2002) Treatment of testicular germ-cell cancer: a cochrane evidence-based systematic review. Cancer Treat Rev 28(5):237–253
2. Dearnaley D, Huddart R, Horwich A (2001) Regular review: managing testicular cancer. BMJ 322(7302):1583–1588
3. Motzer RJ, Agarwal N, Beard C et al (2009) NCCN clinical practice guidelines in oncology: testicular cancer (electronic update 12/13/13). J Natl Compr Cancer Netw 7(6):672–693

4. International germ cell consensus classification: a prognostic factor-based staging system for metastatic germ cell cancers. International germ cell cancer collaborative group (1997) J Clin Oncol 15(2):594–603
5. Saxman SB, Finch D, Gonin R, Einhorn LH (1998) Long-term follow-up of a phase III study of three versus four cycles of bleomycin, etoposide, and cisplatin in favorable-prognosis germ-cell tumors: the Indian University experience. J Clin Oncol 16(2):702–706
6. Adams RB, Aloia TA, Loyer E, Pawlik TM, Taouli B, Vauthey JN (2013) Selection for hepatic resection of colorectal liver metastases: expert consensus statement. HPB (Oxford) 15(2):91–103
7. Abdalla EK, Denys A, Chevalier P, Nemr RA, Vauthey JN (2004) Total and segmental liver volume variations: implications for liver surgery. Surgery 135(4):404–410
8. Shindoh J, Vauthey JN, Zimmitti G et al (2013) Analysis of the efficacy of portal vein embolization for patients with extensive liver malignancy and very low future liver remnant volume, including a comparison with the associating liver partition with portal vein ligation for staged hepatectomy approach. J Am Coll Surg 217(1):126–133
9. Goering JD, Mahvi DM, Niederhuber JE, Chicks D, Rikkers LF (2002) Cryoablation and liver resection for noncolorectal liver metastases. Am J Surg 183(4):384–389
10. Sideras PA, Sofocleous CT, Brody LA, Siegelbaum RH, Shah RP, Taskar NP (2012) Superselective internal radiation with yttrium-90 microspheres in the management of a chemo-refractory testicular liver metastasis. Cardiovasc Intervent Radiol 35(2):426–429
11. Bresadola V, Rossetto A, Adani GL et al (2011) Liver resection for noncolorectal and nonneuroendocrine metastases: results of a study on 56 patients at a single institution. Tumori 97(3):316–322
12. Cordera F, Rea DJ, Rodriguez-Davalos M, Hoskin TL, Nagorney DM, Que FG (2005) Hepatic resection for noncolorectal, nonneuroendocrine metastases. J Gastrointest Surg 9(9): 1361–1370
13. Ercolani G, Grazi GL, Ravaioli M et al (2005) The role of liver resections for noncolorectal, nonneuroendocrine metastases: experience with 142 observed cases. Ann Surg Oncol 12(6): 459–466
14. Adam R, Chiche L, Aloia T et al (2006) Hepatic resection for noncolorectal nonendocrine liver metastases: analysis of 1,452 patients and development of a prognostic model. Ann Surg 244(4):524–535
15. Goulet RJ Jr, Hardacre JM, Einhorn LH et al (1990) Hepatic resection for disseminated germ cell carcinoma. Ann Surg 212(3):290–293; discussion 3–4
16. Harrison LE, Brennan MF, Newman E et al (1997) Hepatic resection for noncolorectal, non-neuroendocrine metastases: a fifteen-year experience with ninety-six patients. Surgery 121(6): 625–632
17. Hartmann JT, Candelaria M, Kuczyk MA, Schmoll HJ, Bokemeyer C (1997) Comparison of histological results from the resection of residual masses at different sites after chemotherapy for metastatic non-seminomatous germ cell tumours. Eur J Cancer 33(6):843–847
18. Elias D, Cavalcanti de Albuquerque A, Eggenspieler P et al (1998) Resection of liver metastases from a noncolorectal primary: indications and results based on 147 monocentric patients. J Am Coll Surg 187(5):487–493
19. Hahn TL, Jacobson L, Einhorn LH, Foster R, Goulet RJ Jr (1999) Hepatic resection of metastatic testicular carcinoma: a further update. Ann Surg Oncol 6(7):640–644
20. Hemming AW, Sielaff TD, Gallinger S et al (2000) Hepatic resection of noncolorectal nonneuroendocrine metastases. Liver Transpl 6(1):97–101
21. Laurent C, Rullier E, Feyler A, Masson B, Saric J (2001) Resection of noncolorectal and nonneuroendocrine liver metastases: late metastases are the only chance of cure. World J Surg 25(12):1532–1536
22. Rivoire M, Elias D, De Cian F, Kaemmerlen P, Theodore C, Droz JP (2001) Multimodality treatment of patients with liver metastases from germ cell tumors: the role of surgery. Cancer 92(3):578–587

23. Weitz J, Blumgart LH, Fong Y et al (2005) Partial hepatectomy for metastases from noncolorectal, nonneuroendocrine carcinoma. Ann Surg 241(2):269–276
24. Hartmann JT, Rick O, Oechsle K et al (2005) Role of postchemotherapy surgery in the management of patients with liver metastases from germ cell tumors. Ann Surg 242(2):260–266
25. O'Rourke TR, Tekkis P, Yeung S et al (2008) Long-term results of liver resection for non-colorectal, non-neuroendocrine metastases. Ann Surg Oncol 15(1):207–218
26. Reddy SK, Barbas AS, Marroquin CE, Morse MA, Kuo PC, Clary BM (2007) Resection of noncolorectal nonneuroendocrine liver metastases: a comparative analysis. J Am Coll Surg 204(3):372–382
27. You YN, Leibovitch BC, Que FG (2009) Hepatic metastasectomy for testicular germ cell tumors: is it worth it? J Gastrointest Surg 13(4):595–601

Liver Metastases in Thyroid Cancer

13

Schelto Kruijff, Anouk N.A. van der Horst-Schrivers, and Koert P. de Jong

13.1 Introduction

Liver metastases from well-differentiated thyroid cancer (WDTC) are rare, with a reported frequency of less than 1 % [1–3]. Liver metastases in medullary thyroid cancer (MTC) are more common with a reported frequency of 21 % [4]. Hepatic involvement in cancer of the thyroid is often multiple and can usually be found with other distant metastases in the lung, bone, and brain [5]. When thyroid cancer-related liver metastases are encountered, patients generally have a poor prognosis [5]. Only a few case reports have been published on patients with liver metastases originating from WDTC and more papers report about hepatic metastases originating from MTC [4]. Thyroid cancer patients with distant metastases in general represent a difficult challenge as there seems to be a lack of definitive cure. Most national guidelines recommend a treatment algorithm with a primary role for radioactive iodine (^{131}I) therapy, rarely followed by surgery [6–9]. For thyroid cancer manifesting with liver metastases specifically, surgical treatment has been assumed to be only beneficial in case of complete curative treatment and oligo-liver metastases [6]. However, today in 2014, several less invasive treatments for metastatic liver disease have become available. Surgical devices have evolved significantly and new approaches have contributed to a safer and more controlled form of liver surgery with a significant reduction of blood loss. More

S. Kruijff (✉) • K.P. de Jong
Department of Hepato-Pancreato-Biliary Surgery and Liver Transplantation, University Medical Centre Groningen, University of Groningen, Hanzeplein 1, 9713 GZ Groningen, The Netherlands
e-mail: s.kruijff@umcg.nl; k.p.de.jong@umcg.nl

A.N.A. van der Horst-Schrivers
Department of Endocrinology, University Medical Centre Groningen, University of Groningen, Hanzeplein 1, 9713 GZ Groningen, The Netherlands
e-mail: s.kruijff@umcg.nl

I. Di Carlo (ed.), *Noncolorectal, Nonneuroendocrine Liver Metastases: Diagnosis and Current Therapies*, DOI 10.1007/978-3-319-09293-5_13

importantly, there is a profound increase in the number of locoregional liver-directed therapies which have supplied the surgeon with a large armamentarium of less invasive, local approaches of liver tumors. Subsequently, the classical surgical resection has lost its sole potential curative status as less invasive treatment modalities are within reach. Therefore, thyroid cancer liver metastases might increasingly be considered for curative or even palliative treatment, possibly reducing symptoms and with a potential impact on outcome. In this chapter an overview of treatment of distant metastases in thyroid cancer is given, with the emphasis on liver-directed interventions in patients with liver metastases from thyroid carcinoma.

13.2 Incidence and Natural History

13.2.1 Thyroid Cancer and Distant Metastases

Thyroid carcinoma is a relatively rare tumor, encompassing only 1 % of all malignancies but representing the most common endocrine type of cancer. Of the WDTC, papillary thyroid cancer (PTC) is the most common followed by follicular thyroid carcinoma (FTC), also including the oncocytic variant (further referred to as Hürthle cell thyroid carcinoma (HTC)) [10, 11]. Other variants of thyroid cancer, including anaplastic thyroid carcinoma (ATC), and MTC have a lower incidence.

Papillary and Follicular Thyroid Cancer (PTC and FTC)

Papillary and follicular thyroid cancer (PTC and FTC) are characterized by a slowly progressive course and indolent behavior. Most patients with PTC or FTC are cured with total thyroidectomy (with or without lymph node dissection), ^{131}I ablation therapy, and suppression of thyroid-stimulating hormone (TSH). The overall 10-year disease-free survival (DFS) is high (80–95 %) despite the presence of cervical lymph node metastases in 40–90 % and a recurrence rate of about 20 % [12–14]. The standard administering of adjuvant ^{131}I ablation therapy in patients with low-risk WDTC is increasingly controversial and is currently being studied in a randomized control trial comparing recurrence in patients not having ^{131}I ablation, with those who do [15, 16]. About 33 % of patients with recurrent PTC or FTC will eventually present with distant metastases [17]. Independent factors predicting distant metastases in WDTC are male gender, follicular and Hürthle cell histology, larger tumors, extrathyroidal growth, and positive regional lymph nodes followed by the quality of initial therapy [18–20]. The occurrence of distant metastases itself is the most significant poor prognostic factor for survival followed by age (>45 years) and multiple organ involvement [19–22]. Patterns of distant metastases in thyroid cancer are shown in Table 13.1 [2, 3, 22–26]. In general, distant metastases occur in lungs in 50 % (more often found in PTC (72 %) than FTC (40 %)), in bones in 25 % (fourfold higher incidence in FTC compared to PTC), and both lungs and bones in 20 % or at other sites in 5 % of the cases, with 10-year-survival rates ranging from 25 to 42 % [21, 27, 28]. Noteworthy, metastasized thyroid cancer survival rates are variable with reported 10-year survival rates up to 92 % [28]. In general the overall

Table 13.1 Overview of the literature of distant metastases with anatomical locations of metastatic spread

	Patients (N)	Tumor type	Lung (%)	Bone (%)	Liver	Other sites/ multiple (%)
Mazaferri and Jhiang [18]	61	WDTC	63	19		19
Shaha et al. [22]	44	PTC/FTC/HTC	53	20	–	16
Haq and Harmer [23]	111	WDTC	49	24	–	27
Durante et al. [24]	444	PTC/FTC	50	26	–	24
Lee and Soh [3]	1,560	WDTC	68	16	1	15
Nixon et al. [25]	52	WDTC	75	25	–	16
Machens and Dralle [4]	117	MTC	34	9	21	36
Lang et al. [26]	51	WDTC	35	14	–	48

PTC papillary thyroid carcinoma, *FTC* follicular thyroid carcinoma, *HTC* Hürthle cell carcinoma, *MTC* medullary thyroid cancer, *WDTC* well-differentiated thyroid carcinoma

risk of synchronous distant metastasis is 4 %, 2 % for PTC, and up to 11 % for FTC [28]. Similarly, the risk of developing metachronous distant disease is lower in PTC (10 %) versus FTC (20 %) [24].

^{131}I treatment can be highly effective in patients with multiple distant metastases with ^{131}I avidity. Especially in micronodular lung metastases, ^{131}I therapy is effective to administer until loss of avidity has been reached [29]. Only for those with limited macronodular lung metastases, resection followed by ^{131}I or external radiotherapy, can be a potentially curative treatment [6, 27, 30]. Patients with non-^{131}I avid metastasis have a significantly worse cancer-specific survival. Therefore, it is not surprising that ^{131}I avidity is a sole independent prognostic factor for survival in distant metastases [26, 29]. For patients with bone metastases, complete remission with only ^{131}I is achieved in only 7 % of patients. Although resection of solitary distant metastases is rare, complete metastasectomy contributes to a better survival [31]. Early in 1986, surgical resection of single bone metastases of thyroid cancer was reported with an estimated cumulative 10-year survival rate of 33 % [32]. Limited numbers of bone metastases can be treated with surgery, usually combined with ^{131}I and external beam radiotherapy [33, 34]. Apparently, resection of distant metastases in thyroid cancer can be a valuable alternative [32]. Given the lack of survival improvement observed over the last two decades of patients with distant metastases, innovative treatments are in dire need [19]. Several targeted drugs influencing tumor growth have been studied in phase II/III studies. Sorafenib, a multi-tyrosine kinase inhibitor (TKI), was recently investigated in a phase III study and is now registered for the treatment of patients with advanced ^{131}I refractory WDTC. The median progression-free survival (PFS) was better in the sorafenib group (10.8 months) versus the placebo group (5.8 months, $p<0.0001$) [35]. In conclusion, even though the presence of distant metastasis in WDTC is rare and associated with a grave prognosis, long-term survival can still be achieved with ^{131}I followed by additional surgical treatment if feasible [22].

Hürthle Cell Carcinoma (HTC)

HTC, first described in 1894 by the pathologist Hürthle, is a rare tumor and is considered an oncocytic variant of FTC, accounting for 3–7 % of all thyroid carcinomas [36]. Little is known about its biological characteristics or clinical behavior. When Hürthle cells comprise more than 75 % of an encapsulated nodule, the lesion is classified as a Hürthle cell neoplasm, either an adenoma or carcinoma. As in FTC, there is no reliable preoperative diagnostic test to differentiate HTC from Hürthle cell adenoma [37]. The low incidence and lack of long-term follow-up data have caused controversy regarding its survival characteristics [38]. This poses a diagnostic and therapeutic challenge. HTC has different biological behavior – usually not observed in FTC – like nodal metastasis, intrathyroidal spread, and poor ^{131}I uptake [39, 40]. The survival is described to be around 74 and 49 % at 5 and 10 years, respectively [40]. Pulmonary metastases are most common, but metastases also occur in the bone, liver, and central nervous system. Literature shows that about 67 % of patients with metastatic HTC have lung metastases, 58 % soft tissue metastases, 33 % nodal metastases, 17 % bone metastases, and 17 % brain metastases [40]. Like patients with PTC and FTC, sorafenib is also active in patients with advanced HTC [35].

Medullary Thyroid Carcinoma

Medullary thyroid carcinoma (MTC) is an oncological entity on its own and accounts for 5–8 % of all thyroid cancers, originating from the calcitonin-secreting C cells of the thyroid [3, 44]. MTC is mainly sporadic in nature, but hereditary patterns (multiple endocrine neoplasia type 2 (MEN type 2) and familial medullary thyroid carcinoma (FMTC)) are present in 20–30 % of patients. These genetic diseases are inherited in an autosomal-dominant pattern and are caused by mutations of the rearranged during transfection (RET) proto-oncogene [41]. The primary treatment of both hereditary and sporadic forms of MTC is surgery by means of total thyroidectomy and extensive lymph node dissection. Locoregional recurrence frequently occurs in MTC, and tumor control may be improved by standard central, bilateral, and upper mediastinal neck dissection [42]. In MTC patients, extrathyroidal extension and stage at diagnosis are the only independent predictors of (recurrence-free) life expectancy. Patients diagnosed in an early stage of disease and patients without detectable recurrence have a favorable life expectancy independent of biochemical cure [43]. Distant metastases are the main cause of death in patients with MTC and in 50 % they present synchronous and at multiple sites [41]. Metastases often simultaneously affect various organs, such as liver, lungs, and bones and, less frequently, brain and skin. Survival is 51 % at 1 year, 26 % at 5 years, and 10 % at 10 years. However, the prognosis can be variable and long-term survival of more than 15–20 years has been described [41, 44]. In the follow-up of MTC, measurements of serum calcitonin and carcinoembryonic antigen (CEA) are of great importance as they reflect the presence of persistent disease. Surgery is the only potential curative treatments for distant metastases but usually multiple distant metastases require systemic therapy [44]. Recently, vandetanib was studied in a phase III trial for advanced MTC and demonstrated therapeutic efficacy with a median PFS of 19.3 months in the placebo group and 30.5 months in the treatment group [45]. When MTC impairs quality of life caused by hyper-calcitonemia-associated diarrhea or pain from local tumor growth, a need might arise for efficient tumor reduction [46]. In patients with predominant liver involvement, thermoablation, embolization, or transarterial chemoembolization (TACE) can reduce tumor mass and ameliorate symptoms [41, 47].

Anaplastic Thyroid Carcinoma

ATC is the most lethal type of thyroid cancer, with an overall median survival time of less than 6 months from diagnosis. Anecdotal cases of long-term survivors have been reported, mainly in patients with intra-thyroid tumors at the time of surgical treatment [48]. Almost all patients are classified as stage IV, with the primary lesion restricted to the thyroid gland in stage IVA; locoregional lymph nodes may exist in IVA/IVB, whereas stage IVC disease is defined by distant metastases [49]. Besic et al. studied the sites of metastases of ATC in an autopsy series of 45 patients and observed metastases in 41 cases (91 %). The most common sites of metastases were the lungs (78 %), intrathoracic lymph nodes (58 %), neck lymph nodes (51 %), pleura (29 %), adrenal glands (24 %), liver (20 %), brain (18 %), heart (18 %), and retroperitoneal lymph nodes (18 %) [50]. Causes of cancer-related mortality are distant metastases in 51.5 % (range 12–68 %), local complications in 23.7 % (5–37 %), or both in 26.2 % of patients (25–51 %) [48, 49, 51]. There is no place for surgery for distant metastases in ATC as it does not contribute to survival. The main aim of treatment focuses on prevention of complications by local tumor progression and can be obtained by palliative treatment, e.g., external beam radiotherapy and possibly surgery.

13.3 Current Strategies for Liver-Directed Therapies of Liver Tumors

The liver is frequently involved by metastatic disease. Although nearly all primary tumors can metastasize to the liver, especially digestive tract tumors often give rise to liver metastases. Drainage of these organs via the portal system directly toward the liver is the major contributing anatomical background. In the early days of liver surgery for metastatic disease, predominantly metastases of colorectal origin were treated by partial liver resection. The paradigm of limited liver involvement, no extrahepatic disease, and "easily" resectable metastases has undergone a dramatic change. Nowadays, unresectable liver tumors are converted into resectable liver tumors by increasing the future liver remnant with portal vein embolization and decreasing size and number by neoadjuvant chemotherapy or by combining partial liver resection with local ablative therapy like radiofrequency ablation (RFA) [52, 53]. Ablation of liver tumors is considered to be a new treatment strategy in comparison to partial liver resection, and as a consequence many require evidence

Table 13.2 Currently available liver-directed therapies in the treatment of liver tumors

	Tumor destruction	
Approach	Mechanism	Technique
Direct puncture	Heat	Radiofrequency ablation Microwave ablation
	Cold	Cryoablation
	Electrical	Irreversible electroporation-perforation
	Chemical	Ethanol injection
Indirect	Ionizing radiation	Stereotactic radiotherapy Proton radiotherapy
Tumor vasculature	*Embolizing*	
	Ionizing radiation	Radio-embolization with beads
	Ischemia	Transarterial embolization
	Ischemia and drugs	Transarterial chemoembolization
Hepatic vasculature	*Non-embolizing*	
	Local drugs	Hepatic artery infusion
	Regional drugs	Isolated liver perfusion

before it can be introduced as a useful strategy. In this respect it is important to realize that thermoablation of liver was published as early as 1961, only 4 years after the first published liver resection [54]. Currently, several interventional approaches are used to treat liver tumors [54]. Since the introduction of less invasive, local or regional, treatment modalities of liver tumors, other more "exotic" metastatic tumor types than colorectal liver metastases are increasingly considered for treatment [55]. Locoregional liver-directed therapies can be classified as depicted in Table 13.2. For many patients with non-colorectal liver metastasis, decision making on the best type of therapy – if any – cannot be based on evidence. For these patients, personalized medicine using clinical reasoning – based on knowledge of tumor biology – and expertise in liver-directed treatments should guide the best therapeutic approach. In this context, the following variables will be of influence: (1) tumor progression ("stable" versus progressive disease); (2) localization (liver-only versus liver-predominant); (3) presence of symptoms (asymptomatic versus symptomatic); (4) the impact and risks of the intended therapy; (5) the aim of therapy (intentionally curative, not curative but aiming at prolongation of life, palliative with the aim to ameliorate symptoms); and (6) the availability, expected response, and toxicity of systemic treatments. In patients with distant metastases of thyroid cancer, reduction of large metastatic tumor masses (debulking) could be useful to make the ^{131}I therapy for other smaller remaining metastases more effective [56]. On the one end of the spectrum is the (theoretical) patient with severe debilitating symptoms from a liver-only, relatively stable, potentially curable liver metastasis which can be treated by a minimal invasive – e.g., percutaneous – thermoablation, for whom the alternative would be a highly toxic systemic treatment. In such an example, the decision for treatment will be relatively straight forward. On the other side of the spectrum is the patient with equally debilitating symptoms, with rapidly progressive, widespread metastatic disease for whom a major liver resection needs to be performed, knowing that this will offer only palliation. These cases will probably be withheld from invasive treatment and will be offered best supportive care. In between these extremes are patients in whom decision making is far more complex and prone to extensive discussions. In conclusion, the benefit-risk ratio has dramatically shifted toward a lower risk for patients with liver metastases when treated by minimal invasive locoregional liver-directed treatments. This paves the way for a more liberal use of these treatments probably also in patients with liver metastases from thyroid cancer.

13.4 Diagnosis and Treatment of Liver Metastases in Thyroid Cancer

Over the last 30 years, 57 patients were reported in 25 case reports for which various treatments were used (Table 13.3) [1, 46, 47, 56–77]. Seven patients were found with liver metastases from FTC, 40 from MTC, six from PTC, and three from HTC.

13.4.1 Papillary Thyroid Carcinoma

There are three case reports describing six patients with PTC and hepatic metastases (Table 13.1) [56–58]. All cases reveal the major limitations of planar imaging and its lack of anatomic precision. They also illustrate the benefit of ^{131}I single-photon emission computed tomography (SPECT)/CT which offers an accurate anatomic localization that planar whole body ^{131}I imaging lacks. ^{131}I SPECT/CT has an important role in clarifying equivocal findings in metastasized PTC as especially the concomitant CT scan, even when low dosed and without contrast, lends SPECT tremendous localizing potential. Therefore, this technique has the potential to alter patient management and provide important clinical information [24]. Well-differentiated thyroid tissue has the capability to take up iodine but is metabolically inactive, while less-differentiated thyroid tissue loses its capability to trap ^{131}I and becomes metabolically more active [63]. This so-called "flip-flop" phenomenon makes position emission tomography (PET) with ^{18}F-fluoro-2-deoxy-D-glucose (^{18}F-FDG) valuable for the detection of ^{131}I negative metastases [74]. In the described cases, several treatment modalities were used; five patients were treated with surgery by means of segment resection, and one patient was treated with RFA [56–58]. RFA should be considered as a potential treatment option next to resection, ^{131}I, external beam radiotherapy, or transarterial (chemo) embolization (TACE). Furthermore, it can also be considered in those patients in whom the metastases have low or no^{131}I uptake or for those who have stopped uptaking ^{131}I after several treatments in the past [24, 74, 78].

Table 13.3 Case reports 1984–2014 reporting hepatic metastases in thyroid cancer

Author	Year of publication	Total pts	Diagnosis	No. liver mets	Therapy	Follow-up (months)
Agriantonis et al. [56]	2009	1	PTC	1	RFA	–
VandenBusche et al. [57]	2011	4	PTC	4	Surgery	–
Mosci et al. [58]	2012	1	PTC	1	Surgery	–
Brown et al. [59]	1984	1	FTC	–	I^{131}	–
Guglielmi et al. [60]	1999	1	FTC	–	Laser coagulation	–
Kondo et al. [61]	2000	1	FTC	1	Surgery and RFA	–
Kelessis et al. [62]	2005	1	FTC	1	I^{131}	14
Kouso et al. [63]	2005	1	FTC	2	Surgery	>24
Mackie et al. [64]	2005	1	FTC	1	I^{131}	6
Salvatori et al. [1]	2004	1	HTC	1	Surgery	22
Oreel et al. [65]	2006	1	HTC	1	Surgery	–
Hui Zhang et al. [66]	2011	1	HTC	>8	Docetaxel and cisplatin	–
Siperstein et al. [67]	1997	1	MTC	1	RFA	2
Curley et al. [68]	1999	1	MTC	–	RFA	–
Machens et al. [69]	2000	1	MTC	–	TACE	0
Siperstein, Berber [70]	2001	6	MTC	–	RFA	–
El Rassi et al. [71]	2002	1	MTC	–	Surgery + RT	–
Lorenz et al. [46]	2005	11	MTC	–	TACE	1–72
Fromigue et al. [47]	2006	12	MTC	–	TACE	15–28
Elvin et al. [72]	2005	2	MTC	2	RFA	38
Iftikhar et al. [73]	2006	1	MTC	>8	No treatment	–
Wertenbroek et al. [74]	2008	3	MTC (FTC)	7	RFA	6–72
Imperiale et al. [75]	2010	1	MTC	1	Surgery	–
Souncess et al. [76]	2013	1	MTC	>8	No therapy reported	–
Waters et al. [77]	2013	1	MTC	1	No therapy reported	240

PTC papillary thyroid carcinoma, *FTC* follicular thyroid carcinoma, *HTC* Hürthle cell carcinoma, *MTC* medullary thyroid cancer, *WDTC* well-differentiated thyroid carcinoma, *RFA* radiofrequency ablation, *TACE* transarterial chemoembolization, *RT* radiotherapy, I^{131} radioactive iodine treatment

13.4.2 Follicular Thyroid Carcinoma

Seven case reports were found with hepatic metastases in FTC (Table 13.3) [59–64, 74]. In one of the cases, it was recommended that the patient should undergo a second operation to remove a liver mass; however, she refused and was therefore managed with ^{131}I [62]. Another case illustrates a patient with a liver mass who was eventually treated successfully with RFA followed by ^{131}I treatment [62].

Furthermore, a segment resection was performed as a tumor debulking procedure which enhanced the effectiveness of ^{131}I postoperatively [56, 67]. In a situation like this, TACE could have been an alternative for the management of a large liver metastasis [62]. This method has been successfully applied in patients with liver metastases from gastrointestinal and other endocrine malignancies, but there is little experience regarding its effectiveness for the treatment of liver metastases from FTC. It is known that TACE is a successful technique in the treatment of various liver tumors. In hepatic arterial anatomy variation, arteriovenous shunting can sometimes make TACE a potential complicated procedure [79]. The rate of major complications after TACE is rather low (5 %) but the postembolization syndrome is reported in up to 90 % of patients [80]. This syndrome consists of fever, abdominal pain, nausea, and vomiting and is the main reason for prolongation of hospital stay after TACE. Both RFA and TACE have weak and strong points; RFA is a very effective local tumor treatment with a low complication rate, and TACE has a more diffuse effect on the liver but is associated with a potentially higher complication rate [47, 48, 80].

13.4.3 Hürthle Cell Carcinoma

Most HTC's show impaired ^{131}I entrapment, which poses a diagnostic and therapeutic challenge [40, 65, 66]. In this tumor type, ^{18}F-FDG PET is of value for diagnosis and follow-up. Nevertheless, it is still worthwhile to evaluate ^{131}I uptake as there are not many other therapeutic options. Although I^{131} has no survival benefit, generally outcomes are still improved by means of adjuvant ablation therapy [81]. Three cases describe a hepatic disseminated HTC [1, 65, 66]. In the first two cases surgical resections were performed, and the last case was withheld from local surgical treatment and administrated docetaxel and cisplatin [1, 66]. Therefore, RFA and cryoablation have also gained clinical interest recently as these procedures may alleviate pain and reduce tumor bulk, even as long survival data are not readily available.

13.4.4 Medullary Thyroid Carcinoma

Forty patients with hepatic metastases from MTC were reported [46, 47, 67–77]. It is well observed that the liver is the second most common organ for metastatic MTC preceded by lung and followed by bone metastases [3]. Hepatic MTC metastases typically present as small and multiple nodules [42, 43]. With this unpredictable clinical course, good palliation of tumor-related symptoms with high efficacy and low rate of side effects can be indicated. Fromigue et al. using TACE showed improved quality of life in two of five patients by reduction of diarrhea [43]. Currently, no consensus exists about the imaging modality that has the highest diagnostic accuracy for the management of patients with metastatic or recurrent MTC. Anatomical imaging techniques include ultrasonography of the neck, CT, and MRI; scintigraphic imaging techniques include 99mTc-V-dimercapto-sulphuricacid (99mTc-V-DMSA),

^{111}In-labeled somatostatin receptor scintigraphy (SRS), and PET-labeled with ^{18}F-FDG and with ^{18}F-dihydroxyphenylalanine (^{18}F-DOPA). The diverse modalities have complementary values depending on different tumor characteristics. ^{18}F-FDG PET/CT has a limited utility if the calcitonin level is less than 500 ng/L [82]. Despite this, ^{18}F-FDG PET is especially useful in tumors with calcitonin doubling time shorter than 12 months, identifying patients with poor survival. ^{18}F-DOPA PET has a reported sensitivity of about 62 %, possibly reflecting the more indolent type of MTC, but combined with CT imaging the reported sensitivities may increase to 94 and 100 % [83–85]. It has to be emphasized that surgical treatment is focused on palliation of symptoms by tumor load reduction. This probably explains why – as summarized in Table 13.3 – only two of the 40 patients underwent surgery and the other patients no treatment or minimal invasive treatments [75]. Furthermore, 11 RFA procedures were performed, three patients could not be treated at all, and in total 24 patients underwent TACE. The diffuse targeting area that goes with TACE is better suited to treat diffusely spread liver metastases compared to the local effect of RFA. In most of the cases, side effects of TACE were mild, and hepatic parameters were always normalized within 4 weeks after the procedure [46, 47, 69, 86]. Lorenz et al. propose a clinical protocol and algorithm based on four categories of patients with metastatic MTC [46]. Patients with resectable liver metastases without micrometastasis can be candidates for liver resection. Patients in whom additional, limited (in number and size) metastases in the contralateral liver lobe are present can be treated with thermoablation in combination with partial liver resection [52]. The third group, according to Lorenz, consists of patients with bilobar, diffusely spread metastases, or large lesions with multiple small liver metastases qualify for TACE. We disagree with Lorenz et al. and think that thermoablation with the aim to obtain symptomatic relief has a better value. Even when metastases are larger than 5 cm, they can be attempted to control by overlapping RFA zones taking care not to damage larger bile ducts because this can result in biliary fistulae, strictures, or abscesses [87].

13.5 Conclusions and Recommendations

Despite a scarcity in literature, this chapter tries to set the stage for an innovative and conceptually different way of thinking about the treatment of liver metastases of thyroid cancer. Based on the perspective of the various biological subtypes of thyroid cancer (PTC, FTC, MTC, HCC, and ATC), new liver-directed treatments are nowadays available which can ameliorate the symptomatic patient and possibly contribute to a better quality of life and – less likely – a better survival. The different thyroid cancer disease entities have genuine different biological characteristics and a thorough understanding of these varieties is essential in organizing a successful treatment. Having said this, in the treatment of liver metastases in general, recently the benefit-risk ratio has dramatically improved toward a lower risk for patients with liver metastases when treated by minimal invasive locoregional liver-directed treatments. Thus, when thyroid cancer disseminates to the liver, patients can also increasingly be considered for curative or palliative treatment options. In general, the aim of applying these liver-directed therapies on liver metastases in thyroid carcinoma is mainly with palliative intent as distant metastases in thyroid cancer are always a reflection of widespread disease. Nevertheless, as metastasized thyroid cancer patients can have a considerable life expectancy, aiming for a good or reasonable quality of life is an important and a realistic goal to achieve. Minimal invasive therapies like RFA should be considered as a cytoreductive modality next to resection, ^{131}I, TKI's, external beam radiotherapy, or transarterial (chemo)embolization (TACE) or combinations of any of these treatment types. It has to be emphasized that a multimodality treatment of these liver-directed therapies in combination with ^{131}I might be more successful rather than choosing either one of them as a single therapy. Hypothetically, surgical tumor bulk reduction before ^{131}I treatment should enhance the effectiveness of ^{131}I treatment, as it prevents ^{131}I to be absorbed completely by one large tumor deposit. After surgical cytoreduction of bulky tumors, ^{131}I could more effectively treat smaller tumor deposits. Liver-disseminated thyroid cancer patients that also seem candidates for the usage of minimal invasive liver-directed therapies are those in whom the metastases have low or no ^{131}I uptake and those who have lost avidity after diverse treatments in the past. For this category, the risk of developing myeloproliferative disorders or a secondary malignancy is at risk and therefore the option of alternative treatment modalities like RFA should always be considered. Also, tumor debulking with the aim to reduce symptoms should be kept in mind as a serious option. Especially in MTC, palliation of tumor-related symptoms with high efficacy and low rate of side effects can add to quality of life, and therapies like RFA and TACE are able to achieve good temporary results [74]. The expertise about liver-directed therapies should be concentrated as much as possible in so-called "centers of expertise" to achieve high-quality and minimal complication rates. In these centers, the threshold for endocrinologists to seek for advice or referral should be kept as low as possible. Also, these centers have the ethical obligation to carefully document generated data and outcomes of these treatments. Internationally organized databases, collecting case series of patients, should provide support for liver-directed minimal invasive locoregional treatments. The recent rapid evolution has not only expanded possibilities but also has supplied us with a task, a task to explore these new barriers. Without doubts, in the following decade the ongoing development of liver-directed therapies will benefit the outcome of patients with liver metastases from any origin and thus also for patients with liver metastases in thyroid carcinoma.

References

1. Salvatori M, Perotti G, Rufini V et al (2004) Solitary liver metastasis from Hürthle cell thyroid cancer: a case report and review of the literature. J Endocrinol Investig 27:52–56
2. Song HJ, Xue YL, Xu YH et al (2011) Rare metastases of differentiated thyroid carcinoma: pictorial review. Endocr Relat Cancer 18:165–174
3. Lee J, Soh EY (2010) Differentiated thyroid carcinoma presenting with distant metastasis at initial diagnosis, clinical outcomes and prognostic factors. Ann Surg 251:114–119

4. Machens A, Dralle H (2013) Prognostic impact of N staging in 715 medullary thyroid cancer patients: proposal for a revised staging system. Ann Surg 257:323–329
5. Pacini F, Castagna MG, Brilli L, Pentheroudakis G (2010) Thyroid cancer: ESMO Clinical Practice Guidelines for diagnosis, treatment and follow-up, on behalf of the ESMO Guidelines Working Group. Ann Oncol 21:v214–v219
6. IKNL; Dutch thyroid cancer guidelines (Richtlijn Schildkliercarcinoom) conceptversion 3.0: 2014. http://www.oncoline.nl/schildkliercarcinoom
7. Dralle H, Musholt TJ, Schabram J et al (2013) German Association of Endocrine Surgeons practice guideline for the surgical management of malignant thyroid tumors. Langenbecks Arch Surg 398:347–375
8. Guidelines for the management of thyroid cancer (2007) 2nd edn. British Thyroid Association, Royal College of Physicians. www.british-thyroid-association.org
9. Cooper DS, Doherty GM, Bryan R et al (2013) Revised American Thyroid Association management guidelines for patients with thyroid nodules and differentiated thyroid cancer. Thyroid 19:1167–1214
10. Lerch H, Schober O, Kuwert T, Saur HB (1997) Survival of differentiated thyroid carcinoma studied in 500 patients. J Clin Oncol 15:2067–2075
11. Davies L, Welch HG (2006) Increasing incidence of thyroid cancer in the United States 1973–2002. JAMA 295:2164–2167
12. Enyioha C, Roman SA, Sosa JA (2013) Central lymph node dissection in patients with papillary thyroid cancer: a population level analysis of 14,257 cases. Am J Surg 205:655–661
13. Kruijff S, Petersen JF, Chen P et al (2014) Patterns of structural recurrence in papillary thyroid cancer. World J Surg 38:653–659
14. Links TP, van Tol KM, Jager PL et al (2005) Life expectancy in differentiated thyroid cancer: a novel approach to survival analysis. Endocr Relat Cancer 12:273–280
15. Kruijff S, Aniss AM, Chen P et al (2013) Decreasing the dose of radioiodine for remnant ablation does not increase structural recurrence rates in papillary thyroid carcinoma. Surgery 154:1337–1344; discussion 1344–5
16. Mallick U, Harmer C, Hackshaw A et al (2012) Iodine or not for low-risk differentiated thyroid cancer: the next UK National Cancer Research Network randomised trial following HiLo. Clin Oncol (R Coll Radiol) 24:159–161
17. Aggarwal V, Bhargav PR, Mishra A et al (2007) Clinico-pathological characteristics and long-term outcome in patients with distant metastases from differentiated thyroid carcinoma. World J Surg 31:246–247
18. Mazzaferri EL, Jhiang SM (1994) Long-term impact of initial surgical and medical therapy on papillary and follicular thyroid cancer. Am J Med 97:418–428
19. Goffredo P, Sosa JA, Roman SA (2013) Differentiated thyroid cancer presenting with distant metastases: a population analysis over two decades. World J Surg 37:1599–1605
20. Elisei R, Molinaro E et al (2010) Are the clinical and pathological features of differentiated thyroid carcinoma really changed over the last 35 years? Study on 4187 patients from a single Italian institution to answer this question. J Clin Endocrinol Metab 95:1516–1527
21. Ruegemer JJ, Hay ID, Bergstralh EJ et al (1988) Distant metastases in differentiated 9487 thyroid carcinoma: a multivariate analysis of prognostic variables. J Clin Endocrinol Metab 67:501–508
22. Shaha AR, Shah JP, Loree TR (1997) Differentiated thyroid cancer presenting initially with distant metastasis. Am J Surg 174:474–476
23. Haq M, Harmer C (2005) Differentiated thyroid carcinoma with distant metastases at presentation: prognostic factors and outcome. Clin Endocrinol 63:87–93
24. Durante C, Haddy N, Baudin E et al (2006) Long term outcome of 444 patients with distant metastases from papillary and follicular thyroid carcinoma: benefits and limits of radioiodine therapy. J Clin Endocrinol Metab 91:2892–2899
25. Nixon IJ, Whitcher MW, Palmer FL et al (2012) The impact of distant metastases at presentation on prognosis in patients with differentiated carcinoma of the thyroid gland. Thyroid 22:884–889

26. Lang BH, Wong KP, Cheung CJ (2013) Evaluating the prognostic factors associated with cancer-specific survival of differentiated thyroid carcinoma presenting with distant metastasis. Ann Surg Oncol 20:1329–1335
27. Schlumberger M, Tubiana M, De Vathaire F et al (1986) Long-term results of treatment of 283 patients with lung and bone metastases from differentiated thyroid carcinoma. J Clin Endocrinol Metab 63:960–967
28. Baudain E, Schlumberger M (2007) New therapeutic approaches for metastatic thyroid carcinoma. Lancet Oncol 8:148–156
29. Schlumberger M, Challeton C, De Vathaire F et al (1996) Radioactive iodine treatment and external radiotherapy for lung and bone metastases from thyroid carcinoma. J Nucl Med 37:598–605
30. Protopapas AD, Nicholson AG, Vini L, Harmer CL, Goldstraw P (2001) Thoracic metastasectomy in thyroid malignancies. Ann Thorac Surg 72:1906–1908
31. Stojadinovic A, Shoup M, Ghossein RA et al (2002) The role of operations for distantly metastatic well-differentiated thyroid carcinoma. Surgery 131:636–643
32. Niederle B, Roka R, Schemper M et al (1986) Surgical treatment of distant metastases in differentiated thyroid cancer: indications and results. Surgery 100:1088–1096
33. Proye CA, Dromer DH, Carnaille BM et al (1992) Is it still worthwhile to treat bone metastases from differentiated thyroid carcinoma with radioactive iodine? World J Surg 16:640–645; discussion 645–6
34. Zettenig G, Fueger BJ, Passler C et al (2002) Long-term follow-up of patients with bone metastases from differentiated thyroid carcinoma – surgery or conventional therapy? Clin Endocrinol 56:377–382
35. Brose MS, Nutting CM, Elisei R et al (2014) Sorafenib in radioacrive iodine refractory locally advanced or metastatic differentiated thyroid cancer: A randomized double blind phase III trial. Lancet 384:319–328
36. Hürthle K (1894) Beiträge zur Kenntnis des Sekretionsvorganges in der Schilddrüse. Arch Ges Physiol 56:1–44
37. Montone KT, Baloch ZW, LiVolsi VA (2008) The thyroid Hürthle (oncocytic) cell and its associated pathologic conditions: a surgical pathology and cytopathology review. Arch Pathol Lab Med 132:1241–1250
38. DeLellis RA, Lloyd RV, Heitz PU, Eng C (2004) WHO classification of tumours, pathology and genetics of tumours of endocrine organs. IARC, Lyon, pp 73–76
39. Sugino K, Kameyama K, Ito K (2013) Does Hürthle cell carcinoma of the thyroid have a poorer prognosis than ordinary follicular thyroid carcinoma? Ann Surg Oncol 20:2944–2950
40. Kushchayeva Y, Duh QY, Kebebew E, Clark OH (2004) Prognostic indications for Hürthle cell cancer. World J Surg 28:1266–1270
41. Pacini F, Castagna MG, Cipri C, Schlumberger M (2010) Medullary thyroid carcinoma, overview. Clin Oncol 22:475–485
42. de Groot JW, Links TP, Sluiter WJ et al (2007) Loco-regional control in patients with palpable medullary thyroid cancer: results of standardized compartment-oriented surgery. Head Neck 29:857–863
43. de Groot JW, Plukker JT, Wolffenbuttel BH et al (2006) Determinants of life expectancy in medullary thyroid cancer: age does not matter. J Clin Endocrinol 65:729–736
44. Van Heerden JA, Grant CS, Gharib H et al (1990) Long-term course of patients with persistent hypercalcitoninemia after apparent curative primary surgery for medullary thyroid carcinoma. Ann Surg 212:395–400
45. Wells SA Jr, Robinson BG, Gagel RF et al (2012) Vandetanib in patients with locally advanced or metastatic medullary thyroid cancer: a randomized, double-blind phase III trial. J Clin Oncol 30:134–141
46. Lorenz K, Brauckhoff M, Behrmann C et al (2005) Selective arterial chemo embolization for hepatic metastases from medullary thyroid carcinoma. Surgery 138:986–993
47. Fromigue J, de Baere T, Baudin E et al (2006) Chemoembolization for liver metastases from medullary thyroid carcinoma. J Clin Endocrinol Metab 91:2496–2499

48. Lim SM, Shin SJ, Chung WY et al (2012) Treatment outcome of patients with anaplastic thyroid cancer: a single center experience. Yonsei Med J 53:352–357
49. Smallridge RC (2012) Approach to the patient with anaplastic thyroid carcinoma. J Clin Endocrinol Metab 97:2566–2572
50. Besic N, Gazic B (2013) Sites of metastases of anaplastic thyroid carcinoma: autopsy findings in 45 cases from a single institution. Thyroid 23:709–713
51. Granata R, Locati L, Licitra L (2013) Therapeutic strategies in the management of patients with metastatic anaplastic thyroid cancer: review of the current literature. Curr Opin Oncol 25:224–228
52. de Jong KP (2007) Review article: multimodality treatment of liver metastases increases suitability for surgical treatment. Aliment Pharmacol Ther 26:161–169
53. de Jong KP, Wertenbroek MW (2011) Liver resection combined with local ablation: where are the limits? Dig Surg 28:127–133
54. de Jong KP (2011) What is new in liver surgery? Focus on thermoablation and the relevance of the inflammatory response. Minerva Chir 66:561–572
55. van Laarhoven S, van Baren R, Tamminga RYJ, de Jong KP (2012) Radiofrequency ablation in the treatment of liver tumors in children. J Pediatr Surg 47:e7–e12
56. Agriantonis DJ, Hall L, Wilson MA (2009) Utility of SPECT/CT as an adjunct to planar whole body I-131 imaging. Liver metastasis from papillary thyroid cancer. Clin Nucl Med 34:247–248
57. VandenBusche CJ, Cocke CD, Kay LQ (2011) Fine needle aspiration of metastatic papillary thyroid carcinoma found in the liver. Diagn Cytopathol 41:418–421
58. Mosci C, Mc Dougall IR, Jeffrey RB, Iagaru A (2012) ^{18}F-FDG PET/CT demonstration of a liver metastasis in a patient with papillary thyroid cancer. Clin Nucl Med 37:234–236
59. Brown AP, Greening WP, McCready VR, Shaw HJ, Harmer CL (1984) Radioiodine treatment of metastatic thyroid carcinoma: the Royal Marsden Hospital experience. Br J Radiol 57:323–327
60. Guglielmi R, Pacella CM, Dottorini ME et al (1999) Severe thyrotoxicosis due to hyperfunctioning liver metastasis from follicular carcinoma: treatment with I and interstitial laser ablation. Thyroid 9:173–177
61. Kondo T, Katoh R, Omata K et al (2000) Incidentally detected liver metastasis of well differentiated follicular carcinoma of the thyroid, mimicking ectopic thyroid. Pathol Int 50:509–513
62. Kelessis NG, Prassis PE, Dimitra DV et al (2005) Unusual metastatic spread of follicular carcinoma: report of a case. Surg Today 35:300–303
63. Kouso H, Ikegami T, Ezaki T et al (2005) Liver metastasis from thyroid carcinoma 32 years after resection of the primary tumor: report of a case. Surg Today 35:480–482
64. Mackie GC, Shulkin BL (2005) Amiodarone-induced hyperthyroidism in a patient with functioning papillary carcinoma of the thyroid and extensive hepatic metastases. Thyroid 15:1337–1340
65. Oreel MA, Tiel-van Buul MMC, de Bruin PC, Koelemij R, Verzijlbergen JF (2006) Hürthle cell carcinoma with a giant cystic liver metastasis imaged with 18F-labeled fluorodeoxyglucose-positron emission tomography. Thyroid 16:195–196
66. Zhang H, Zeng L, Liang C et al (2012) Successful treatment of Hürthle cell thyroid carcinoma with lung and liver metastasis using docetaxel and cisplatin. Jpn J Clin Oncol 42:1086–1090
67. Siperstein AE, Rogers SJ, Hansen PD, Gitomirsky A (1997) Laparoscopic thermal ablation of hepatic neuroendocrine tumor metastases. Surgery 122:1147–1154
68. Curley SA, Izzo F, Delrio P et al (1999) Radio frequency ablation of unresectable primary and metastatic hepatic malignancies: results in 123 patients. Ann Surg 230:1–8
69. Machens A, Behrmann C, Dralle H (2002) Chemoembolization of liver metastases from medullary thyroid carcinoma. Ann Intern Med 132:596–597
70. Siperstein AE, Berber (2001) Cryoablation, percutaneous alcohol injection, and radiofrequency ablation for treatment of neuroendocrine liver metastases. World J Surg 25:693–696

71. El Rassi ZS, Ferdinand L, Mohsine RM et al (2002) Primary and secondary liver endocrine tumors: clinical presentation, surgical approach and outcome. Hepatogastroenterology 49:1340–1346
72. Elvin A, Skogseid B, Hellman P (2005) Radiofrequency ablation of neuroendocrine liver metastases. Abdom Imaging 30:427–434
73. Iftikhar A, Johns W, Gupta SM (2006) Visualization of hepatic metastases of medullary thyroid carcinoma on Tc-99m MDP bone scintigraphy. Clin Nucl Med 31:611–613
74. Wertenbroek MWJLAE, Links TP, Prins TR et al (2008) Radiofrequency ablation of hepatic metastases from thyroid carcinoma. Thyroid 18:1105–1110
75. Imperiale A, Greget M, Chabrier G et al (2010) Solitary hepatic metastasis from medullary thyroid carcinoma mimicking atypical hemangioma insights from multimodality diagnostic approach by MRI, F-18 FDG and F-18 FDOPA PET/CT. Clin Nucl Med 35:434–437
76. Souncess BD, Schembri GP (2013) ^{68}Ga-dotatate avid medullary thyroid cancer with occult liver metastases. Clin Nucl Med 39:87–90
77. Waters KM, Syed ZA, Erozan YS, Olson MT (2014) Smoldering medullary thyroid carcinoma liver metastasis 37 years after resection of an organ-confined tumor. Diagn cytopath E pub ahead of print
78. Rubino C, De VF, Dottorini ME et al (2003) Second primary malignancies in thyroid cancer patients. Br J Cancer 89:1638–1644
79. Liu DM, Salem R, Bui JT et al (2005) Angiographic considerations in patients undergoing liver-directed therapy. J Vasc Interv Radiol 16:911–935
80. Leung DA, Goin JE, Sickles C et al (2001) Determinants of postembolization syndrome after hepatic chemoembolization. J Vasc Interv Radiol 12:321–326
81. Lopez-Penabad L, Chiu AC, Hoff AO et al (2003) Prognostic factors in patients with Hürthle cell neoplasms of the thyroid. Cancer 97:1186–1194
82. Mahnken AH, Pareire PL, de Baère T (2013) Interventional oncologic approaches to liver metastases. Radiology 266:407–430
83. Hoegerle S, Altehoefer C, Ghanem N et al (2001) 18F-DOPA positron emission tomography for tumour detection in patients with medullary thyroid carcinoma and elevated calcitonin levels. Eur J Nucl Med 28:64–71
84. Koopmans KP, de Groot JW, Plukker JT et al (2008) 18F-dihydroxyphenylalanine PET in patients with biochemical evidence of medullary thyroid cancer: relation to tumor differentiation. J Nucl Med 49:524–531
85. Luster M, Karges W, Zeich K et al (2010) Clinical value of 18-fluorine-fluorodihydroxyphenylalanine positron emission tomography/computed tomography in the follow-up of medullary thyroid carcinoma. Thyroid 20:527–533
86. Kress O, Wagner HJ, Wied M et al (2003) Transarterial chemoembolization of advanced liver metastases of neuroendocrine tumors—a retrospective single center experience. Digestion 68:94–101
87. Elias D, Sideris L, Pocard M, Dromain C et al (2004) Intraductal cooling of the main bile ducts during radiofrequency ablation prevents biliary stenosis. J Am Coll Surg 198:717–721

Liver Metastases from Ureteral and Bladder Cancer

14

Manabu Tatokoro and Kazunori Kihara

14.1 Incidence

14.1.1 Epidemiology and Risk Factors of Urothelial Cancers

Urothelial cancers are the fourth most common tumors after prostate (or breast), lung, and colorectal cancer [1]. They are classified as lower urinary tract (bladder and urethra) or upper urinary tract (renal pelvis and ureter). Bladder cancers account for over 90 % of urothelial cancers [2]. Renal pelvic cancers are about twice as common as ureteral cancers. In 17 % of cases with upper urinary tract cancers, concurrent bladder cancers are present [3].

Smoking is the most common risk factor for them. Occupational exposure to aromatic amines and polycyclic aromatic hydrocarbons are other important risk factors. The impact of diet and environmental pollution is less evident [4]. There are familial cases of upper urinary tract cancers associated with hereditary nonpolyposis colorectal carcinoma [5].

14.1.2 Metastatic Pattern and Liver Metastases of Urothelial Cancers

While urothelial cancers spread to any organ, the most common metastatic locations are lymph nodes, lung, liver, and bone. Shinagare et al. evaluated the metastatic pattern of muscle-invasive bladder cancer [6]. Of 150 patients with

M. Tatokoro • K. Kihara
Department of Urology, Tokyo Medical and Dental University Graduate School, 1-5-45, Yushima, Bunkyo, Tokyo 113-8519, Japan
e-mail: tatokoro.uro@tmd.ac.jp

I. Di Carlo (ed.), *Noncolorectal, Nonneuroendocrine Liver Metastases: Diagnosis and Current Therapies*, DOI 10.1007/978-3-319-09293-5_14

metastatic urothelial cancer, the most common metastatic sites were lymph nodes (69 %), bone (47 %), lung (37 %), liver (26 %), and peritoneum (16 %). Ninety percent of the patients with liver metastases had multiple lesions, but only 10 % had a solitary liver metastatic lesion. Five percent of patients with liver metastasis had portal venous thrombosis [6]. Wallmeroth et al. investigated the metastatic behavior of bladder cancers with autopsies of 367 patients with muscle-invasive bladder cancer [7]. Metastases were found in 68 % of them and the most common metastatic sites were regional lymph nodes (90 %), liver (47 %), lung (45 %), and bone (32 %).

Shinagare et al. investigated the metastatic pattern of upper urinary tract cancers [8]. Of 52 patients with metastatic upper urinary tract cancer, lymph nodes (75 %), lung (65 %), liver (54 %), bone (39 %), and peritoneum (19 %) were the most common metastatic sites. Tumor location within the upper urinary tract has no effect on metastatic pattern. Ninety-two percent of the patients with liver metastases had multiple lesions, whereas only 7 % had a solitary liver metastasis.

Although liver metastases from urothelial cancers are common, those are considered a systemic disease associated with a dismal prognosis.

14.2 Natural History

14.2.1 Histology of Urothelial Cancers

More than 95 % of urothelial cancers are derived from the urothelium [1]. Morphological variants such as micropapillary, clear cell, neuroendocrine, and lymphoepithelial variants are associated with high-grade cancers [1]. Squamous cell carcinoma is associated with chronic inflammatory and infectious disease mainly associated with urolithiasis [9]. Other histological subtypes are adenocarcinomas, small cell carcinomas, and sarcomas [10].

14.2.2 Advanced/Metastatic Urothelial Cancers

At the initial diagnosis of bladder cancer, 30 % of cases are diagnosed as muscle-invasive disease and approximately 30 % of patients diagnosed with muscle-invasive disease have undetected metastases [11]. In contrast to bladder cancers, 60 % of upper urinary tract cancers are invasive at diagnosis [12].

Median survival in patients with locally advanced or metastatic urothelial cancer treated with chemotherapy was approximately 14 months and a 5-year survival rate was 14 %. Patients with visceral metastases had a median overall survival of 10 months and a 5-year survival rate of 6.8 % [13]. Especially, Abe et al. reported the median survival of those patients with visceral metastases beyond the lung was only 7 months [14].

14.2.3 Prognosis and Risk Factor of Metastatic Urothelial Cancers

Some investigators reported that the presence of visceral metastasis was of independent significance. Bajorin et al. reported Karnofsky performance status of <80 % and presence of visceral metastases were independent prognostic factors of poor survival after treatment with the standard chemotherapy [15]. Abe et al. demonstrated that absence of liver, bone, and local recurrence and resection of metastasis were independent significant predictors of prolonged survival [14].

14.3 Diagnosis

14.3.1 The Radiological Evaluation of Liver Metastases from Urothelial Cancers

Although liver metastases are common in patients with disseminated urothelial cancer, there is little data to suggest specific imaging features that enable metastases of urothelial cancers to be distinguished from other hypovascular liver metastases [16]. Computed tomography is the diagnostic techniques of choice to detect metastases to liver [17]. On CT imaging, the liver metastases of urothelial cancers were usually of low attenuation [6]. When there is uncertainty regarding the interpretation of CT, MRI or positron emission tomography CT may be employed [16]. T2-weighted MRI image of liver metastases usually demonstrates multiple foci of T2 hyperintensity. Gd-enhanced T1-weighted image demonstrates peripheral enhancement of these metastatic liver lesions [18]. Fludeoxyglucose positron emission tomography/CT is reported to improve staging because of its higher sensitivity for metastatic disease [19].

14.4 Treatment

14.4.1 Treatment Strategy for Metastatic Urothelial Cancers

Metastatic urothelial cancers, even if limited to a single site, are considered disseminated disease, and therefore systemic therapy is the mainstay of treatment.

According to the European Association of Urology (EAU) guideline [1, 17], the current mainstay of treatment for patients with metastatic urothelial cancer is systemic combination chemotherapy. Urothelial cancers are chemosensitive tumors and respond to several active agents, but recurrence after response to chemotherapy is inevitable.

Nearly half of patients diagnosed with metastatic urothelial cancer will eventually develop liver metastases [7]. As other distant metastases, the treatment strategy for liver metastases of urothelial cancer is systemic combination chemotherapy. Role of liver-directed therapies including surgery and interventional radiology has remained controversial in metastatic urothelial cancer.

14.4.2 Chemotherapy

Standard First-Line Chemotherapy

Combination chemotherapy including cisplatin has been the standard chemotherapy regimen for metastatic urothelial cancers since the late 1980s. Methotrexate, vinblastine, doxorubicin, and cisplatin (MVAC) regimen has been proven superior to cisplatin monotherapy [20]. In the late 1990s, some phase II trials of gemcitabine in combination with cisplatin (GC) demonstrated a response rate of over 40 % in the treatment of chemotherapy-naive patients with metastatic urothelial cancer [21, 22]. A randomized phase III study showed similar efficacy with response rate (GC, 49.4 %; MVAC, 45.7 %); however, a better safety profile was observed with GC [23]. In the updated analysis of the trial, overall survival was similar in both regimens with a median survival of 14.0 months for GC and 15.2 months for MVAC and the 5-year overall survival rates were 13.0 and 15.3 %, respectively [13]. Currently, the lower toxicity of GC has been a new standard regimen. As the further intensified chemotherapy, PCG regimen (paclitaxel, cisplatin, and gemcitabine) did not result in a significant improvement in overall survival in a randomized phase III trial, comparing PCG to GC, although the overall response rate was higher with PCG [24].

According to the EAU guideline, GC, PCG, MVAC, or high-dose MVAC with granulocyte colony-stimulating factor are recommended for above patients with normal renal function [17]. For patients with impaired renal function or whose performance status is unsatisfactory, using carboplatin is recommended instead of cisplatin.

Second-Line Chemotherapy

Second-line chemotherapy regimen for metastatic urothelial cancers remains controversial. Above all, vinflunine (VFL), a microtubule inhibitor, seems to be a reasonable second-line option for patients with progression after a platinum-containing regimen. In a randomized phase III study of VFL and best supportive care (BSC) versus BSC alone [25], VFL demonstrates a survival advantage in the eligible patient population without any harmful effect on quality of life. Currently, VFL is the only European Medicines Agency-approved agent in the second-line setting [17].

14.4.3 Surgery

Although role of surgery for liver metastases from colon cancer is well established [26], it is controversial in patients with metastatic non-colorectal cancer including urothelial cancers. Although a few cases of surgical intervention for liver metastasis, including a case of resection of solitary liver metastases without prior chemotherapy [27], have been reported, it is not generally considered the standard practice.

Post-chemotherapy Surgery for Residual Tumors

Although several investigators have indicated the importance of surgery for residual tumors after achieving a major clinical response to chemotherapy [28–30, 14], the impact on survival remains controversial. Moreover, selection of patients who receive benefits from post-chemotherapy surgery is not well established.

Of the 30 patients whose residual metastases were completely resected resulting in a complete response (CR) to MVAC chemotherapy plus surgery, 33 % remained alive at 5 years, similar to results attained for patients achieving a CR to chemotherapy alone [28]. Investigators at the MD Anderson Cancer Center observed 31 patients with metastatic urothelial cancer (lung in 24 cases, distant lymph nodes in 4, brain in 2) undergoing metastasectomy, with the intent of rendering these patients free from disease [30]. The median overall survival time from diagnosis of metastases was 31 months and they suggested that post-chemotherapy surgery for residual metastases is feasible and could contribute to long-term disease control, when integrated with effective chemotherapy and the tumor was considered surgically resectable with clear margins. Abe et al. reported 12 patients underwent metastasectomy (7 patients received lobectomy) of 48 patients with metastatic urothelial cancer underwent systemic chemotherapy [14]. The median overall survival in this group was 42 months, whereas that in patients without metastasectomy was 10 months. They described that lung metastases would be one of the good indications whereas; patients with liver metastasis did not seem to be likely candidates for metastasectomy because they usually had other sites of metastases.

Recently, a long-term multi-institutional retrospective study, including 42 patients who underwent resection of metastases from urothelial cancer, was reported. Metastasectomy included lymph node dissection in 20, pulmonary resection in 12, and, especially, liver resection in 1. Median overall survival was 26 months and the overall 5-year survival rate from metastasectomy was 31 % [31].

Although a CR to chemotherapy alone or chemotherapy plus surgery is the best correlate of prolonged survival, the majority of patients in those reports were treated with resection of the lymph nodes or lung.

14.4.4 Interventional Radiology

Liver metastases from urothelial cancer are usually multiple and diffuse, therefore candidates for local therapies are only in less than 10 % of those patients [8, 6]. As mentioned above, patients with liver metastases are not candidates for metastasectomy, and there is no report regarding the efficacy of surgery for liver metastases from urothelial cancers.

However, patients with a solitary or only several liver lesions after achieving a major clinical response to chemotherapy may receive benefits from liver-directed therapies. There are many patients who are not suitable for the surgery either because of comorbidity, tumor location, or inadequate hepatic reserve [32]. To my knowledge, there is no trial investigating the efficacy of an interventional radiology in patients with liver metastases from urothelial cancer. Scattered reports of the interventional radiology including some cases of hepatic arterial infusion chemotherapy [33, 34] in the management of focal metastatic lesions of urothelial cancer have appeared.

In current liver-directed therapies for liver malignancies, the most popular and widely practiced local treatment modality is radiofrequency thermal ablation (RFA) [35]. RFA is the most commonly used ablation technique and an effective therapy for primary and metastatic liver cancers, particularly for liver metastases from colorectal cancer [36].

On the basis of the results obtained with RFA in the treatment of liver metastases from colorectal cancer, Yasuda et al. treated a patient suffering from two liver metastases from ureteral cancer [37]. After three courses of GC chemotherapy, one tumor disappeared and another achieved a partial response. The patient underwent RFA for the residual mass followed by GC. More than 3 years after surgery, the patient has achieved a high quality of life. The findings have suggested RFA against hepatic metastases could contribute to long-term disease control when integrated with effective chemotherapy.

References

1. Roupret M, Babjuk M, Comperat E, Zigeuner R, Sylvester R, Burger M, Cowan N, Bohle A, Van Rhijn BW, Kaasinen E, Palou J, Shariat SF (2013) European guidelines on upper tract urothelial carcinomas: 2013 update. Eur Urol 63(6):1059–1071
2. Ploeg M, Aben KK, Kiemeney LA (2009) The present and future burden of urinary bladder cancer in the world. World J Urol 27(3):289–293
3. Cosentino M, Palou J, Gaya JM, Breda A, Rodriguez-Faba O, Villavicencio-Mavrich H (2013) Upper urinary tract urothelial cell carcinoma: location as a predictive factor for concomitant bladder carcinoma. World J Urol 31(1):141–145
4. Burger M, Catto JW, Dalbagni G, Grossman HB, Herr H, Karakiewicz P, Kassouf W, Kiemeney LA, La Vecchia C, Shariat S, Lotan Y (2013) Epidemiology and risk factors of urothelial bladder cancer. Eur Urol 63(2):234–241
5. Roupret M, Yates DR, Comperat E, Cussenot O (2008) Upper urinary tract urothelial cell carcinomas and other urological malignancies involved in the hereditary nonpolyposis colorectal cancer (lynch syndrome) tumor spectrum. Eur Urol 54(6):1226–1236
6. Shinagare AB, Ramaiya NH, Jagannathan JP, Fennessy FM, Taplin ME, Van den Abbeele AD (2011) Metastatic pattern of bladder cancer: correlation with the characteristics of the primary tumor. AJR Am J Roentgenol 196(1):117–122
7. Wallmeroth A, Wagner U, Moch H, Gasser TC, Sauter G, Mihatsch MJ (1999) Patterns of metastasis in muscle-invasive bladder cancer (pT2-4): an autopsy study on 367 patients. Urol Int 62(2):69–75
8. Shinagare AB, Fennessy FM, Ramaiya NH, Jagannathan JP, Taplin ME, Van den Abbeele AD (2011) Urothelial cancers of the upper urinary tract: metastatic pattern and its correlation with tumor histopathology and location. J Comput Assist Tomogr 35(2):217–222
9. Olgac S, Mazumdar M, Dalbagni G, Reuter VE (2004) Urothelial carcinoma of the renal pelvis: a clinicopathologic study of 130 cases. Am J Surg Pathol 28(12):1545–1552
10. Saxman SB, Propert KJ, Einhorn LH, Crawford ED, Tannock I, Raghavan D, Loehrer PJ Sr, Trump D (1997) Long-term follow-up of a phase III intergroup study of cisplatin alone or in combination with methotrexate, vinblastine, and doxorubicin in patients with metastatic urothelial carcinoma: a cooperative group study. J Clin Oncol 15(7):2564–2569

11. Prout GR Jr, Griffin PP, Shipley WU (1979) Bladder carcinoma as a systemic disease. Cancer 43(6):2532–2539
12. Margulis V, Shariat SF, Matin SF, Kamat AM, Zigeuner R, Kikuchi E, Lotan Y, Weizer A, Raman JD, Wood CG (2009) Outcomes of radical nephroureterectomy: a series from the Upper Tract Urothelial Carcinoma Collaboration. Cancer 115(6):1224–1233
13. von der Maase H, Sengelov L, Roberts JT, Ricci S, Dogliotti L, Oliver T, Moore MJ, Zimmermann A, Arning M (2005) Long-term survival results of a randomized trial comparing gemcitabine plus cisplatin, with methotrexate, vinblastine, doxorubicin, plus cisplatin in patients with bladder cancer. J Clin Oncol 23(21):4602–4608
14. Abe T, Shinohara N, Harabayashi T, Sazawa A, Maruyama S, Suzuki S, Nonomura K (2007) Impact of multimodal treatment on survival in patients with metastatic urothelial cancer. Eur Urol 52(4):1106–1113
15. Bajorin DF, Dodd PM, Mazumdar M, Fazzari M, McCaffrey JA, Scher HI, Herr H, Higgins G, Boyle MG (1999) Long-term survival in metastatic transitional-cell carcinoma and prognostic factors predicting outcome of therapy. J Clin Oncol 17(10):3173–3181
16. Berry J, MacVicar D (2008) Carcinoma of the bladder. Contemporary issues in cancer imaging. Cambridge University Press, New York
17. Witjes JA, Comperat E, Cowan NC, De Santis M, Gakis G, Lebret T, Ribal MJ, Van der Heijden AG, Sherif A (2014) EAU guidelines on muscle-invasive and metastatic bladder cancer: summary of the 2013 guidelines. Eur Urol 65(4):778–792
18. Scardino P, Linehan M, Zelefsky M, Vogelzang N (2011) Comprehensive textbook of genitourinary oncology, 4th edn. Lippincott Williams & Wilkins, Philadelphia
19. Mertens LS, Fioole-Bruining A, Vegt E, Vogel WV, van Rhijn BW, Horenblas S (2013) Impact of (18) F-fluorodeoxyglucose (FDG)-positron-emission tomography/computed tomography (PET/CT) on management of patients with carcinoma invading bladder muscle. BJU Int 112(6):729–734
20. Sternberg CN, Yagoda A, Scher HI, Watson RC, Geller N, Herr HW, Morse MJ, Sogani PC, Vaughan ED, Bander N et al (1989) Methotrexate, vinblastine, doxorubicin, and cisplatin for advanced transitional cell carcinoma of the urothelium. Efficacy and patterns of response and relapse. Cancer 64(12):2448–2458
21. Kaufman D, Raghavan D, Carducci M, Levine EG, Murphy B, Aisner J, Kuzel T, Nicol S, Oh W, Stadler W (2000) Phase II trial of gemcitabine plus cisplatin in patients with metastatic urothelial cancer. J Clin Oncol 18(9):1921–1927
22. von der Maase H, Andersen L, Crino L, Weinknecht S, Dogliotti L (1999) Weekly gemcitabine and cisplatin combination therapy in patients with transitional cell carcinoma of the urothelium: a phase II clinical trial. Ann Oncol 10(12):1461–1465
23. von der Maase H, Hansen SW, Roberts JT, Dogliotti L, Oliver T, Moore MJ, Bodrogi I, Albers P, Knuth A, Lippert CM, Kerbrat P, Sanchez Rovira P, Wersall P, Cleall SP, Roychowdhury DF, Tomlin I, Visseren-Grul CM, Conte PF (2000) Gemcitabine and cisplatin versus methotrexate, vinblastine, doxorubicin, and cisplatin in advanced or metastatic bladder cancer: results of a large, randomized, multinational, multicenter, phase III study. J Clin Oncol 18(17):3068–3077
24. Bellmunt J, von der Maase H, Mead GM, Skoneczna I, De Santis M, Daugaard G, Boehle A, Chevreau C, Paz-Ares L, Laufman LR, Winquist E, Raghavan D, Marreaud S, Collette S, Sylvester R, de Wit R (2012) Randomized phase III study comparing paclitaxel/cisplatin/gemcitabine and gemcitabine/cisplatin in patients with locally advanced or metastatic urothelial cancer without prior systemic therapy: EORTC Intergroup Study 30987. J Clin Oncol 30(10):1107–1113
25. Bellmunt J, Theodore C, Demkov T, Komyakov B, Sengelov L, Daugaard G, Caty A, Carles J, Jagiello-Gruszfeld A, Karyakin O, Delgado FM, Hurteloup P, Winquist E, Morsli N, Salhi Y, Culine S, von der Maase H (2009) Phase III trial of vinflunine plus best supportive care compared with best supportive care alone after a platinum-containing regimen in patients with advanced transitional cell carcinoma of the urothelial tract. J Clin Oncol 27(27):4454–4461

26. Wong SL, Mangu PB, Choti MA, Crocenzi TS, Dodd GD 3rd, Dorfman GS, Eng C, Fong Y, Giusti AF, Lu D, Marsland TA, Michelson R, Poston GJ, Schrag D, Seidenfeld J, Benson AB 3rd (2010) American Society of Clinical Oncology 2009 clinical evidence review on radiofrequency ablation of hepatic metastases from colorectal cancer. J Clin Oncol 28(3):493–508
27. Gallagher HJ, Redmond HP, Deasy J, McLean PA (1998) Hepatic resection of solitary metastasis from transitional cell carcinoma of the bladder. J Urol 159(3):986
28. Dodd PM, McCaffrey JA, Herr H, Mazumdar M, Bacik J, Higgins G, Boyle MG, Scher HI, Bajorin DF (1999) Outcome of postchemotherapy surgery after treatment with methotrexate, vinblastine, doxorubicin, and cisplatin in patients with unresectable or metastatic transitional cell carcinoma. J Clin Oncol 17(8):2546–2552
29. Miller RS, Freiha FS, Reese JH, Ozen H, Torti FM (1993) Cisplatin, methotrexate and vinblastine plus surgical restaging for patients with advanced transitional cell carcinoma of the urothelium. J Urol 150(1):65–69
30. Siefker-Radtke AO, Walsh GL, Pisters LL, Shen Y, Swanson DA, Logothetis CJ, Millikan RE (2004) Is there a role for surgery in the management of metastatic urothelial cancer? The M. D. Anderson experience. J Urol 171(1):145–148
31. Abe T, Kitamura H, Obara W, Matsumura N, Tsukamoto T, Fujioka T, Hara I, Murai S, Shinohara N, Nonomura K (2013) Outcome of metastasectomy for urothelial carcinoma: a multi-institutional retrospective study in Japan. J Urol
32. Gillams AR (2005) The use of radiofrequency in cancer. Br J Cancer 92(10):1825–1829
33. Kobayashi M, Kinouchi T, Kinoshita T, Hatano H, Ueda T, Inoue H, Takada T, Hara T, Yamaguchi S (2011) A case of renal pelvic cancer with hepatic metastasis where hepatic arterial infusion chemotherapy (HAIC) proved effective: a case report. Hinyokika kiyo Acta Urol Jpn 57(11):627–631
34. Inoue T, Ohyama C, Horikawa Y, Togashi H, Matsuura S, Tsuchiya N, Satoh S, Sato K, Habuchi T, Saito S, Hoshi S, Arai Y, Kato T (2004) Active chemotherapy with gemcitabine, carboplatin and docetaxel for three patients with MVAC-resistant liver metastasis of urothelial carcinoma. Hinyokika kiyo Acta Urol Jpn 50(4):273–277
35. Gannon CJ, Curley SA (2005) The role of focal liver ablation in the treatment of unresectable primary and secondary malignant liver tumors. Semin Radiat Oncol 15(4):265–272
36. Gazelle GS, McMahon PM, Beinfeld MT, Halpern EF, Weinstein MC (2004) Metastatic colorectal carcinoma: cost-effectiveness of percutaneous radiofrequency ablation versus that of hepatic resection. Radiology 233(3):729–739
37. Yasuda Y, Tatokoro M, Yokoyama M, Koga F, Saito K, Masuda H, Fujii Y, Kawakami S, Kihara K (2010) Successful long-term management of hepatic and lymph nodes metastases of ureteral cancer by multimodal treatment including radiofrequency ablation. Nihon Hinyokika Gakkai Zasshi Jpn J Urol 101(7):758–763

Liver Metastases from Prostate Cancer 15

Jiao Zhang, HaiTao Wang, and YanHong Yao

Clinically, liver metastases (LM) originating from prostate cancer is uncommon and remains poorly understood. Despite improvements in diagnosis, surgical techniques, and chemotherapies, most deaths of prostate cancer patients occur due to disease progression and metastasis. Patients with LM have been reported to be usually a rather late event in the course of the disease, and LM most often occurs in patients after extensive therapy with hormone and/or chemotherapy. They usually present a subset of patients with a poor prognosis. Prostate cancer with LM is frequently associated with neuroendocrine characteristics. Diagnostic methods are

The study was supported in part by NSFC (81071787) and Tianjin Municipal Science and Technology Commission (08JCYBJC10300)

J. Zhang
Department of Interventional Oncology, Tianjin Medical University
Cancer Institute and Hospital, National Clinical Research
Center for Cancer, Tianjin, China

Department of Interventional Oncology, Tianjin Key Laboratory of Cancer Prevention
and Therapy, Tianjin, China

H. Wang (✉)
Department of Interventional Oncology, Tianjin Key Laboratory of Cancer Prevention
and Therapy, Tianjin, China

Department of Interventional Oncology, Tianjin Medical University Cancer Institute and
Hospital, National Clinical Research Center for Cancer, Tianjin, China

Medical Oncology, Research Group of Evidence-based Clinical Oncology, Tianjin, China
e-mail: peterrock2000@126.com

Y. Yao
Department of Interventional Oncology,
Tianjin Medical University Cancer Institute and Hospital,
National Clinical Research Center for Cancer, Tianjin, China

Research Group of Evidence-based Clinical Oncology, Tianjin, China

I. Di Carlo (ed.), *Noncolorectal, Nonneuroendocrine Liver Metastases: Diagnosis and Current Therapies*, DOI 10.1007/978-3-319-09293-5_15

increasingly sensitive and provide improved early detection and monitoring of treatment response. Treatment of LM from prostate cancer should be individualized based on the patient's clinical course, extent of disease, and symptoms. Multimodality therapy is often employed in the management of metastatic disease in the liver. The purpose of this chapter is to present the incidence, natural history, diagnosis, and treatment of LM from prostate cancer.

15.1 Incidence

Metastatic prostate cancer to the liver is not an uncommon finding at autopsy, being the third most common site after bone and lung. In a large autopsy series of 1,589 patients with hormone refractory prostate cancer (HRPC), Bubendorf et al. [1] reported 25 % of cases had metastases to the liver, and the likelihood of LM was increased when the primary tumor was greater than 8 cm. Prostate cancer with clinical LM is uncommon and has not been well reported. One series of over 345 metastatic prostate cancer patients at the Montpellier Cancer Center between 1995 and 2005 yielded an incidence of 8 % [2]. One recent study retrospectively reviewed 1,050 metastatic castration-resistant prostate cancer (mCRPC) patients, 59 cases of LM were identified with an incidence of 5.62 % [3]. Another study of 629 metastatic prostate cancer patients in Tianjin prostate cancer database from 2005 to 2012 reported an incidence of liver metastasis was 4.29 % (27/629) [4].

All these results showed that the prevalence of LM was quite lower than the autopsy result. The disparity in the incidence of LM of prostate cancer between autopsy and clinical studies is due in part to the limitations of current liver imaging techniques; autopsy series included cases with microscopic metastases that are not detectable by ultrasonography (US) or computed tomography (CT). Additionally, in patients who have severe systemic disease, the possible diagnosis of LM may not have been pursued due to the overall poor prognosis of the patients.

15.2 Natural History

An understanding of the optimal treatment strategies in patients with prostate cancer with LM requires an understanding of the natural history of prostate metastases to the liver. An important goal of the ongoing investigation into the natural history of this disease is to better evaluate the prognosis of patients with prostate cancer with LM. The clinical characteristics of reported liver metastasis in literature were shown in Table 15.1. The Figs. 15.1 and 15.2 showed the initial hormone-sensitive prostate cancer with LM and CRPC with LM respectively.

Table 15.1 Clinical characteristics of reported liver metastasis in literature

Author	Year	Patients (n)	LMs (n)	Diagnosis tool	Treatment	Hormone status		Time since PC diagnosis (mon)		Survival after LM diagnosis (mon)	
						HSPC	CRPC	HSPC	CRPC	HSPC	CRPC
Wang	2013	27	NA	US/CT/MRI/B	ADT/CT/RT	8	19	NA	14	38	6
Pouessel	2007	28	NA	US/CT/B	HT/CT	1	27	NA	NA	NA	6
Kelly	2012	59	NA	NA	D, P with either B or placebo		59	NA	NA	NA	NA
Pezaro	2014	71	NA	CT	NA		71	55.2	19.2	NA	NA
Shakir	2008	1	M	CT, A	SC	1		NA		NA	
Marech	2013	1	M	CT	AA and P/ZA/Ca		1		51		NA
Batty	2013	1	NA	CT	Ca/Cy and P/AA/Mi		1		20		6

HSPC hormone-sensitive prostate cancer, *CRPC* castration-resistant prostate cancer, *NA* not available, *US* ultrasonography, *CT* computed tomography, *MRI*, magnetic resonance imaging, *B* biopsy, *ADT* androgen deprivation therapy, *CT* chemotherapy, *RT* radiotherapy, *HT* hormone therapy, *D* docetaxel, *P* prednisone, *B* bevacizumab, *A* autopsy, *M* multiples, *SC* supportive care, *AA* abiraterone acetate, *ZA* zoledronic acid, *Ca* cabazitaxel, *Cy* cyclophosphamide, *Mi* mitoxantrone

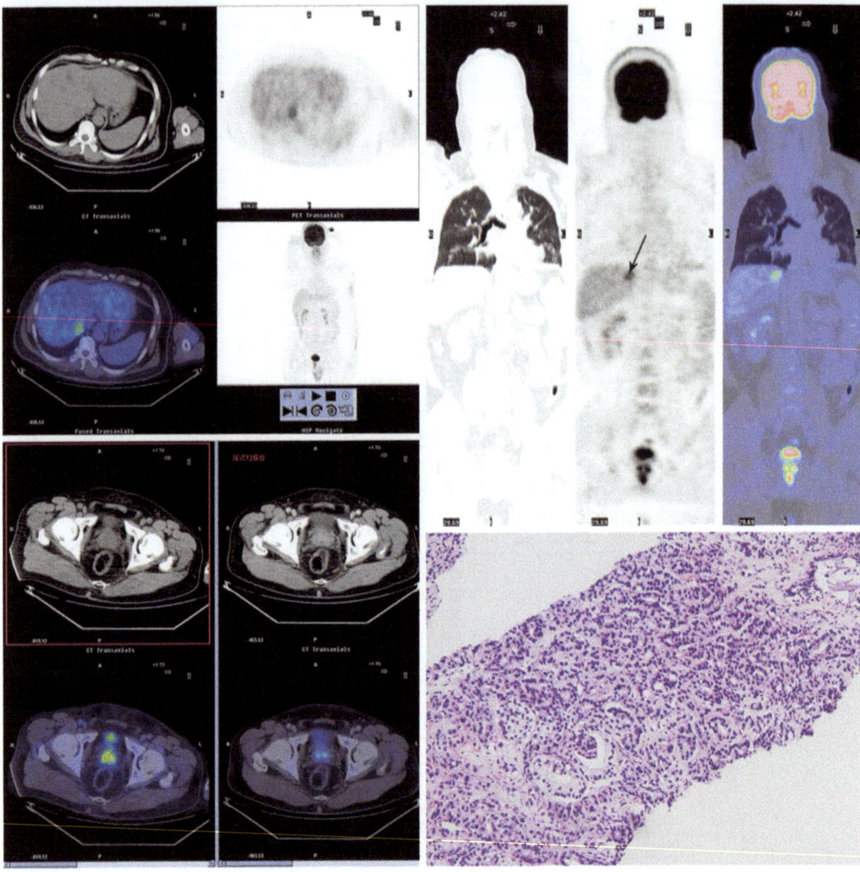

Fig. 15.1 F18 fluorodeoxyglucose positron emission tomography/computed tomography images in a prostate cancer patient with solitary liver metastasis. Axial positron emission tomography and fusion images show increased activity in prostate (*down left*) and solitary hepatic metastases (*upper left*). Maximum intensity projection image (*upper right*) also shows solitary liver metastasis and prostate cancer. Focally increased activity (*arrow*) is seen in liver. The prostate biopsy showed the low differentiated prostate adenocarcinoma (*down right*)

15.3 The Prognosis Difference Between Liver Metastases and Non-liver Metastases

CRPC patients with LM usually represent a poor prognosis. Armstrong et al. [5] reported that 640 CRPC patients had received chemotherapy; in their multivariable analysis, LM was associated with post-progression survival (hazard ratio (HR) = 1.48, 95 % confidence interval (CI) 0.94–2.30, $P = 0.089$). Kelly et al. [3] announced a set of data in ASCO Annual Meeting in 2012, data from 1,050 men treated with docetaxel (D) and prednisone (P) with either bevacizumab (B) or placebo. Patients were chemotherapy naïve and had evidence of progressive mCRPC despite castrate testosterone levels and antiandrogen withdrawal, ECOG

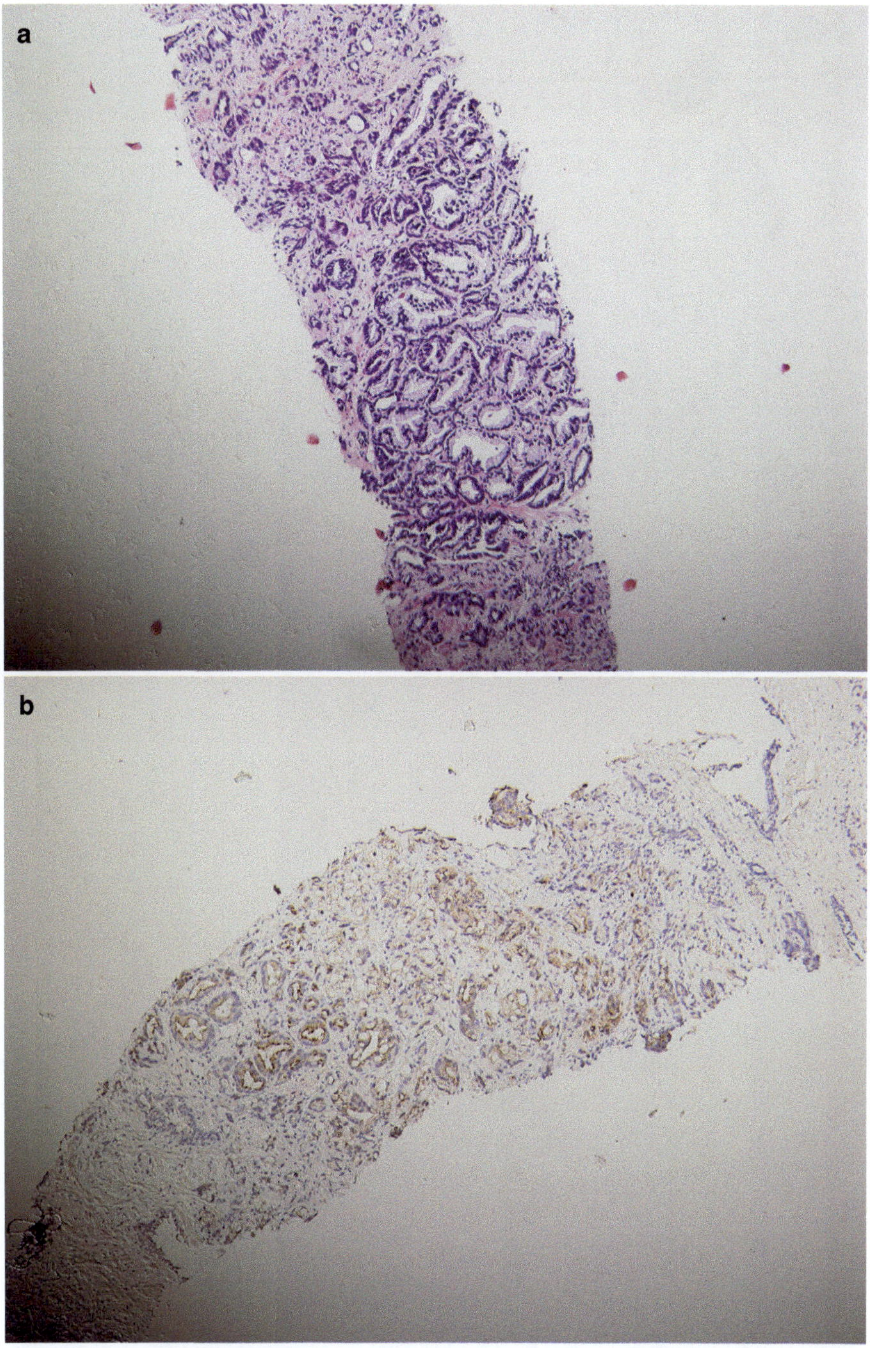

Fig. 15.2 A patient's tumor tissue at initial pretreatment prostate biopsy (**a. b.**) and liver biopsy (**c–e**) at liver metastasis for CRPC with hematoxylin-and-eosin-stained material showing histologic changes from initial biopsy (**a**) to liver biopsy at CRPC with immunohistochemical staining for P504S and Ki67 on liver biopsy at CRPC (**d, e.**) and P504S on initial biopsy (**b**)

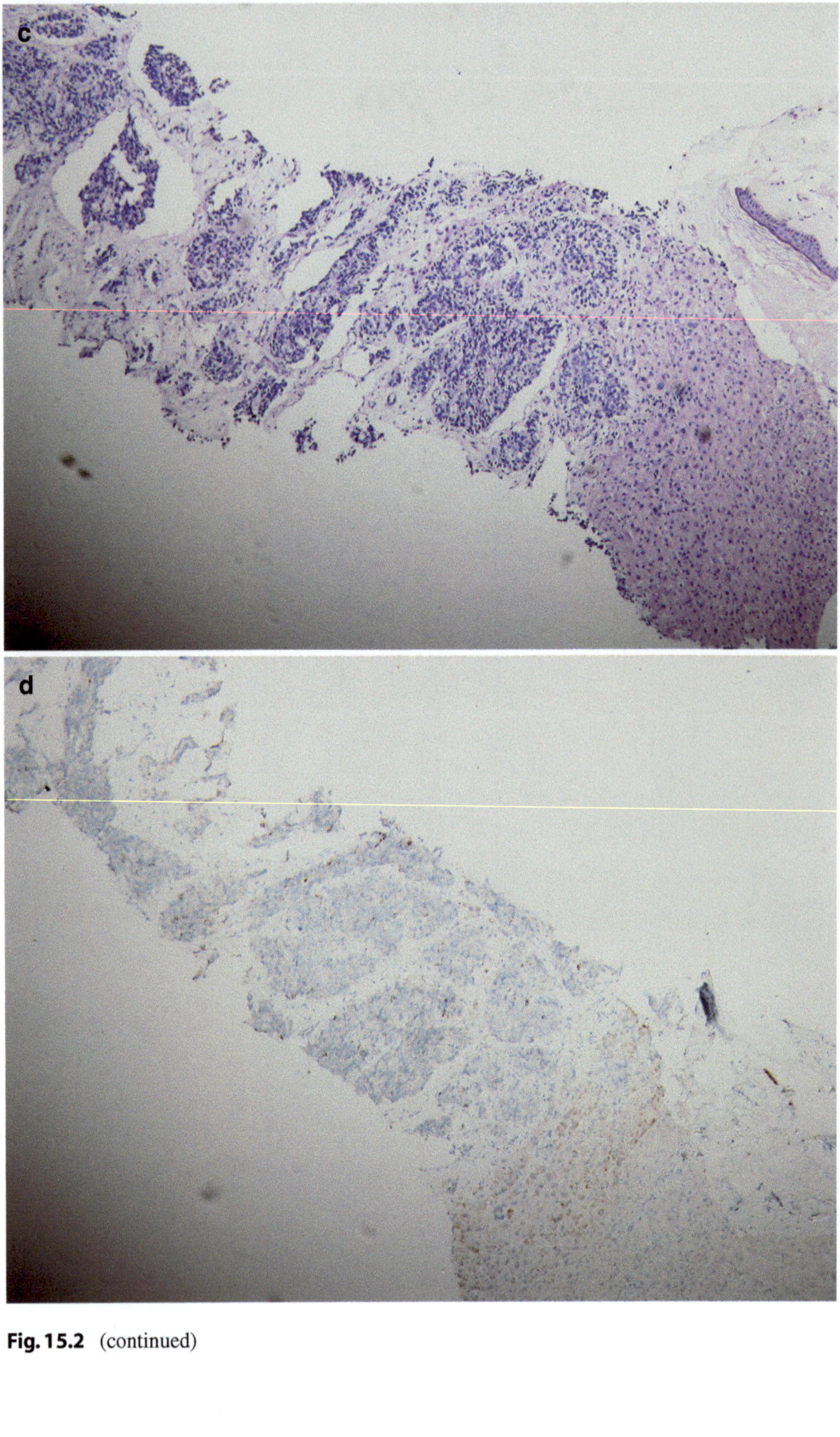

Fig. 15.2 (continued)

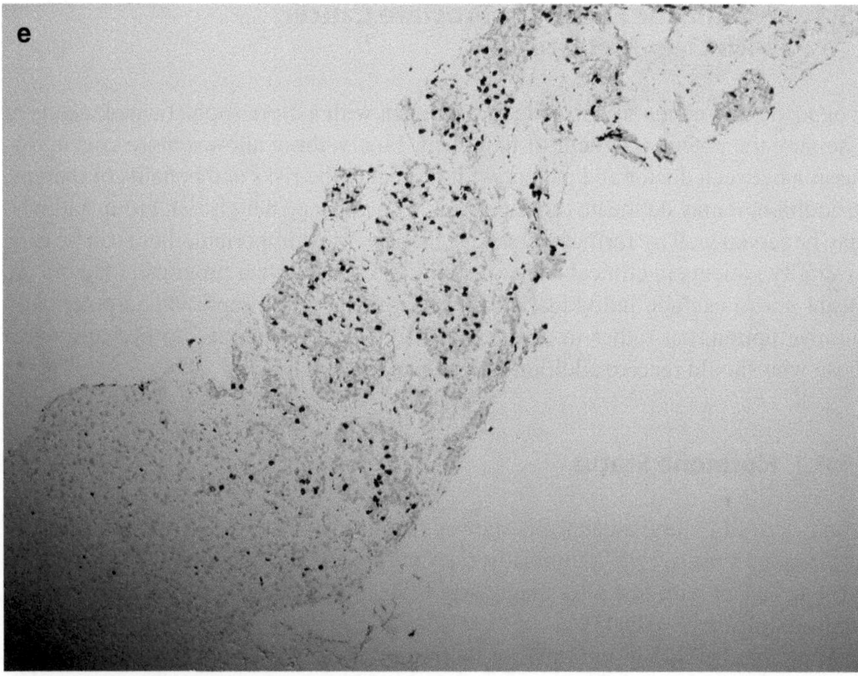

Fig. 15.2 (continued)

performance status ≤2, and adequate bone marrow, hepatic, and renal functions. The median overall survival (OS) time in LM patients was 14.4 compared to 22.6 months, with a HR of 1.4. The HR for treatment effect (DP+B vs. DP) for LM was not statistically significant for either group. Compared to patients without LM, mCRPC patients with LM have a poor OS despite having similar progression-free survival (PFS) and objective biochemical response to docetaxel-based therapy. In these cases, CRPC with LM was reported to be associated with poor prognosis.

However, Pezaro et al. [6] reported that CRPC patients with visceral metastases (VM) may not represent a more aggressive disease phenotype. The association with worse outcome may instead relate to the increased prevalence of VM as overall disease burden increases. Their study also showed that VM involved the liver (20 %) in 359 CRPC patients. Patient outcome differed based on the degree of bone involvement at detection of VM, with a median survival of 18.2 months in men with no evident bone disease ($n=12$; interquartile range [IQR]: 24.9; $P=0.001$ vs. more than six lesions), 8.1 months in those with moderate bone involvement (fewer than six lesions; $n=18$; IQR: 25.6; $P=0.049$ vs. six or more lesions), and 6.1 months in those with more extensive bone involvement (six or more lesions; $n=84$; IQR: 8.9). Wang et al. [4] reported that LM does not necessarily predict a worse outcome when seen as synchronous LM at the diagnosis of prostate cancer; when seen as a site of progressive CRPC, prognosis was worse.

15.4 Prognostic Factors in Prostate Cancer with Liver Metastasis

Prognostic factors mainly provide the clinician with a more sophisticated means of assessing the potential benefit of treatment. Firstly, these allow a more cogent discussion between doctor and patient with respect to the risks and benefits of therapy. In addition, it may delineate those patients who make up a high-risk group and who may be served well by further aggressive therapy. Most important, these can be used to stratify patients in clinical trials. It should be stressed that prognostic factors are meant not to exclude individuals from given therapy that represents a potentially curative option, but rather to assess the risk of progression and to perhaps select those who should receive additional treatment.

15.4.1 Hormone Status

Wang et al.'s [4] survival analysis showed that hormone status (hormone refractory or hormone sensitive) is a clinically relevant predictor of poor overall survival in prostate cancer with LM after diagnosis of LM and has demonstrated to be statistically significant ($P=0.003$).

Wang et al. also reported that in the hormone-sensitive group, the median OS after LM diagnosis was 38 months and half of the patients were still alive at the latest follow-up [4]. This compares with published median survivals between 28 and 52 months for large series employing androgen deprivation for treatment of patients with minimal or extensive metastatic prostate cancer [7]. While in the hormone refractory group, the median OS after LM diagnosis was only 6 months. Pouessel et al. [2] reported the median OS was 6 (1–27) months, confirming the results of Wang et al. [4]. Thus, prostate cancer with LM does not mean poor outcome, it also needs to take into account other factors, including hormonal status.

15.4.2 Neuroendocrine Differentiation

The neuroendocrine pattern is in agreement with the concept of progression from normal prostate to adenocarcinoma and finally to small-cell carcinoma during prostatic tumorigenesis [8]. Neuroendocrine differentiation (NED) in prostate cancer appears to be a poor prognostic factor [8]. In GETUG P01 trial [9], 55 mCRPC patients present with at least one of the following: those with VM (lung, liver, or lymph node involvement) except bone metastases or any elevated neuroendocrine serum marker (chromogranin (CgA) or neuron-specific enolase (NSE)) of ≥1.5-fold normal value, who received the association of etoposide and carboplatin with a median of four treatment cycles, and those with VM with or without neuroendocrine serum markers have an OS 8.9 months, 95 % CI (5.9–9.6), and 11.7 months, 95 % CI (8.7–18.4), respectively. Wang et al.'s study [4] also confirmed the results of GETUG P01 trial. In their study, the NSE level at LM

≥12.5 ng/ml, the median survival was 4 months, 95 % CI (1.228, 6.772); NSE level at LM <12.5 ng/ml, the median survival was 9.6 months, 95 % CI (not evaluable, 19.802), $P=0.042$.

NED in prostate cancer is uncommon and highly aggressive with a tendency to systemically metastasize and thus has a poor prognosis, possibly related to the increasing degree of dedifferentiation, resistance to hormonal therapy, and growth stimulation of the tumor by neurosecretory products [10]. Pouessel et al.'s [2] study showed that LM was associated with the NED. NED is known to occur in prostate cancer where it associates with poorly differentiated disease with VM and/or secretion of neuroendocrine serum tumor markers (NSE and CgA) [11]. Wang et al.'s [4] univariable analysis showed that in the hormone-refractory group, high concentration of serum NSE is one of the factors that predict poor survival after LM. In their study, the concentrations of NSE were available after the diagnosis of liver metastases in 14/27 patients. Eight of 14 patients received chemotherapy. During the course of chemotherapy, of the seven patients followed up serially, NSE was raised in all two patients who had normal NSE prior to chemotherapy. Out of five patients with elevated NSE levels, four showed a fall in NSE. In two of the latter, it became normal and all the four patients with a decrease of NSE during the course of chemotherapy showed radiologically assessed partial response ($n=3$) or stable disease ($n=1$).

Pouessel et al. [2] reported 28 patients with metastatic prostate cancer with LM. Serum measurement of neuroendocrine markers showed high level of CgA and NSE in 84 and 44 % of patients, respectively. For the six patients who had liver biopsies and two were neuroendocrine carcinomas, one of which was poorly differentiated, with a small-cell carcinoma pattern. For immunohistochemistry (IHC), all adenocarcinomas were positive for prostate-specific antigen (PSA), whereas none of the neuroendocrine carcinomas expressed PSA. Conversely, neuroendocrine tumors expressed specific markers such as synaptophysin (Syn), CgA, or neural cell adhesion molecule (N-CAM). Notably, CgA was detected in only one case of neuroendocrine tumor, and thyroid transcription factor 1 (TTF1) was positive in the poorly differentiated neuroendocrine component.

In summary, we may consider that NED is correlated closely with poor prognosis of prostate cancer with LM.

15.4.3 Previous Chemotherapy

Wang et al. [4] also reported that another important prognostic factor for survival is the previous chemotherapy. In their study, five patients with previous chemotherapy, the median survival time was 2 months, 95 % CI (not evaluable, 4.147); 14 patients without previous chemotherapy, the median survival time was 9.6 months, 95 % CI (2.266, 16.934), $P<0.001$. But they found that in the previous chemotherapy, a significant prognostic factor does not mean that chemotherapy itself makes survival worse. The possible reason is that those with previous chemotherapy have no or few effective options for chemotherapy left after LM occurred.

15.5 Diagnosis

A variety of modalities, including clinical manifestations, laboratory tests, tumor markers, radiologic examinations, and invasive techniques, are relevant in diagnosing patients with prostate cancer with LM.

15.5.1 Clinical Manifestations

Prostate cancer with LM has been reported to be usually a late manifestation of systemic disease and most often occurs in patients after extensive therapy with hormone and/or chemotherapy [2]. Prostate cancer with LM may present asymptomatically during a metastatic screen or may present with specific symptoms. The most common specific symptoms were as follows: upper abdominal pain, jaundice, and distention of abdomen. Wang et al. [4] reported that 40.74 % had symptoms specific to the liver during the onset of LM, while 59.26 % did not have symptoms specific to the liver. In severe cases with rapidly growing tumors, patients can present with fulminant hepatic failure (FHF) and subsequent multisystem organ failure as a result of homogenous infiltration of the liver by metastatic disease. Shakir et al. [12] presented a case of metastatic prostate adenocarcinoma in which a 68-year-old man presented with FHF. An abdominal CT scan revealed hepatomegaly without focal lesions, and Doppler ultrasound showed hepatomegaly and hepatic steatosis. The patient's condition rapidly declined, with multiorgan system failure necessitating emergent ICU interventions. Autopsy revealed an enlarged liver weighing 3,478 g, with the biopsy showing intravascular and intraparenchymal widespread metastatic prostatic adenocarcinoma.

15.5.2 Laboratory Tests

When hepatic involvement occurs with tumors, the degree of hepatic enzyme elevation varies upon presentation but is often found to correlate with the degree of intrasinusoidal hepatic involvement. Wang et al.'s [4] study showed that liver function tests are deranged in 13 patients (48 %) at presentation with ALP and AST being the most commonly elevated enzymes.

15.5.3 Tumor Markers

Pouessel et al.'s [2] study showed that LM is associated with the NED. In their study, 28 patients with metastatic prostate cancer with LM, serum measurement of neuroendocrine markers showed high level of CgA and NSE in 84 and 44 % of patients, respectively. Wang et al.'s study [4] also confirmed the results of Pouessel et al.'s. In their study, the concentrations of NSE were available after the diagnosis of LM in 14 patients (52 %). Cussenot et al. [13] reported CgA appears to be the best marker of NED and a correlation has been found between neuroendocrine serum markers and the incidence of distant metastases. Pezaro et al.'s [6] study also demonstrated a patient with LM developed widespread metastatic liver disease despite very low levels of PSA; the biopsy revealed small-cell carcinoma morphology with negative IHC staining for PSA and androgen receptor (AR). Thus, plasma neuroendocrine markers can be used as predictive markers associated with prostate cancer with LM.

15.5.4 Imaging Modality

Ultrasonography

Conventional transabdominal US is routinely used as the first-line imaging modality for the detection of liver metastases, and it also plays a substantial role in the intra-procedural localization of lesions during biopsy and therapeutic interventions such as thermal ablation, providing real-time imaging with no ionizing radiation to the operator.

The reported sensitivity of US is much lower than that of CT or magnetic resonance imaging(MRI), ranging from 40 to 77 %, and can drop to 20 % for small lesions (<1 cm) or for lesions that are isoechoic compared with the surrounding liver parenchyma [14, 15]. Thus, detection of hepatic lesions with US frequently initiates a request for an imaging study with greater accuracy, such as CT or MRI.

The development of new ultrasound contrast agents and sonographic techniques has considerably improved the US detection of hepatic metastases and the evaluation of response to therapeutic procedures. Contrast-enhanced ultrasound (CEUS) has improved the sensitivity for detecting LM to 80–90 %, which is not statistically different than the diagnostic performance of CT, and is especially useful for LM smaller than 10 mm [14]. CEUS alone was reported sufficient to classify 89.0 % of focal liver lesions as benign or malignant, which served as a one-stop diagnostic test for 80.8 % of patients, reducing the need for CT and MRI scans, and provided savings in terms of radiation exposure, time, and money [16].

Computed Tomography

In clinical practice, CT is the mainstay of oncological imaging because of its excellent availability, good patient tolerance, and reproducibility. As metastatic hepatic lesions are usually hypovascular, the optimal CT strategy is helical scanning during the portal venous phase of enhancement. This technique improves lesion identification by increasing the attenuation of normal liver tissue, and occasionally rim enhancement of a hypoattenuating metastasis can be seen [17].

The advent of multidetector row computed tomography (MDCT) effectively replaced computed tomography during arterial portography for diagnosis of hepatic metastases. MDCT is highly accurate for evaluating staging, especially for the detection of lymph node enlargement and distant metastases. The accuracy of MDCT for overall M staging is 85.6 %, and for identifying LM the sensitivity is

80.0 % [18]. CT is a standard test for the detection of the LM; however, the reported sensitivity for small metastases (<1.5 cm) is low [19]. A recent comparison between total liver-volume perfusion CT (CTP) and four-phase CT revealed that CTP increased the sensitivity for the detection of LM to 89.2 % from 78.4 % ($P=0.046$) and specificity to 82.6 % from 78.3 % ($P=0.074$), indicating that CTP is a noninvasive, quantitative, and feasible technique [20].

Magnetic Resonance Imaging

MRI is considered to be the optimal diagnostic modality for evaluation of suspected LM, with a reported sensitivity of 80–100% and specificity up to 97 % [21]. The diagnostic performance of MRI for small lesions (<1.0 cm) has been shown to be superior to helical CT [22]. Modern comprehensive liver imaging protocols generally use a variety of sequences to optimize lesion detection and characterization. Diffusion-weighted (DW)-MRI has been found to be sensitive for the detection of small liver lesions (<1 cm) that mimic small intrahepatic vessels; however, as there is an overlap of apparent diffusion coefficient (ADC) values between different types of lesions, the predominant limitation of the DW-echo planar imaging (EPI) sequence is the differentiation between benign and malignant lesions [23]. Contrast-enhanced MRI can demonstrate tissue-specific physiological information, thereby facilitating liver lesion characterization, which may facilitate the accurate diagnostic workup of patients in order to avoid invasive procedures for lesion characterization, such as biopsy. Gadolinium-enhanced T2-weighted images and superparamagnetic iron oxide (SPIO)-enhanced T2-weighted MRI have been reported to have the ability to differentiate primary malignant, metastatic, and benign lesions in the liver [24]. However, with the increasing awareness of the potential risks of contrast material administration in patients with severe renal failure, there is a strong clinical need for methods to diagnose LM without exogenous contrast materials. Nasu et al. [25] retrospectively compared the accuracy of respiratory-triggered DW-EPI in combination with unenhanced T1- and T2-weighted imaging versus SPIO-enhanced imaging and found that there was no significant difference of sensitivity and specificity between the two imaging methods. DW-MRI combined with unenhanced T1- and T2-weighted imaging is a reasonable alternative to contrast-enhanced MRI for the detection of LM [25].

Positron Emission Tomography (PET)

18F-FDG PET and FDG-PET with CT (PET/CT) have the added advantage over MRI and CT of providing not only anatomic but also functional information. The major advantages of PET are the ability to detect extrahepatic disease and to evaluate therapeutic response early. One series found that FDG-PET had a sensitivity and specificity of 85 and 74 %, respectively, for the detection of LM originating from gastric cancer [26]. A recent study demonstrated that the detection rate of liver lesions was significantly lower for PET/CT than for gadolinium-ethoxybenzyl-diethylenetriamine pentaacetic acid-enhanced MRI (64 % vs. 85 %, respectively; $P=0.002$), which is especially relevant in small LM ($\leq$1 cm in diameter) [27].

15.5.5 Invasive Techniques

The tumor biopsy is presently defined by standard clinical and pathologic features of patients and their cancers. When metastasizing to liver from prostate cancer, they tend to form discrete lesions that are easily identified by standard radiographic methods, including MRI and CT. However, when the tumor radiographically blends with the normal organ parenchyma or micrometastases that imaging methods cannot detect, the diagnosis of metastatic disease can be difficult. Thus, extensive workup can ensue until a tissue biopsy is obtained. But the physician must pay special attention to the potential risk of bleeding postprocedure when the organ involved is the liver. In summary, quick recognition of this diagnosis and confirmatory biopsy will usually lead to the best available outcome for the patient.

Clinical manifestations and laboratory findings usually are late manifestations in patients with LM. The ideal radiologic approach to screening for LM from prostate cancer remains to be established. However, a variety of modalities, including imaging modality and biopsy, are relevant in diagnosing patients with prostate cancer with LM. Each imaging modality has its relative benefits in the evaluation of prostate cancer with LM. Helical multidetector CT is widely available and can accurately diagnose larger lesions, whereas MRI has superior performance versus helical CT in the detection and characterization of small liver metastases. US is frequently used as a guiding technology for percutaneous lesion sampling and therapeutic interventions. PET-CT is superior for the detection of extrahepatic disease. CEUS is a noninvasive and promising tool for detecting LM, as well as for guidance and the evaluation of response of therapeutic procedures early. Tissue biopsy is the gold standard for diagnosis.

15.6 Treatment

After the patient has been evaluated for the LM from prostate cancer, a number of therapeutic options are available. These include hormone therapy; systemic chemotherapy; abiraterone; surgical resection; other local ablative procedures, such as cryosurgery and hepatic artery embolization; and regional infusion chemotherapy.

15.6.1 Hormone-Sensitive Prostate Cancer with LM

Clinically, the treatment of metastatic prostate cancer is based on castration and androgen deprivation therapy (ADT). For patients with hormone-sensitive prostate cancer (HSPC) with LM, hormone therapy (by orchiectomy, gonadotropin-releasing agonists, or antagonists with the early addition of antiandrogens) is the main strategy.

Castration Therapy

Luteinizing hormone-releasing hormone (LHRH) agonists have become the standard of care in castration therapy because these agents have the potential of reversibility and enable the use of intermittent ADT, avoid the physical and psychological discomfort associated with orchiectomy, have a lower risk of cardiotoxicity than observed with diethylstilbestrol, and result in equivalent oncologic efficacy [28, 29].

In contrast to the agonists, LHRH antagonists result in a rapid decrease in luteinizing hormone, follicle-stimulating hormone, and testosterone levels without any flare. In a recent prospective randomized phase 3 trial, 610 men with prostate cancer requiring ADT were randomized to receive degarelix or leuprolide for 12 months [30]. At the end of the observation period, degarelix was not inferior to leuprolide but achieved a more rapid suppression of testosterone within the first 3 days and avoided any flare phenomenon. In an additional analysis of secondary endpoints, a significantly lower risk of PSA progression and prostate cancer-specific death in favor of degarelix was described for patients with advanced disease and high baseline PSA levels [31]. However, only 11 % of the patients treated with leuprolide have received flare protection with bicalutamide, and the number of patients included in the subgroup analysis is too small to draw any clinically relevant conclusions. The positive data of the C21 trial were maintained in a phase 3 extension trial where 385 patients of the C21 trial either were kept on degarelix or were switched from leuprolide to degarelix [32]. Switching from leuprolide to degarelix resulted in a significant decrease of the PSA PFS hazard rate from 0.20 events during year 1 to 0.08 events annually thereafter (chi-square test $P=0.003$). Also, in patients with PSA >20 ng/ml at the initiation of treatment, a significant decrease of PSA PFS hazard rate from 0.38 events annually to 0.19 events annually was achieved after the switch (chi-square test $P=0.031$).

The rapid and effective castration of LHRH antagonists primarily plays an important role in patients with symptomatic locally advanced or metastatic disease. Its benefit in other clinical situations remains to be proven.

Antiandrogen

ADT is the mainstay initial systemic treatment for advanced prostate cancer. Both nonsteroidal antiandrogens, nilutamide and flutamide, have produced conflicting results so these agents do not play a clinically important role in the hormonal treatment of prostate cancer as monotherapy.

As primary antiandrogen monotherapy, bicalutamide 150 mg/day was compared with medical or surgical castration in two large prospective randomized trials with identical study design including a total of 1,435 patients with locally advanced M0 or M1 prostate cancer [33]. A pooled analysis showed a significant improvement in OS with castration [34] in M1 patients.

Maximum Androgen Blockade

Maximum androgen blockade (MAB) has long been the gold standard for androgen stimulated metastatic prostate cancer and is used frequently in men who have experienced biochemical failure after local therapy. From the most recent systematic reviews and meta-analyses, it appears that at a follow-up of 5 year, MAB with nonsteroidal antiandrogens provides a small but statistically significant survival advantage (<5 %) compared with LHRH monotherapy [35, 36]. However, it has to be recognized that patients under MAB experience a significant impairment of quality of life (QoL) in the terms of sexuality, cognitive function, and thermoregulation [37].

Intermittent Androgen Deprivation

The optimal timing, duration, and schedule of ADT remain an active area of research. Given the many potential side effects of MAB, intermittent administration is becoming an increasingly popular alternative to continuous administration. Intermittent androgen deprivation (IAD) alternates androgen blockade with treatment cessation to allow hormonal recovery between treatment cycles, thus potentially improving tolerability and QoL [38]. Hussain et al. [39] conducted the SWOG 9346 trial to evaluate intermittent and continuous ADT in metastatic patients. Eligibility criteria included a new diagnosis of metastatic, androgen-stimulated prostate cancer; performance status of 0–2; and PSA level of 5 ng/mL or higher. After 7 months of induction ADT, 1,535 patients whose PSA decreased to 4 ng/mL or below (thereby showing androgen sensitivity) were randomized to intermittent or continuous ADT. In the intermittent group, ADT was reinitiated when the PSA level reached 20 ng/mL and stopped after 7 months if PSA decreased to 4 ng/mL or below. At a median follow-up of 9.8 years, median survival was 5.1 years for the intermittent ADT arm and 5.8 years for the continuous ADT arm. The HR for death with intermittent ADT was 1.10 with a 90 % CI between 0.99 and 1.23, which exceeded the prespecified upper boundary of 1.20 for noninferiority. The authors stated that the survival results were inconclusive and that a 20 % greater mortality risk with the intermittent approach cannot be ruled out. The study showed better erectile function and mental health in patients receiving intermittent ADT at 3 months, but the difference became insignificant thereafter.

The NCCN Prostate Cancer Panel considers that intermittent ADT requires close monitoring of PSA and testosterone levels, especially during off-treatment periods, and patients may need to switch to continuous therapy on signs of disease progression. Even in metastatic disease, intermittent ADT seems appropriate, in that survival is similar to that seen with ADT administered continuously in all studies comparing the two strategies thus far, and QoL is better with intermittent ADT in most studies [39, 40].

15.6.2 Castration-Resistant Prostate Cancer with LM

Presently, docetaxel in combination with prednisone at 3-week intervals as the standard first-line chemotherapy regime of CRPC patients. But those who experienced remission after a period of time and eventually develop disease progression or distant metastasis, additional therapies are needed. Treatment of advanced mCRPC has dramatically improved in recent years, due to the availability of new chemotherapeutic agents, including cabazitaxel, and of new antiandrogens, such as abiraterone. It has been demonstrated that prostate cancer maintains a certain degree of hormonal dependence even following failure to respond to treatment with MAB. In particular, new antiandrogens, including abiraterone, interfere with adrenal, testicular, and intra-tumoral androgen synthesis (in addition to blocking AR) [41–43].

Systemic Chemotherapy

LM is a late development in prostate cancer, especially those that were CRPC. For the vast majority of prostate cancer patients, liver involvement may reflect generalized disease. Local control may not be sufficient, especially for those with metastatic disease. Systemic chemotherapy is an appropriate option with the hope of prolonged survival. Chemotherapy improves the median OS of patients with hormone-refractory prostate cancer [44, 45].

Based on the prospective randomized phase 3 TAX 327 trial [44], docetaxel at 75 mg/m^2 at 3-week intervals in combination with prednisone represents the cytotoxic regime of choice in men with CRPC resulting in a median survival benefit of 3 months and a significant improvement of pain and QoL compared with weekly docetaxel and mitoxantrone. The most appropriate indication for chemotherapy might be the clinical scenario of symptomatic or extensive metastases, rapid PSA doubling time (PSADT), high Gleason score, or short-term response to primary ADT considering the inclusion criteria of the COU-302, IMPACT, and TAX327 trial [46]. However, despite the initial response, CRPC eventually develops drug resistance and additional therapies are needed [44, 47–49]. Several therapeutic options are now available, including second-line chemotherapy involving cabazitaxel and alkylating agent such as cyclophosphamide.

Cabazitaxel, a novel taxane agent, was approved by the FDA in 2010 based on the TROPIC trial, as a second-line agent in combination with low-dose prednisone for the treatment of patients with mCRPC who have already undergone docetaxel-based therapy. Cabazitaxel is the only chemotherapeutic agent to have demonstrated survival in a second-line mCRPC setting [50]. In the TROPIC trial, OS for patients treated with cabazitaxel was 15.1 months compared with 12.7 months for the mitoxantrone-treated patients, a 30 % relative risk reduction (HR 0.70; 95 % CI, 0.59–0.83; $P<0.0001$. Secondary endpoints also favored cabazitaxel. PFS was longer in duration for patients administered with cabazitaxel vs. mitoxantrone (2.8 vs. 1.4 months, respectively; HR 0.74; 95 % CI, 0.64–0.86; $P<0.0001$). Tumor response, PSA response, time to tumor progression, and time to PSA progression were also significantly superior with cabazitaxel compared with mitoxantrone. The number of patients with visceral disease was not higher than 25 % in either the cabazitaxel or mitoxantrone arms. Additionally, the response rate to VM was not revealed. However, the authors demonstrated that there was no difference in the OS of patients with VM between cabazitaxel-treated or mitoxantrone-treated patients [50].

For patients with LM, cyclophosphamide may also be a possible therapeutic option. Batty et al. [51] reported a 43-year-old man with rapidly progressing CRPC that responded initially to docetaxel and did not tolerate cabazitaxel. Then he subsequently received a third line of chemotherapy with cyclophosphamide and prednisone and experienced a dramatic clinical and radiographic response in his LM. This shows the potential use of cyclophosphamide in patients with CRPC, particularly in those with LM. In conclusion, in order to identify the role of cyclophosphamide in those with liver metastases, there is a great need for further investigation.

Though systemic chemotherapy is an appropriate option and can prolong survival time in patients with CRPC with LM, there is no optimal chemotherapy regimen currently, especially for patients who experienced failure in both first- and second-line chemotherapy regimes. Further investigations are needed to optimize the management of patients with prostate cancer with LM.

Abiraterone

For patients with advanced prostate cancer who failed first-line docetaxel-based chemotherapy, abiraterone is also a good choice. The lyase inhibitor abiraterone acetate (Cyp17 inhibitor) plus prednisone was approved for treatment of asymptomatic and mildly symptomatic mCRPC patients based on the results of the COU-302 trial [52] in 2012. But the most recent update to the NCCN treatment guidelines notes that abiraterone is one of several options among treatments for CRPC patients with symptomatic and/or visceral disease for whom chemotherapy is contraindicated and also is one of several second-line options for patients who have failed docetaxel therapy [53]. The pivotal phase III trial of abiraterone showed that OS was 14.8 months for those treated with abiraterone significantly longer ($P<0.001$) than the 10.9 months OS seen in the placebo group (HR 0.65; 95 % CI, 0.54–0.77) [52].

It is noteworthy that in patients with advanced prostate cancer, visceral involvement is not frequent. In fact, in the SWOG 99-16 and TAX 327 studies, the majority of patients had only bone disease (80–90 %), whereas visceral involvement was present in only 18–22 % of patients [44, 45]. The NCT00638690 phase III trial, comparing abiraterone with a placebo in docetaxel-resistant patients, enrolled 11 % of patients with LM in an abiraterone arm and 8 % in a placebo arm. Although the authors did not reveal the response rate to abiraterone in this subgroup of patients, the forest plot for survival demonstrated that these patients significantly benefited from abiraterone rather than the placebo [52].

Marech et al. [54] presented a case of a 65-year-old male prostate cancer with liver and node metastasis who was resistant to docetaxel and was treated with abiraterone. Abiraterone achieved a partial response, according to Response Evaluation Criteria in Solid Tumors (RECIST) criteria, and was achieved relatively quickly, as demonstrated by the first reevaluation CT scan performed after treatment for 2 months, which revealed a significant reduction in the retroperitoneal nodes and liver lesions; the maximum diameter of the nodes was 2.5 cm, as compared with 5 cm in the basal examination, and that of the lesions was 1.8 cm, as compared with 3 cm in the basal examination. Notably, the patient demonstrated a reduction in the level of PSA after 1 month (from 500 to 350 ng/ml). Moreover, the patient's pain was greatly reduced. The treatment was well tolerated and the serum biochemistry was normal. In addition, the response obtained in the visceral disease was maintained for 7 months, and the disease was only considered to be in progression due to the rising PSA level and the appearance of two new lesions during the bone scan, while the liver and lymph node lesions consistently exhibited shrinkage, as compared with the basal measurement. This demonstrated a high activity of abiraterone also in VM.

For patients with progressive CRPC with LM, abiraterone is a good choice. To further study the role of abiraterone in patients with LM, there is a great need for prospective studies.

Hepatic Metastasectomy

Hepatic resection is accepted as the treatment of choice when all hepatic disease can be removed and when there is no evidence of extrahepatic metastatic disease. The number of metastases in the liver affects the outcome: patients with solitary metastases fare better than those with multiple metastases. The vast majority of LM from prostate cancer is multiple. Therefore, many patients with liver metastases are not suitable candidates for hepatic resection, even if only a solitary hepatic metastasis (i.e., some patients' cancer may rapidly progress during a short period of observation, indicating that their tumors are biologically unfavorable and not amenable to benefit from surgical resection) is involved. Resection of prostate cancer with LM is rarely indicated. However, in highly selected patients with a long disease-free interval, resection may be reasonable, and prolonged survival may be achieved. Resection can be offered irrespective of the patient's age and the number, location, and size of metastases. Presently, the indications for hepatic resection for metastases have not been established and there are no firm guidelines regarding the resection for prostate cancer with LM. Therefore, the challenge for the future is to select patients for resection in the best manner.

Ablative Therapy

As most prostate cancer patients with LM are not candidates for resection, local ablative therapies have emerged as a possible alternative or complement to resection. Ablative techniques include radiofrequency thermal ablation (RFA), microwave ablation (MWA), and cryoablation. But no data exist to suggest that any of these modalities is the treatment gold standard. The application of these methods remains limited by tumor size and location. Lesions adjacent to major vascular structures cannot be completely ablated. Details of these approaches need further prospective study. The increasing complexity of decision making in patients with LM underscores the benefit of a multidisciplinary planning conference to optimize the planning of treatment for individual patients.

Transarterial Therapy

Transarterial therapy may be a useful treatment option in patients with unresectable disease and possibly as an adjuvant treatment after liver resection, which include hepatic arterial infusion chemotherapy and embolization. One of the advantages of transarterial therapy is the first-pass effects of cytotoxic agents, delivering a higher local drug concentration to unresectable liver tumors with fewer significant systemic toxicity. It can be used for liver-only metastases patients as an effective method of local control or be performed as part of a neoadjuvant therapeutic regimen, with the intent of tumor size reduction so that the lesion can later be effectively ablated or resected. Additionally, it can also be used in combination with intravenous chemotherapy as a palliative measure in cases of extrahepatic spread or post-surgical recurrence. Transarterial administration of anticancer drugs combined with vascular occlusive agents can achieve higher tissue drug concentrations, which may elicit an increased antitumor response. Though there is no data that suggest the role of transarterial therapy in prostate cancer with LM, based on the above advantages, there is a rationale for transarterial therapy which can be used as an effective treatment for LM.

15.6.3 Small-Cell Prostate Carcinoma with LM

Small-cell prostate carcinoma (SCPC) is very rare and has a poor prognosis. It constitutes less than 1 % of all prostate cancers [55]. The clinical behavior of SCPC is characterized by extensive local disease, visceral disease, and low PSA levels despite large metastatic burden. It clinically behaves like small-cell carcinoma of the lung and is classified as diffuse and limited disease. Even at the time of diagnosis, nearly 75 % of patients are at advanced stage. SCPC can be pure or combined as a component of the prostatic acinar adenocarcinoma [56]· In nearly half of all cases, there is a co-occurrence between SCPC and adenocarcinoma [57].

SCPC has similar features with small-cell lung cancer [58]. Therefore, chemotherapy is generally viewed as the backbone of treatment for metastatic SCPC; similar cisplatin-based cytotoxic agents to small-cell carcinoma of the lung are usually applied such as irinotecan (CPT-11) + cisplatin (CDDP) or etoposide (VP-16)+cisplatin (CDDP) [59]. According to small-cell lung carcinoma treatment experience, cisplatin and etoposide are the most commonly recommended agents. Cyclophosphamide, vincristine, taxanes, and ifosfamide have also been added to cisplatin in various combinations [60, 61]. Carboplatin combined with etoposide or taxanes has also been administered instead of cisplatin. On the other hand, chemotherapy using docetaxel and CDDP for conventional androgen-independent prostate carcinoma had limited response for neuroendocrine marker [59]. Papandreou et al. [62] reported 38 patients with histologically proven SCPC (pure or mixed) and no prior treatment with doxorubicin, etoposide, or cisplatin were treated every 4 weeks with doxorubicin 50 mg/m^2 as a 24-h intravenous (IV) infusion followed by etoposide 120 mg/m^2/day and cisplatin 25 mg/m^2/day IV on days 2–4. Median time to progression and OS time were 5.8 months and 10.5 months, respectively. Regarding irradiation, no exact guidelines for total dose and irradiation volume have been given.

For SCPC with LM, the role of hormonal treatment is controversial. For patients with mixed adenocarcinoma/SCPC with LM, the standard treatment regimen includes hormonal therapy (by orchiectomy, gonadotropin-releasing agonists, or antagonists with the early addition of antiandrogens) in combination with systemic etoposide/cisplatin chemotherapy [63]. In cases of pure SCPC with LM, hormonal therapy is not recommended, as the prostatic neuroendocrine cells are deprived of androgen receptors [56]. A retrospective review done in 1992 showed immediate chemotherapy with or without hormonal therapy for both pure SCPC and mixed adenocarcinoma of the prostate resulted in longer clinical remissions, although none survived [64].

Commonly, the emergence of the SCPC occurs in patients with high-grade adenocarcinoma who are often treated with ADT. Whether the androgen ablation therapy should be continued or not in patients with adenocarcinoma whose tumors undergo NED is a crucial matter. Considering that prolonged hormonal ablation therapy may enhance the selection and progression of NED, androgen-independent tumor cells through processes of transdifferentiation or clonal selection [65] in combination with the antiandrogen withdrawal effect, it is recommended that the antiandrogens are discontinued before initiation of chemotherapy. As the number of cases so far is limited, optimal therapy for SCPC with LM has still not to be defined.

Currently, the treatment of SCPC is imitating the treatment model of small-cell lung cancer. To improve the management of SCPC and prolong the survival time of patients with SCPC with LM, further research needed to carry out to find effective molecular markers for early diagnosis and monitoring of treatment response.

15.6.4 Neuroendocrine Differentiation in Prostate Cancer with LM

NED is one of the unique features of prostate cancer. NED is often characterized by scattered clusters of differentiated neuroendocrine cells among a predominant population of adenocarcinoma cells, except for rare cases of total NED of prostate cancer (i.e., small-cell carcinoma or carcinoid). Controversially, the prevalence of neuroendocrine cells has been correlated with higher-grade malignancy and poor prognosis.

For patients with NED with LM disease, hormonal therapy should be used combined with chemotherapy. Cisplatin-based chemotherapy was reported to have significant activity in patients with poorly differentiated neuroendocrine tumors other than prostate cancer [66, 67]. In malignant neuroendocrine cells, production of ectopic neuropeptides has been reported. Thus, neuroendocrine-targeted therapy (somatostatin analogs, bombesin antagonist, serotonin antagonist, mTOR inhibitor) also should be used for treatment.

In conclusion, LM usually occurs late in the course of the disease in most patients. Early detection and characterization of LM are crucial for the treatment and prognosis of prostate cancer patients. Improved understanding of related genes and gene products such as the vascular endothelial growth factor (VEGF) family, HGF/met signal pathway, and E-cadherin will assist in the development of promising tumor markers for the early detection of patients with a high risk of LM. Moreover, it will also lead to the development of targeted therapies and perhaps for predictive markers of chemosensitivity. Optimal treatment strategies should be based on the clinicopathological and biological characteristics of each patient. Results from prospective studies or detailed meta-analyses are necessary to determine which patients will have the greatest benefits from each treatment strategy. Therefore, multimodality therapies and strategies are necessary for patients with LM. Multidisciplinary team discussions are required to evaluate the extent of the disease and the feasibilities and benefits of each treatment modality.

References

1. Bubendorf L et al (2000) Metastatic patterns of prostate cancer: an autopsy study of 1,589 patients. Hum Pathol 31(5):578–583
2. Pouessel D et al (2007) Liver metastases in prostate carcinoma: clinical characteristics and outcome. BJU Int 99(4):807–811
3. Kelly WK et al (2012) Liver metastases (LM) to predict for short overall survival (OS) in metastatic castration-resistant prostate cancer (mCRPC) patients (pts). in J Clin Oncol: Am Soc Clin Oncol 2318 Mill Road, STE 800, Alexandria, VA 22314 USA
4. Wang H et al (2014) Clinical characteristics and prognostic factors of prostate cancer with liver metastases. Tumor Biol 35(1):595–601
5. Armstrong AJ et al (2010) Prediction of survival following first-line chemotherapy in men with castration-resistant metastatic prostate cancer. Clin Cancer Res 16(1):203–211
6. Pezaro CJ et al (2014) Visceral disease in castration-resistant prostate cancer. Eur Urol 65(2):270–273
7. Eisenberger MA et al (1998) Bilateral orchiectomy with or without flutamide for metastatic prostate cancer. N Engl J Med 339(15):1036–1042
8. Vashchenko N, Abrahamsson P (2005) Neuroendocrine differentiation in prostate cancer: implications for new treatment modalities. Eur Urol 47(2):147–155
9. Flechon A et al (2011) Phase II study of carboplatin and etoposide in patients with anaplastic progressive metastatic castration-resistant prostate cancer (mCRPC) with or without neuroendocrine differentiation: results of the French Genito-Urinary Tumor Group (GETUG) P01 trial. Ann Oncol 22(11):2476–2481
10. Berruti A et al (2000) Circulating neuroendocrine markers in patients with prostate carcinoma. Cancer 88(11):2590–2597
11. Yuan T, Veeramani S, Lin M (2007) Neuroendocrine-like prostate cancer cells: neuroendocrine transdifferentiation of prostate adenocarcinoma cells. Endocr Relat Cancer 14(3):531–547
12. Shakir FA et al (2008) Metastatic prostatic carcinoma presenting as fulminant hepatic failure. South Med J 101(10):1049–1050
13. Cussenot O et al (1996) Plasma neuroendocrine markers in patients with benign prostatic hyperplasia and prostatic carcinoma. J Urol 155(4):1340–1343
14. Quaia E et al (2006) Comparison of contrast-enhanced ultrasonography versus baseline ultrasound and contrast-enhanced computed tomography in metastatic disease of the liver: diagnostic performance and confidence. Eur Radiol 16(7):1599–1609
15. Bartolotta TV et al (2009) Focal liver lesions: contrast-enhanced ultrasound. Abdom Imaging 34(2):193–209
16. Cokkinos DD et al (2007) Can contrast-enhanced ultrasonography characterize focal liver lesions and differentiate between benign and malignant, thus providing a one-stop imaging service for patients? J Ultrasound 10(4):186–193
17. Lim JS et al (2006) CT and PET in stomach cancer: preoperative staging and monitoring of response to therapy. Radiographics 26(1):143–156

18. Pan Z et al (2010) Determining gastric cancer resectability by dynamic MDCT. Eur Radiol 20(3):613–620
19. Ward J et al (2005) Liver metastases in candidates for hepatic resection: comparison of helical CT and gadolinium-and SPIO-enhanced MR imaging 1. Radiology 237(1):170–180
20. Meijerink MR et al (2008) Total-liver-volume perfusion CT using 3-D image fusion to improve detection and characterization of liver metastases. Eur Radiol 18(10):2345–2354
21. Hussain SM, Semelka RC (2005) Hepatic imaging: comparison of modalities. Radiol Clin North Am 43(5):929–947
22. Liu PS, Francis IR (2010) Hepatic imaging for metastatic disease. Cancer J 16(2):93–102
23. Bruegel M, Rummeny EJ (2010) Hepatic metastases: use of diffusion-weighted echo-planar imaging. Abdom Imaging 35(4):454–461
24. Ba-Ssalamah A et al (2009) Clinical value of MRI liver-specific contrast agents: a tailored examination for a confident non-invasive diagnosis of focal liver lesions. Eur Radiol 19(2): 342–357
25. Nasu K et al (2006) Hepatic metastases: diffusion-weighted sensitivity-encoding versus SPIO-enhanced MR imaging 1. Radiology 239(1):122–130
26. Yoshioka T et al (2003) Evaluation of 18F-FDG PET in patients with advanced, metastatic, or recurrent gastric cancer. J Nucl Med 44(5):690–699
27. Donati OF et al (2010) Value of retrospective fusion of PET and MR images in detection of hepatic metastases: comparison with 18F-FDG PET/CT and Gd-EOB-DTPA–enhanced MRI. J Nucl Med 51(5):692–699
28. Mcleod DG (2003) Hormonal therapy: historical perspective to future directions. Urology 61(2 Suppl 1):3–7
29. Seidenfeld J et al (2000) Single-therapy androgen suppression in men with advanced prostate cancer: a systematic review and meta-analysis. Ann Intern Med 132(7):566–577
30. Klotz L et al (2008) The efficacy and safety of degarelix: a 12-month, comparative, randomized, open-label, parallel-group phase III study in patients with prostate cancer. BJU Int 102(11):1531–1538
31. Tombal B et al (2010) Additional analysis of the secondary end point of biochemical recurrence rate in a phase 3 trial (CS21) comparing degarelix 80 mg versus leuprolide in prostate cancer patients segmented by baseline characteristics. Eur Urol 57(5):836–842
32. Crawford ED et al (2011) A phase III extension trial with a 1-arm crossover from leuprolide to degarelix: comparison of gonadotropin-releasing hormone agonist and antagonist effect on prostate cancer. J Urol 186(3):889–897
33. Kaisary AV et al (2001) Is there a role for antiandrogen monotherapy in patients with metastatic prostate cancer? Prostate Cancer Prostatic Dis 4(4):196–203
34. Tyrrell CJ et al (1998) Casodex 10–200 mg daily, used as monotherapy for the treatment of patients with advanced prostate cancer. An overview of the efficacy, tolerability and pharmacokinetics from three phase II dose-ranging studies. Casodex Study Group. Eur Urol 33(1):39–53
35. Schmitt B et al (2001) Combined androgen blockade with nonsteroidal antiandrogens for advanced prostate cancer: a systematic review. Urology 57(4):727–732
36. Moul JW (2009) Twenty years of controversy surrounding combined androgen blockade for advanced prostate cancer. Cancer 115(15):3376–3378
37. Cruz GN (2009) Outcomes from the use of maximal androgen blockade in prostate cancer at health area with reference hospital type 2 (1st part). Quality of life: application of EORTC QLQ-C30 instrument. Arch Esp Urol 62(6):431–457
38. Abrahamsson PA (2010) Potential benefits of intermittent androgen suppression therapy in the treatment of prostate cancer: a systematic review of the literature. Eur Urol 57(1):49–59
39. Hussain M et al (2013) Intermittent versus continuous androgen deprivation in prostate cancer. N Engl J Med 368(14):1314–1325
40. De Leval J et al (2002) Intermittent versus continuous total androgen blockade in the treatment of patients with advanced hormone-naive prostate cancer: results of a prospective randomized multicenter trial. Clin Genitourin Cancer 1(3):163–171

41. Singh SM, Gauthier S, Labrie F (2000) Androgen receptor antagonists (antiandrogens) structure-activity relationships. Curr Med Chem 7(2):211–247
42. Attard G et al (2009) Antitumor activity with CYP17 blockade indicates that castration-resistant prostate cancer frequently remains hormone driven. Cancer Res 69(12): 4937–4940
43. Attard G et al (2009) Selective inhibition of CYP17 with abiraterone acetate is highly active in the treatment of castration-resistant prostate cancer. J Clin Oncol 27(23):3742–3748
44. Tannock IF et al (2004) Docetaxel plus prednisone or mitoxantrone plus prednisone for advanced prostate cancer. N Engl J Med 351(15):1502–1512
45. Petrylak DP et al (2004) Docetaxel and estramustine compared with mitoxantrone and prednisone for advanced refractory prostate cancer. N Engl J Med 351(15):1513–1520
46. Mottet N et al (2011) EAU guidelines on prostate cancer. Part II: treatment of advanced, relapsing, and castration-resistant prostate cancer. Actas Urol Esp 35(10):565–579, English Edition
47. Nelius T et al (2010) Clinical outcome of patients with docetaxel-resistant hormone-refractory prostate cancer treated with second-line cyclophosphamide-based metronomic chemotherapy. Med Oncol 27(2):363–367
48. Oudard S et al (2005) Multicenter randomized phase II study of two schedules of docetaxel, estramustine, and prednisone versus mitoxantrone plus prednisone in patients with metastatic hormone-refractory prostate cancer. J Clin Oncol 23(15):3343–3351
49. Nelius T et al (2005) Characterization of prognostic factors and efficacy in a phase-II study with docetaxel and estramustine for advanced hormone refractory prostate cancer. Onkologie 28(11):573–578
50. de Bono JS et al (2010) Prednisone plus cabazitaxel or mitoxantrone for metastatic castration-resistant prostate cancer progressing after docetaxel treatment: a randomised open-label trial. Lancet 376(9747):1147–1154
51. Batty N, Yarlagadda N, Pili R (2013) Major response to cyclophosphamide and prednisone in recurrent castration-resistant prostate cancer. J Natl Compr Canc Netw 11(8):911–915
52. De Bono JS et al (2011) Abiraterone and increased survival in metastatic prostate cancer. N Engl J Med 364(21):1995–2005
53. Small EJ et al (2006) Placebo-controlled phase III trial of immunologic therapy with sipuleucel-T (APC8015) in patients with metastatic, asymptomatic hormone refractory prostate cancer. J Clin Oncol 24(19):3089–3094
54. Marech I et al (2013) Partial response of liver metastases treated with abiraterone in castration-resistant prostate cancer: a case report. Oncol Lett 5(6):1877–1880
55. Abbas F et al (1995) Small cell carcinoma of the bladder and prostate. Urology 46(5):617–630
56. di Sant'Agnese PA (1992) Neuroendocrine differentiation in carcinoma of the prostate. Diagnostic, prognostic, and therapeutic implications. Cancer 70(1 Suppl):254–268
57. Aygun C (1997) Small cell carcinoma of the prostate: a case report and review of the literature. Md Med J 46(7):353–356, Baltimore, Md.: 1985
58. Tĕtu B et al (1987) Small cell carcinoma of the prostate part I a clinicopathologic study of 20 cases. Cancer 59(10):1803–1809
59. Noda K et al (2002) Irinotecan plus cisplatin compared with etoposide plus cisplatin for extensive small-cell lung cancer. N Engl J Med 346(2):85–91
60. Palmgren JS, Karavadia SS, Wakefield MR (2007) Unusual and underappreciated: small cell carcinoma of the prostate. in Seminars in Oncology: Elsevier
61. Amato RJ et al (1992) Chemotherapy for small cell carcinoma of prostatic origin. J Urol 147(3 Pt 2):935–937
62. Papandreou CN et al (2002) Results of a phase II study with doxorubicin, etoposide, and cisplatin in patients with fully characterized small-cell carcinoma of the prostate. J Clin Oncol 20(14):3072–3080
63. Network, N.C.C. (2013) The NCCN clinical practice guidelines in oncology 2011: prostate cancer version 1: clinical practice guidelines in oncology

64. Moore SR, Reinberg Y, Zhang G (1992) Small cell carcinoma of prostate: effectiveness of hormonal versus chemotherapy. Urology 39(5):411–416
65. Abrahamsson PA (1999) Neuroendocrine differentiation in prostatic carcinoma. Prostate 39(2):135–148
66. Mitry E et al (1999) Treatment of poorly differentiated neuroendocrine tumours with etoposide and cisplatin. Br J Cancer 81(8):1351
67. Fjällskog MLH et al (2001) Treatment with cisplatin and etoposide in patients with neuroendocrine tumors. Cancer 92(5):1101–1107

Liver Metastases from Brain Tumors

16

Adriana Toro, Luigi Manfré, and Isidoro Di Carlo

16.1 Introduction

Primary tumors of the brain are divided into glial tumors (Table 16.1) and nonglial tumors (Table 16.2). Astrogliomas, including glioblastoma multiforme (GBM), meningiomas, pituitary adenomas, and metastatic tumors, represent the most frequent brain tumors in adults [1]. Extracranial metastases of brain tumors are uncommon and have been reported in the lungs, lymph nodes, pleura, mediastinum, liver, diaphragmatic muscle, and bone [2], with a frequency between 2 and 3.8 % [3, 4].

16.2 Epidemiology

Until now, the rarity of extraneural metastases has not had a clear explanation. The most current hypotheses are because (1) there is an absence of lymphatic vessels in the central nervous system (CNS); (2) the intracranial perivascular spaces do not communicate with the extracranial fluid space; (3) connections between the subarachnoid space and extracranial lymphatic vessels are rare; (4) intracerebral veins walls are thin and they probably collapse from compression

A. Toro, MD, PhD
Department of Surgery, Taormina Hospital, Messina, Italy
e-mail: atoroct@gmail.com

L. Manfré, MD
Department of Minimal Invasive Spinal Therapy, Cannizzaro Hospital,
Via Messina, 826, Catania, Italy

I. Di Carlo, MD, PhD, FACS (✉)
Department of Surgical Sciences, Organ Transplantation, and Advanced Technologies,
University of Catania, Cannizzaro Hospital, via Messina 826, Catania 95126, Italy
e-mail: idicarlo@unict.it

I. Di Carlo (ed.), *Noncolorectal, Nonneuroendocrine Liver Metastases: Diagnosis and Current Therapies*, DOI 10.1007/978-3-319-09293-5_16

Table 16.1 Neuroepithelial tumors of the CNS

Astrocytic tumors
Astrocytoma
Anaplastic (malignant) astrocytoma
Glioblastoma
Pilocytic astrocytoma
Subependymal giant cell astrocytoma
Pleomorphic xanthoastrocytoma
Oligodendroglial tumors
Oligodendroglioma
Anaplastic (malignant) oligodendroglioma
Ependymal cell tumors
Ependymoma
Anaplastic ependymoma
Myxopapillary ependymoma
Subependymoma
Mixed gliomas
Mixed oligoastrocytoma
Anaplastic (malignant) oligoastrocytoma
Others
Neuroepithelial tumors of uncertain origin
Polar spongioblastoma
Astroblastoma
Gliomatosis cerebri
Tumors of the choroid plexus
Choroid plexus papilloma
Choroid plexus carcinoma (anaplastic choroid plexus papilloma)
Neuronal and mixed neuronal–glial tumors
Gangliocytoma
Dysplastic gangliocytoma of cerebellum (Lhermitte–Duclos)
Ganglioglioma
Anaplastic (malignant) ganglioglioma
Desmoplastic infantile ganglioglioma
Central neurocytoma
Dysembryoplastic neuroepithelial tumor
Olfactory neuroblastoma (esthesioneuroblastoma)
Pineal parenchyma tumors
Pineocytoma
Pineoblastoma
Mixed pineocytoma/pineoblastoma
Tumors with neuroblastic or glioblastic elements (embryonal tumors)
Medulloepithelioma
Primitive neuroectodermal tumors with multipotent differentiation (medulloblastoma — cerebral primitive neuroectodermal tumor)
Neuroblastoma
Retinoblastoma
Ependymoblastoma

Table 16.2 Other CNS neoplasms

Other CNS neoplasms
Tumors of the sellar region
Pituitary adenoma
Pituitary carcinoma
Craniopharyngioma
Hematopoietic tumors
Primary malignant lymphomas
Plasmacytoma
Granulocytic sarcoma
Others
Germ cell tumors
Germinoma
Embryonal carcinoma
Yolk sac tumor (endodermal sinus tumor)
Choriocarcinoma
Teratoma
Mixed germ cell tumors
Tumors of the meninges
Meningioma
Atypical meningioma
Anaplastic (malignant) meningioma
Non-meningothelial tumors of the meninges
Benign mesenchymal
Malignant mesenchymal
Primary melanocytic lesions
Hemopoietic neoplasms
Tumors of uncertain histogenesis
Tumors of cranial and spinal nerves
Schwannoma (neurinoma, neurilemmoma)
Neurofibroma
Malignant peripheral nerve sheath tumor (Malignant schwannoma)
Local extensions from regional tumors
Paraganglioma (chemodectoma)
Chordoma
Chondroma
Chondrosarcoma
Carcinoma
Metastatic tumors
Unclassified tumors
Cysts and tumor-like lesions
Rathke cleft cyst
Epidermoid
Dermoid
Colloid cyst of the third ventricle
Enterogenous cyst

(continued)

Table 16.2 (continued)

Neuroglial cyst
Granular cell tumor (choristoma, pituicytoma)
Hypothalamic neuronal hamartoma
Nasal glial heterotopia
Plasma cell granuloma

before a tumor penetrates them; (5) meningeal tumors grow on the dura mater but remain only on the surface; and (6) dural veins are protected by a dense connective tissue [5].

An additional hypothesis regarding the pathogenesis of the brain metastases has suggested that the metastatic potential of the GBM might be correlated with particular molecular features, such as *P53* gene mutations and differential clonal selection [6]. In fact, some metastases arise from genetically altered subclones of the primary tumor. Several biological and molecular studies have shown an overexpression of insulin growth factor and a decrease of DNA-PK (a DNA-dependent protein kinase involved in DNA repair mechanisms) genetic expression. The first probably plays a role in tumor progression; the second contributes to the malignant transformation of the glioma. One study suggested that distant dissemination is the consequence of direct infiltration of tumor cells into extracranial blood vessels [6].

A review of 128 patients affected by GBM with extra-CNS metastases found 19 patients who had liver metastases (14.8 %) [7]. The total numbers of patients reported in the literature as affected by hepatic metastases from brain primary tumors are reported in Table 16.3.

16.3 Diagnosis

The diagnosis of liver metastases from cancer of the brain may be sincronous or metacronous. The discovery of the liver metastases can be also absolutely incidentally and can be prodromic for the diagnosis of the primary tumor in the brain. Liver metastases are often completely asymptomatic. Abdominal computed tomography (CT) scan is the most common diagnostic method. The use of biopsy to stage the tumor has not been reported in the literature.

16.4 Treatment

Although these tumors do not have much tendency to metastasize, reports of metastases of these tumors have increased over time. In fact, between 1928 and 1967, only 21 cases of GBM extra-CNS metastases were reported in the literature; and between 1968 and 2006, 107 cases were reported. The percentage of extracranial metastases has consequently increased from 0.44 %, reported by Smith et al. in 1969 [9], to the current value of 2 % [4]. The increase in reports is probably

Table 16.3 Patients with liver metastases from brain cancer

Author	Year	Type of tumors	Number of patients	Sex M/F	Age (years)	Synchronous/ metachronous	Number of hepatic MTS	Other MTS	Therapy	Disease-free interval (months)	Survival (months) after diagnosis of primary brain cancer	Outcome	Causes
Thiry [8]	1959	Glioblastoma	1	F	57		Multiple	NA	NA	NA	>60	Dead	NA
Smith [9]	1969	Glioblastoma	6	M	43	met	NA	no	NA	NA	6	Dead	NA
				M	45	met	NA	no	NA	NA	6	Dead	NA
				M	58	met	NA	no	NA	NA	6	Dead	NA
				M	49	met	NA	no	NA	NA	8	Dead	NA
				M	49	met	NA	yes	NA	NA	16	Dead	NA
				M	64	met	NA	yes	NA	NA	10	Dead	NA
		Medulloblastoma	2	F	24	met	NA	yes	NA	NA	49	Dead	NA
Anzil [10]	1970	Glioblastoma	1	F	53	PM	5	yes	NA	NA	13	Dead	GCDR
Johnson [11]	1974	Glioblastoma	1	M	46	NA	NA	yes	NA	NA	36	Dead	NA
Montaut [12]	1976	Glioblastoma	1	M	23	NA	NA	yes	NA	NA	14	Dead	NA
Pasquier [13]	1980	Glioblastoma	1	F	21	PM	3	no	NA	NA	5	Dead	GCDR
Ogata [14]	1987	Glioblastoma	1	M	68	NA	NA	yes	NA	NA	8	Dead	NA
Matsuyama [15]	1989	Meningioma	1	M	68	PM	Multiple	yes	NA	NA	5	Dead	NA
Shuto [16]	1995	Glioblastoma	1	F	42	met	Multiple	no	NA	NA	NA	NA	NA
Greif [17]	1998	Glioblastoma	1	M	51	syn	Multiple	yes	NA	NA	7	Dead	GCDR
Widiaja [18]	2000	Glioblastoma	1	M	58	met	5	NA	CMT	NA	NA	NA	NA
Ueda [6]	2003	Glioblastoma	1	M	42	PM	Multiple	yes	NA	NA	41	Dead	GCDR
Astner [19]	2006	Glioblastoma	1	M	54	met	Multiple	NA	CMT	12	36	Dead	LDP

Table 16.3 (continued)

Author	Year	Type of tumors	Number of patients	Sex M/F	Age (years)	Synchronous/ metachronous	Number of hepatic MTS	Other MTS	Therapy	Disease-free interval (months)	Survival (months) after diagnosis of primary brain cancer	Outcome	Causes
Beaumont [20]	2007	Gliosarcoma	1	M	47	met	Multiple	NA	NA	NA	19	Dead	NA
Robert [21]	2008	Glioblastoma	1	F	45	met	Multiple	NA	NA	NA	NA	NA	NA
Piccirilli [7]	2008	Glioblastoma	1	F	74	NA	NA	no	resection	NA	26	Dead	NA
Garcia-Conde [22]	2009	Meningioma	1	M	44	met	Multiple	NA	NA	NA	7	Dead	Hepatic failure
Chan [23]	2010	Hemangiopericytoma	1	F	42	met	Multiple	NA	CMT	NA	NA	NA	NA
Schonsteiner [24]	2011	Glioblastoma	1	M	69	met	Multiple	NA	NA	NA	24	Dead	Hepatic failure
Surov [25]	2013	Meningioma	15	NA	NA	NA	NA	NA	NA	NA	NA	NA	NA
Total			41										

M male, *F* female, *MTS* metastases, *met* metachronous, *syn* synchronous, *CMT* Chemotherapy, *PM* post mortem, *GCDR* general condition deteriorated rapidly, *LDP* local disease progression, *NA* not available

reflective of earlier diagnoses because of improvements in neuroimaging techniques and the use of multimodality treatments, and the consequent longer patient survival times.

Little is known about successful treatment of extracranial metastases, including liver metastases. In the literature, just one case of hepatic resection for GBM metastases has been reported, with 8 months survival [7]. Systemic chemotherapy has led to partial remission of liver metastases, but all patients die within 2 years of the discovery of metastases [6].

References

1. Black PM (1991) Brain tumors. N Engl J Med 324:1471–1476
2. Newton HB, Henson J, Walker RW (1992) Extraneural metastases in ependymoma. J Neurooncol 14:135–142
3. Nakamura K, Hawkin S, Aizawa M, Maekubo H, Kobayashi N, Ozasa T, Kunieda Y, Hokari I, Matsushima T, Miyazaki T et al (1986) Extracranial metastases of brain tumors–a case report and survey of patients with extracranial metastasis sampled from a report on pathological autopsy cases in Japan. Gan No Rinsho 32:281–286
4. Terheggen HG, Müller W (1977) Extracerebrospinal metastases in glioblastoma. Case report and review of the literature. Eur J Pediatr 124:155–164
5. Bouillot-Eimer S, Loiseau H, Vital A (2005) Subcutaneous tumoral seeding from a glioblastoma following stereotactic biopsy: case report and review of the literature. Clin Neuropathol 24:247–251
6. Ueda S, Mineta T, Suzuyama K, Furuta M, Shiraishi T, Tabuchi K (2003) Biologic characterization of a secondary glioblastoma with extracranial progression and systemic metastasis. Neuro Oncol 5:14–18
7. Piccirilli M, Brunetto GM, Rocchi G, Giangaspero F, Salvati M (2008) Extra central nervous system metastases from cerebral glioblastoma multiforme in elderly patients. Clinico-pathological remarks on our series of seven cases and critical review of the literature. Tumori 94:40–51
8. Thiry S, Betz EH, Dewart L (1959) A case of cerebral glioma with hepatic metastases. Neurochirurgie 5:321–326
9. Smith DR, Hardman JM, Earle KM (1969) Metastasizing neuroectodermal tumors of the central nervous system. J Neurosurg 31:50–58
10. Anzil AP (1970) Glioblastoma multiforme with extracranial metastases in the absence of previous craniotomy. Case report. J Neurosurg 33:88–94
11. Johnson RP, Guillan RA (1974) Glioblastoma multiforme with remote extracranial metastases. J Kans Med Soc 75:169–172
12. Montaut J, Metaizeau JP, Gerbaux A, Renard M (1976) Extracranial metastasis of primary brain tumours. Neurochirurgie 22:653–669
13. Pasquier B, Pasquier D, N'Golet A, Panh MH, Couderc P (1980) Extraneural metastases of astrocytomas and glioblastomas: clinicopathological study of two cases and review of literature. Cancer 45:112–125
14. Ogata A, Tashiro K, Abumiya T, Abe H, Matsuno Y, Nakamura K, Kashiwaba T (1987) Glioblastoma multiforme with extracranial metastases without previous surgery: demonstration of extracranial metastases by peroxidase antiperoxidase staining and clinicopathological study. No To Shinkei 39:679–685
15. Matsuyama J, Mori T, Hori S, Nakano T, Yamada A (1989) Gliosarcoma with multiple extracranial metastases. Case report. Neurol Med Chir (Tokyo) 29:938–943
16. Shuto T, Fujino H, Inomori S, Nakayama S, Satoh H, Ideguchi H, Tashiro Y (1995) Glioblastoma multiforme with liver metastasis–case report. No To Shinkei 47:772–777

17. Greif J, Horovitz M, Marmor S (1998) Pleuropulmonary metastasis from an intracranial glioblastoma. Lung Cancer 20:135–137
18. Widjaja A, Mix H, Gölkel C, Flemming P, Egensperger R, Holstein A, Rademaker J, Becker H, Hundt M, Wagner S, Manns MP (2000) Uncommon metastasis of a glioblastoma multiforme in liver and spleen. Digestion 61:219–222
19. Astner ST, Pihusch R, Nieder C, Rachinger W, Lohner H, Tonn JC, Molls M, Grosu AL (2006) Extensive local and systemic therapy in extraneural metastasized glioblastoma multiforme. Anticancer Res 26:4917–420
20. Beaumont TL, Kupsky WJ, Barger GR, Sloan AE (2007) Gliosarcoma with multiple extracranial metastases: case report and review of the literature. J Neurooncol 83:39–46
21. Robert M, Wastie M (2008) Glioblastoma multiforme: a rare manifestation of extensive liver and bone metastases. Biomed Imaging Interv J 4:e3
22. Garcia-Conde M, Roldan-Delgado H, Martel-Barth-Hansen D, Manzano-Sanz C (2009) Anaplastic transformation of an atypical intraventricular meningioma with metastases to the liver: case report. Neurocirugia (Astur) 20:541–549
23. Chan WS, Zhang J, Khong PL (2010) 18F-FDG-PET-CT imaging findings of recurrent intracranial haemangiopericytoma with distant metastases. Br J Radiol 83:e172–e174
24. Schönsteiner SS, Bommer M, Haenle MM, Klaus B, Scheuerle A, Schmid M, Mayer-Steinacker R (2011) Rare phenomenon: liver metastases from glioblastoma multiforme. J Clin Oncol 29:e668–e671
25. Surov A, Gottschling S, Bolz J, Kornhuber M, Alfieri A, Holzhausen HJ, Abbas J, Kösling S (2013) Distant metastases in meningioma: an underestimated problem. J Neurooncol 112:323–327

Index

I. Di Carlo (ed.), *Noncolorectal, Nonneuroendocrine Liver Metastases: Diagnosis and Current Therapies*, DOI 10.1007/978-3-319-09293-5

MIX
Papier aus verantwortungsvollen Quellen
Paper from responsible sources
FSC® C105338

If you have any concerns about our products,
you can contact us on
ProductSafety@springernature.com

In case Publisher is established outside the EU,
the EU authorized representative is:
Springer Nature Customer Service Center GmbH
Europaplatz 3, 69115 Heidelberg, Germany

Printed by Libri Plureos GmbH
in Hamburg, Germany